INTERNATIONAL SERIES OF MONOGRAPHS ON
PURE AND APPLIED BIOLOGY

Division: **ZOOLOGY**

GENERAL EDITOR: G. A. KERKUT

VOLUME 8

THE BRAIN AS A COMPUTER

OTHER TITLES IN THE ZOOLOGY DIVISION

General Editor: G. A. KERKUT

THE BRAIN
AS A COMPUTER

F. H. GEORGE

Department of Cybernetics
Brunel University

PERGAMON PRESS

OXFORD · NEW YORK · TORONTO · SYDNEY · BRAUNSCHWEIG

Pergamon Press Ltd., Headington Hill Hall, Oxford

Pergamon Press Inc., Maxwell House, Fairview Park, Elmsford,
New York 10523

Pergamon of Canada Ltd., 207 Queen's Quay West, Toronto 1

Pergamon Press (Aust.) Pty. Ltd., 19a Boundary Street,
Rushcutters Bay, N.S.W. 2011, Australia

Vieweg & Sohn GmbH, Burgplatz 1, Braunschweig

First edition 1961

Second edition 1973

Library of Congress Cataloging in Publication Data

George, Frank Honywill.

    The brain as computer.

    (International series of monographs on pure and applied biology.
Division: Zoology, v. 8)

    Bibliography: p.

    1. Cybernetics.   I. Title.

Q310.G43 1973   001.53   73-89

ISBN 0-08-017022-6

Printed in Hungary

TO MY WIFE

CONTENTS

CONTENTS

FOREWORD TO THE SECOND EDITION

IT IS a special privilege to have the opportunity to revise any book. Especially is it a privilege in the case of a book which contains some of the most important ideas that I feel I have had on the subject of cybernetics.

The first edition of *The Brain as a Computer* appeared in 1961 and the book itself was written over a period of some five years or more prior to 1961. I was conscious in reading it afterwards that there were many things in it that I would have written differently and there were many emphases that I would have changed in some measure, and above all I felt that all the different sections had not been 'brought to the boil' at exactly the same time.

I cannot think that it could have been otherwise since the range of the book is considerable. One criticism of any such wide-ranging book is that because of its range it may lack depth and this provides one of the oldest and most difficult problems in the world to solve, particularly in a field like cybernetics which covers such a wide variety of topics. The answer must be that some people must devote their time to as much of the depth as they can but make their primary target the range of the subject with a view to integrating different facets of it, while others can concentrate wholly on a particular problem, or some particular problems, while being aware of the general range. I feel clear that I belong to the first category.

Apart from any methodological doubts which I felt about the first edition of *The Brain as a Computer*, there were, of course, obvious changes going on all the time which made me feel that it would be pleasing to have the opportunity to up-date the book. At the same time as carrying out the up-dating I would try to correct some of the errors that I was aware had crept into the first edition. So it was doubly pleasurable to be invited by Pergamon Press to write this second edition and I have been given, by the publishers, complete freedom to rewrite the text as I please.

The problem of rewriting itself occupied me for some period of time, far longer than I expected, since it seemed likely that it would be the last chance I would get to produce a book in terms of my full breadth of interests in the field of cybernetics, and with the added advantage of having done much of the 'donkey work' before. My decisions have been to try to edit the book from start to finish, eliminating errors, and re-stating opinions which have now changed, and at the same time maintaining most of the original information.

Admittedly some of what was included originally would have been omitted if I had tried to write a new book, but it seemed important to maintain continuity with the first edition of the book and thus most of what was there before has remained, and only a few sections have been eliminated on the grounds that they now seem less relevant than they did at the time. At the same time I have tried to up-date the various sections of the book and in particular, I felt that a new chapter was required to deal with heuristic programming, natural language programming, inference making and the general field of artificial intelligence, as well as a new chapter on the theory of games.

In the case of automata theory, and the methodological background of cybernetics, quite a number of changes have been made and I have taken a completely new look at the basic description of computers. It seems to me that, of all the sections, that on digital computers was the most out-of-date and perhaps this is natural in view of the fast-moving nature of the subject. This leaves the very difficult sections on physiology and psychology occupying the central part of the book and also representing fields with which I have been in less contact in the last decade.

The choice here was to omit them altogether, and this seemed to defeat the whole purpose of the book, or to make a great effort to catch up with what has been done in the fields on neurophysiology and experimental psychology which related to the integrated idea of *The Brain as a Computer*. I chose the second course and have tried to bring in the latest information which shows, basically, that there has been little change, or so it seems to me, in either of these two fields; what has occurred is only the emergence of a great deal of additional information. Nothing has happened that substantially changes the principles described and the views originally expressed.

One further difficulty remained. This is a result of a critic of the first edition who pointed out that whereas there may have been merit in the development of neurophysiology and experimental psychology and cybernetics as an overall integrating factor, this was not, as far as the book was concerned, wholly successful because the integration had not been carried through. This I was aware of at the time and recognized the tremendous difficulty involved in such as undertaking. But having this second opportunity to produce a new edition I have given my thoughts to this particular point more than any other single one. To give a detailed integration at the level, as it were, of the neuron or even at the level of the stimulus–response in all its ramifications as studied by experimental psychologists working in the field of cognition, is perhaps too much to ask. But enough has been done, or so I hope, to make much clearer the value of providing an integrating factor in the form of cybernetics to weld neurophysiology, psychology and mathematics together as part of the totality of cybernetics on one hand and the behavioural sciences on the other.

Another feature which I would now want to emphasize, which had not perhaps been sufficiently emphasized before, was that for me, science is a contextual matter in which particular questions are given particular answers. Science, of course, is also concerned with general theory and a framework in which these questions may be answered, but the idea that science is to try to discover the nature of reality seems somewhat dreamy-eyed at this moment in time. As a result, it is important to recognize that any particular type of activity has a particular purpose, or should have.

This matter of context is particularly relevant when a mathematician looks at a book, such as those on cybernetics or biology, and is inclined to say that mathematically they are trivial. This criticism is largely based on the fact that the book does not treat the subject as a mathematician would; it does not provide a rigorous edifice of theorems and the like. The answer is, of course, that the biologists, the cyberneticians and others who are using mathematics are using it for a different end. They are using it as a means to clarify their ideas and to short-circuit their descriptions and to possibly prepare the way for an integration with mathematics as a descriptive language. Hence they would often look at mathematical work and say that whereas it may be mathematically interesting, it supplies nothing of the slightest interest to us in our search to try to develop our own fields such as biology, cybernetics and the like. This is a sort of misunderstanding that has been growing in science over the years and I would like to emphasize that it is absolutely vital to try to understand the purposes for which we are doing anything at any particular time and judge its effects in terms of whether it achieves those purposes or not. There still remains the question as to whether the purposes are sufficiently worth-while but it is at least a separate question from whether the effort made achieves the purpose.

At the same time as carrying through this job of re-editing and correcting, extending and reformulating with new emphases, it was obvious that I would wish to extend the bibliography. Once more I followed the principle of including everything that was included originally in the bibliography and the book as a whole is somewhat larger than what was already a large book. The only excuse that I can offer is that it seems to be a subject that merits it.

I perhaps should add at the very least that I did not for a second suppose that this is a definitive description of cybernetics. On the contrary, I think of it as dealing with one of the central aspects of cybernetics, the extent to which we can use rigorous methods and models, of a self-adapting and feedback kind, to help us to get a clearer understanding and a more rigorous formulation of problems involving human and humanlike intelligence and human and humanlike abilities in general, especially in the cognitive field.

F. H. GEORGE

CHAPTER 1

THE ARGUMENT

IN THIS book an attempt will be made to outline the principles of cybernetics and relate them to what we know of behaviour, both from the point of view of experimental psychology and also from the point of view of neurophysiology.

The title of the book, *The Brain as a Computer*, is intended to convey something of the methodology involved; the idea is to regard the brain itself *as if* it were a computer-type of control system, in the belief that by so doing we are making *explicit* what for some time has been *implicit* in the biological and behavioural sciences.

Neither the chapters on experimental psychology, which are explicitly concerned with cognition, nor the chapters on neurophysiology, which are intended to outline the probable neurological foundations of cognitive behaviour, are complete in any sense; they are intended to be read and understood as illustrative of a point of view. It is clear, from the speed at which all these subjects are developing, and from the vast bulk of knowledge that we now have, that a detailed analysis would provide a lifetime's work for many people. The emphasis is primarily on the cybernetic approach, by which we shall mean simply an attempt to reconsider the biological evidence in terms of mathematical precision, and with the idea of constructing effective models as a foundation for biological theory. This implies no radical departure from much of biological tradition; it is no panacea, but it provides some indication of the possibility of constructing a somewhat different conceptual framework, especially one allowing the application of relatively precise methods, not only because of the need for precision in science and for the positive benefits of quantification, but also in order to avoid the messiness and vagueness implicit in ordinary language when used for the purposes of scientific description.

Cybernetics is a new science, at least in name; it is a new discipline that overlaps traditional sciences, and proposes a new attitude towards those sciences. Although it has had its own historical evolution, the views of modern cyberneticians are both distinctive and novel. The word 'Cybernetics' has been derived from the Greek word for 'steersman', and this underlines the essential properties of control and communication.

In some respects Cybernetics certainly represents a very old point of view dressed in a new garb, since its philosophical forebears are the materialists of early Greek thought, such as Democritus, and the Mechanistic Materialists of the eighteenth century. This ancestry is, however, no more than the bare evolutionary thread of a materialistic outlook, and we are not primarily concerned here with the philosophical aspects of its development. It should, indeed, be quite possible for those who are radically opposed to the Mechanistic Materialists and their modern counterparts to accept some part of cybernetics for its methodology and pragmatic value alone.

We will now outline the main ideas of cybernetics, and say something of its importance for the behavioural and biological sciences.

Cybernetics might be briefly described as the science of control and communication systems, although it must be admitted that such a general definition, while correct, is not very helpful.

Cybernetics is concerned primarily with the construction of theories and models in science, without making a hard and fast distinction between the physical and the biological sciences. The theories and models occur both in symbols and in hardware, and by 'hardware' we shall mean a machine or computer built in terms of physical or chemical, or indeed any fabric at all. Most often we shall think of hardware as meaning electronic parts such as transistors and relays. Cybernetics insists, also, on a further and rather special condition that distinguishes it from ordinary scientific theorizing: it demands a certain standard of *effectiveness*. In this respect it has acquired some of the same motive power that has driven research on modern logic, and this is especially true in the construction and application of artificial languages and the use of operational definitions. Always the search is for precision and effectiveness, and we must now discuss the question of *effectiveness* in some detail. It should be noted that when we talk in these terms we are giving pride of place to the theory of automata at the expense, at least to some extent, of feedback and information theory.

The concept of an effective procedure springs primarily from mathematics, where it is called an algorithm. It has been an important mathematical and mathematical–logical question to ask whether parts, or even the whole, of mathematics is effectively derivable. Is it possible to derive all theorems of classical mathematics in a purely machine-like manner? The theorems of Gödel (1931) and Church (1936), and the work of Turing (1937) on the Turing machine, as it is called, gave answers to these questions as far as mathematics was concerned. It was possible to show that all of classical mathematics could *not* be reproduced in this manner, although most of it could. These results have actually led to misinterpretation outside mathematics, in that they were thought to imply that there were some mathematical operations that could not be performed by a *machine*, whereas they could be performed by a human being. This is a mistake, and certainly does not follow from any work done on decision procedures. What does follow is that, in order to deal with certain mathematical operations (for example, those involving the choice of new branches for development), a machine would need to be able to compute probabilities, and to make inductions. It must necessarily be agreed, however, that the machine may make some mistakes in its computations, though we must not overlook the fact that these are exactly the sort of conditions that would apply to a human being performing the same operations.

Within this framework a decision procedure is to be viewed as a mechanical method, of a deductive kind, for deciding what follows from a particular set of axioms or a simple routine procedure that a person can follow even though he does not understand the purpose of the operation. Let us illustrate the point.

If the problem to be solved is one of finding two from a finite set of numbers that have a certain property *A*, say, then we can enumerate all the numbers to which the property might apply until we either find or do not find two numbers with the said property. This procedure is clearly one that could be carried out by an unintelligent helpmate who knows, and can follow, no more than the simplest routine procedures. There are many such algorithms in mathematics, and very nearly all classical mathematics can be shown to follow a similar routine pattern; but his leaves untouched the problem of how mathematical theories were constructed in the first place.

By 'effective', then, we shall mean the construction of a theory that can be translated into a particular blueprint form, from which an actual hardware model could, if necessary, be constructed. It has some of the same properties that we associate with operational definitions. To avoid ambiguity over the terms of our scientific description we insist that they be clear and precise enough for us to draw up a hardware system from them.

The other main feature, apart from effectiveness, that we shall be concerned with is the notion of a *heuristic*. Heuristics are rough-and-ready rules of thumb, or approximations, or successive approximations, or generalized guides. In some respects a heuristic is much like a hypothesis in that it is not sufficiently confirmed to become a law of the system. If it were a law then it would come somewhere near to being an algorithm, and this represents the difference between heuristics and algorithms. It is probable that heuristics and algorithms differ only as a matter of degree, although this is not by any means certain. The main point is that we have algorithms for many aspects of those systems with which we are concerned and thus we can ensure that there is an effective model building procedure. However, we must also bear in mind that there are methods for short-circuiting the algorithms which still allow us to make 'good decisions' in terms of information which is incomplete. This short-circuiting makes use of heuristics, which are also used in circumstances where it is uneconomic to use algorithms, even where such algorithms exist.

The use of heuristics, which are essential to human thinking and problem solving, is a reminder that cybernetics is very closely concerned with artificial intelligence, in all its ramifications and applications.

The principal aims of cybernetics may be listed under three headings:

(1) To construct an effective theory, with or without actual hardware models, such that the principal functions of the human organism can be realized.
(2) To produce the models and theory in a manner that realizes the functions of human behaviour by the same logical means as in human beings. This implies the simulation of human operations by machines, whether in hardware or with pencil and paper.
(3) To produce models which are constructed from the same colloidal chemical fabrics as are used in human beings.

The methods by which these three aims are collectively realized are manifold, and can be summarized by the following list: (1) Information theory, (2) Finite Automata, (3) Infinite Automata, including, especially, Turing machines, (4) Logical Nets, which are particular finite automata, (5) The programming of general purpose digital computers, (6) Various theories, of games (7) The construction of all the models, in any fabric, which might collectively be called 'special purpose computers', and may be both digital and analog, and may be 'pre-wired', involve growth processes, or involve both. All these methods will be discussed later in the book, and more especially those concerned with finite automata.

All these approaches need to be developed together, and also it seems to be the case that we have lots of partial models that need to be translated into some common form. We shall try to show how the various stages of our machine can be built up, using various different descriptive languages; but first we must consider what is meant by an inductive machine and, by implication, a deductive one.

There is no point as yet in trying to give a precise definition of the inductive process but it can be characterized easily in various special terms. In the business of language translation, the problem of translating from one language to another is, at least in principle, strictly deductive, provided that both languages are already known; all that is needed is a dictionary and a grammar. If, however, one of the languages is not known, then the problem is inductive, at least until such time as a dictionary and a grammar can be constructed. In the same way it looks as if there are two phases in learning: firstly, the finding of a solution of the problem presented; secondly, the application of that solution in performance. The application, after the problem has been solved, is a deductive process, although the recognition of the appropriate place to supply a solution is an inductive one. By inductive we mean something like *heuristic* and by deductive we mean something like *algorithmic*.

There are many other examples, such as in games, where in learning the tactics one is behaving inductively although, *having learned* the tactics, their application is a purely deductive procedure. In other words, the notion of 'induction' is dependent upon the transfer of information from one point (or person) to another.

These matters themselves contribute to a new view of what is involved in the learning process, and we shall attempt to utilize this knowledge in framing a clearer picture of what we are searching for under the names 'learning', 'perception', 'conception' and 'cognition' generally.

Information theory is a precise language, and a part of the theory of probability. It is capable of giving a precise definition of the flow of information in any sort of system or model whatever. It has been used already to describe various psychological and biological models, especially those of the special senses. It can also be used in the study of learning and problem solving, and it is, in fact, an alternative description of these processes.

Information theoretic descriptions are, broadly speaking, interchangeable with descriptions that are couched in logical net terms. Sometimes one is the more convenient and sometimes the other, and sometimes both may be used together (Rapoport, 1955).

The concept of a *finite automaton* requires more careful attention. This is another effective method of defining any system that is constructed from a finite number of parts, which we may call elements, or cells. Each of these elements may be capable of being in only one of a finite number of different states at any given time. The system or model (these words are synonymous here), which is connected according to certain rules, has an input and an output, for we are concerned with the structure of the automaton which is defined by a specified set of rules, and has a specified output for a particular input.

If we allow the number of states or parts to be infinite, then we should be describing an infinite automaton. A well-known example of an infinite automaton is a Turing machine, which is made up of an infinite tape which is ruled off into squares, a reading head, and a control. The control scans one square at a time in turn according to the instructions which make up the programme. It can move either to the left one square on the tape, or to the right one square on the tape, and it can write a symbol on the square or erase an existing symbol which is already on the square. It was with such a theoretical machine that Turing was able to show the effective computability of a large class of mathematical functions (Turing, 1937), and his machines will be described more fully in Chapter 3.

Whereas Turing machines are concerned with systems which are capable of being in an infinite number of states, and therefore are sometimes referred to as infinite, or non-finite, automata, it should be remembered that there is a possibility of a finite but potentially infinite machine. A potentially infinite automaton is one which at any particular moment in time has only a finite number of possible states and symbols, yet if it runs off one end of the tape it is always possible to put more tape on. In other words, we can always go on moving along the tape indefinitely in either left or right direction but should we run off we will always be prepared to put more tape on and this means at any particular moment in time the amount of tape is finite, hence we talk about 'potentially infinite' Turing machines as opposed to either infinite or non-finite Turing machines.

Logical nets, which are of special interest in the biological context, are paper and pencil blueprints, couched in the notation of mathematical logic. They are effectively reproducible in hardware, and will be used to describe the class, or some sub-class, of finite automata.

The general purpose digital computer is a hardware machine made up principally of an input and an output system, a storage, and an arithmetic unit. A control system is also included. It can be described in logical net terms as a finite automaton and is equivalent to a Turing machine in its capacity provided that it always has access to all the information it has used in the past.

We should mention that as far as computers are concerned, we have already gone through the eras of the first- and second-generation computers and we have now arrived at the third generation of computers which has such properties as multi-access and multi-programming, and is far larger and faster than the first and second generations. The third-generation computer is also much more nearly universal in its ability to take languages of various kinds such as COBOL, ALGOL, FORTRAN, etc., without bias. It must be borne in mind, of course, that fourth-generation computers will soon be on the scene and they will have an even greater versatility. In fact, one of our main problems from the computer point of view is to decide how to design a fourth generation of computers so that they have all that is needed by way of constraints of languages and stucture and still have enough versatility to meet the needs of the future.

Finally, by special purpose machines we mean the class of all machines, whether in hardware or in paper and pencil, that can be used to exemplify any process whatever. Here we are especially interested in the class of finite automata which, when synthesized, might be described as special purpose computers. We are also particularly interested in systems that are not fully defined, or have the property of growth, or both. By a combination of all these techniques we may hope ultimately to simulate human behaviour in most of its aspects.

In constructing our models of behaviour, we cannot always meet the exacting criteria demanded by those scientists—mostly those who do not themselves construct theories and models—when they ask that models should be predictive and testable. In fact, models must usually start from more modest beginnings, but *eventually* they must meet these criteria of testability.

It would seem appropriate now to say a word about the sort of analysis this book attempts, especially in so far as it may seem to differ from other works which, while having similar ends, proceed differently in keeping to a policy of deriving particular models from specific sets of experiments. A fairly recent book by Broadbent (1958) may be said to represent the best sort of example of this alternative approach.

In general, the aim of the cybernetic type of analysis attempted here is to provide a conceptual framework for both experimental psychology and experimental biology. It does so by careful analysis of concepts provided by experimental scientists, and it tries to bring them together, seeking by various means to see what is necessary to our model making, and what is incidental. This could be described in part as a meta-theoretical procedure, and one aiming to interest the mathematician and the philosopher as well as the strictly experimental scientist. This is not to be taken as meaning in any sense that the vital role of experiment is being denied, but rather by way of emphasizing that experiment must be seen as part of a broader undertaking, involving the effective synthesis of many different lines of thought.

The view expounded differs from that of such works as Broadbent's only in emphasis, the emphasis having shifted somewhat away from the immediate evidence, and immediate *ad hoc* models, to slightly more general forms of model construction, emphasizing rigour even if at the expense of some immediate reality in the theory itself. Both ways of carrying out research in the behavioural science seem equally valid and necessary, and the writer regards them as being complementary to each other.

At the same time as the cybernetician—at least this particular one—is searching for an analysis of concepts, principles and methods, a theory is being provided at varying levels of generality, and this seems to be an apposite place to state a fairly basic assumption that underlies this work. The assumption is that science does *not* proceed *only* by observing and stating empirical results and observing again, eventually to generalize. Those many writers who have said that it is necessary to describe behaviour before we can hope to explain it are surely—while in one sense stating the obvious—missing an important point, the point being that in constructing models and theories, and in analysing theories and concepts from various points of view, one is able to contribute to the science itself. The assumption here is that the method of presentation of so-called facts is as important as the facts themselves; or to put it more crudely, languages and the references of languages are almost inextricably bound together.

A little more discussion in the field of methodology will be found in Chapters 3 and 14, for the bulk of the book is concerned with the methods of cybernetics and the modelling of behaviour, human and otherwise.

It is because of the belief that methods and findings are intermingled that much can come from a logical and a philosophic type of analysis of existing models, based directly on experimental data, or a scientific analysis based directly on the data themselves. Everyone knows that it is fairly easy to carry out experiments as such in psychology, but the problem arises over the appropriate interpretation of the results. This view has sometimes been mistakenly interpreted to mean that scientific theories can be built without any reference to empirical fact—which is nonsensical—or that logic is being boosted as a source of empirical knowledge in the same way as immediate observation. The wiser opinion is surely that they should be undertaken together, as being complementary to each other.

In saying that one of the next big undertakings of the cybernetician involves analyses of cognitive operations in terms of views proposed by philosophers such as Price (1953), Wittgenstein (1953), Körner (1959) and Ryle (1949), among others, we may possibly be furthering the misunderstanding, so let us say at once that we do not intend to imply that we shall ignore experimental results; on the contrary, experimental results are still our basic material, and the other forms of logical analysis are necessary to increase our understanding of that basic experimental material. Indeed, this is precisely a point where cybernetics and experimental psychology have common ground—since models, either of a paper and pencil or of a hardware kind, are constructable—to make *precise* what is being asserted. This is done in such a manner that it is clear both to the psychologist who wishes to use the results and to the logician who wishes to analyse the methods and their implications.

One of the features that we shall be trying to simulate or synthesize will be that of concept formation (Banerji, 1964, 1968; Sherman, 1959;

Wason and Johnson-Laird, 1968) since the formulation of concepts, whether derived from other concepts or *ab initio*, is not a factor which either increases or decreases their merit. There may be some doubt about whether concepts can be derived other than from old concepts, and in so far as they can, it seems to demand that new input domains must be made available to the system. Even then though the new input domain may well be only capable of interpretation in concepts already familiar to the interpreter. We go from concept to hypothesis formation and this in turn brings us into the field of inductive logic and heuristics which will be a subject for discussion in later sections of this book.

To avoid confusions of language, and in order to broaden the outlook of the experimental scientist, we hope to carry out a model making analysis of experimental results. This means that we should pay attention to the forms of linguistic analyses of logicians, and bear in mind the efforts made towards precise linguistic construction by such writers as Woodger (1939, 1952).

Indeed, the development of artificial formal languages is intimately bound up with cybernetics, since they *can* be regarded as blueprint languages from which actual hardware models can be made.

In the same way we shall bear in mind the distinction made by Braithwaite (1953) between models and theories, and we shall think of them as having a sort of twofold relation to each other, where the theory is an interpretation of the model, and the model is a formalization of the theory. Anything whatever could be taken to be an interpretation of a model (i.e. a theory), and anything could be taken to be a model of a the relation between the two. At the same time we shall, of course, consider certain well-defined models, always with an eye to the intended interpretation.

Generating schemes such as those of Solomonoff (1957), the heuristics of Minsky (1959), and the various attempts to meet the criteria of human thought, are to be derived in a series of stages from a set of conceptual models which start from the concept of ostensive rules (Körner, 1951). The ideas of classes, relations, properties, order, process, etc., which are fundamental to our ways of regarding the empirical world, will be derived similarly; and this book can be no more than a link in the long and complex chain. Initially, the main objects will be both methodological and behavioural; as we progress, the emphasis will change increasingly from the first to the second.

Naturally we shall draw on ready-made techniques, such as Theory of games, Linear Programming, Dynamic Programming, Operational Research, Games against Nature, and the like, since they all represent structural and functional features of the conceptual world from which the empirical world must be reconstructed.

Neurophysiologically, we continue to wait for highly predictive models, and this primary analysis is intended as a basis for model constructions of neurophysiological utility; what it does not claim to do is to supply them in any detail, for that is something that lies beyond the compass of the present analysis.

It is important that it should be clearly understood that this book is not about cognition as such, nor indeed about neurophysiology as such. It is concerned with models of behaviour which include cognitive and neurological data, and of course some attention is paid to modelling these foundation subjects. At the same time it should be said that the main aim is methodological; we want to show the power and usefulness of formalized methods of theory construction, and yet we do not wish to pretend that these supplant experimental data; they are secondary to them. But it is also thought important that methods of constructing theories should themselves be the subject of analysis and experiment; it is by such means that comparisons between theories are facilitated, and the implications of a model are made more lucid.

Many criticisms have been levelled at the hypothetico-deductive method, but although it is sometimes unwieldy, and certainly there are other possible, and quite valid, approaches, it should be remembered that cybernetic ideas are largely built up around axiomatic systems. They are easier to check in axiomatic form, and even models which are apparently useless and unwieldy, like Hull's hypothetico-deductive model of rote learning (1940), are of the greatest use because the reader will bear in mind that, in the age of the computer, it is possible to take a system that looks completely and hopelessly obscure and complicated, and yet derive its logical consequences. In fact, the learning programs that are discussed in Chapter 7 look very complicated in the flow chart form, but any models that purport to explain behaviour in any important sense will be far more complicated than even the Hullian set of postulates. We must not, therefore, set our face against the hypothetico-deductive method; rather, we must find a way of using it, and the digital computer supplies one such way. Logical nets, of the kind we shall be discussing, supply yet another way, but it must be admitted that more research has still to be done if such models are going to be handleable on a large scale, for otherwise precision degenerates quickly into more verbal discussion which, while useful, and even essential, is thought to be inadequate to the task of setting up behavioural models at various levels sufficiently rich and precise to permit the standard of prediction we are seeking; indeed this provides an alternative route to the computer.

In outlining the sections of this book, it may be said that the first section, contained in Chapters 1 to 7 inclusive, is about cybernetic models. First they are summarized in a general way, and then we pay special attention to finite automata, and particularly finite automata in logical net form, which seem especially useful to the modelling of behaviour. Actually there are many cases in which other forms of model are more suitable for particular purposes, but we shall talk largely in logical net terms, although it will be understood that translation into other terms will usually be possible.

Chapter 3 is rather a special chapter. It is about logic and methods of a quasi-philosophical kind. It is almost in the nature of an appendix, but there are a number of models and theories there which might be regarded as being of behavioural interest, and they are a source of many ideas used at other points in the book.

It is not thought that philosophy can contribute greatly to the subject matter of psychology, but a sophistication over linguistic matters seems to be absolutely essential. The writer believes that much that philosophers discuss could be decided, or at least clarified, by experimental methods, but also that care and thoughtfulness over concepts and language is vital in any science, and that philosophy of science is vital to science. Thus every scientist should have something of the philosopher about him, and vice versa.

In Chapter 4 we have outlined a very general and loosely constructed model which is to be used for experimental purposes, by analysing the existing empirical data from cognition. At the end of Chapter 7 we start to introduce some examples of learning.

Chapter 8 summarizes learning theory, and more space is given to the traditional theories of Hull and Tolman, and less to the current and more burning issues on methods of reinforcement. The reason for this is again that the book hopes to find readers who are not already familiar with cognitive problems, and whose interest may be largely methodological.

Chapters 9, 10 and 11 deal with neurological matters, although Chapter 11 represents an all-round approach to the perceptual side of cognition. Chapter 9 is, in particular, an attempt to summarize the main relevant facts of the neurophysiology of nervous function, and although it tries to make the explanations simple—and certainly it is not addressed to the specialist in neurophysiology—it can be better understood by those who have already carried out some previous reading on the subject.

Chapter 12 pays lip service to thinking, and also says some more about perception. The writer is very conscious of the relatively sketchy nature of the treatment he has given to many of the problems discussed in the book, but his main hope has been to persuade experimental scientists that there is much to be said for a greater concentration on matters of methodology, especially from the cybernetic point of view, while continuing to develop experimental methods, which the writer thoroughly believes should still be their chief aim.

Chapter 13 is concerned with artificial intelligence in general and deals with the total reconstruction of conceptual and other processes. It especially emphasizes inference making on computers and this brings into the computer context, and therefore the cybernetic context, the ability to draw inferences of a deductive or inductive kind as well as formulate concepts, reorganize concepts, and the formulation of hypotheses which is in fact an inductive step. It is also concerned with natural language programming which is an essential step in the ability to derive information by description as well as acquaintance. Finally, Chapter 14 is a summary of the general processes discussed in the book with a sort of foreword as to likely future developments.

Summary

This first chapter is intended to outline the general purpose of the book, which is both methodological, and provides a beginning to a model-theory construction process based on the methods of cybernetics. It is in essence an attempt to utilize to the full our concepts, whether from philosophy, logic or science, and to construct a conceptual world in terms of machine analogs, from which we may ultimately derive more precise theories of behaviour, and theories of the internal organization of the human being, especially at the level of the nervous system.

CHAPTER 2

CYBERNETICS

'CYBERNETICS' is a word that was first used in this context by Norbert Wiener (1948), and has since become widely accepted as designating the scientific study of control and communication, as applied equally to *inanimate* and to *living* systems.

Wiener's basic idea was that humans and other organisms are not essentially different from any other type of control and communication system. The principle of negative feedback is characteristic of organisms and closed-loop control systems in general, and this suggests that organisms could be substantially mimicked by electronic switching devices which are controlled by negative feedback.

The word 'cybernetics', although a recent addition to our vocabulary, in fact refers to much that went on for many years before in various fields such as electrical engineering, mathematics, psychology, physiology and other disciplines. The actual area covered by cybernetics is perhaps vague, and certainly very large. It cuts across many of the accepted divisions of science, and this means that cybernetics has many different aspects that will be of interest to scientists working in various branches of scientific endeavour. The main emphasis in this book will be focused on the interests of the experimental psychologist and the biologist, although it is believed that it should also have an appeal to those concerned with many different sides of science.

We shall now say a little about the mathematical and historical background of cybernetics.

Mathematics

The primary interest of mathematics to cybernetics is due not only to the direct relevance of mathematical logic and questions involving the foundations of mathematics and axiomatic methods, but also because of the design of computing machines.

First let us briefly consider the history of mathematical thought and the problem raised for the foundation of mathematics.

We should begin by reminding ourselves of the important fact that mathematics is a language or language form. It is, indeed, a highly precise and abstract language that handles—or is capable of handling —any of the structural relations that actually exist, or are theoretically capable of existing. An example of this can be drawn from geometry.

The geometry of the world in which we live appears to be four-dimensional—that is, from the relativistic point of view; but from the purely mathematical point of view we can develop geometry in any dimensions whatsoever, and the user of the n-dimensional geometry can choose whatever value of n is necessary or relevant to his particular problem. This is an example of the imposition of a theory on to a model.

Pure mathematicians develop mathematical systems (models) that may have no application whatever; it is like the development of the grammar of a potential language, and the constructions follow simply from the various possible sets of rules. At the same time it is a fact that a great deal of the mathematics that has been developed has quickly been turned to practical account. One of the reasons for this is of course the fact that mathematicians keep their eyes on the problems that scientists are dealing with, and a new line of development with no applications tends to fade out very quickly.

The power of the mathematical language lies partly in the fact that its constituents have a well organized structure, and partly in the fact that the notion of number seems to be basic to our descriptions of the world. Mathematics, though, is not always numerical; there are branches of mathematics, such as those dealing with shapes and relations of a geo-metrical kind, that go under the name of topology; there is also mathe-matical logic, which deals with properties and propositions which are not numerical. Indeed, the main feature of mathematics is that it tries to pick out the most general structural relations in any situation capable of description. It is thus a very general language, and a provides a powerful form of model making.

One possible misconception should be mentioned. Much that is symbolic and put in terms of algebraic symbols where these symbols represent real or complex numbers, is not mathematics, or certainly may not be mathematics of any importance; whereas much that is written in longhand *is* mathematics. Mathematics is a language that is ideally a shorthand, but *also* it is a powerful system for making deductions, and carrying out reasoning processes, because of the ease with which it is possible to see the form of the deductive or inductive argument. In ordinary, everyday language this is hardly ever the case if the description is complicated.

Our interest in mathematics is directly associated with cybernetics, for mathematics is concerned with the whole development of precision, which is also the concern of cybernetics. In particular, it has been in the search for mechanical methods of computation, and for proof that mathematics has played an important part in the evolution of 'thinking' machines.

We should say in the context of mathematics that cybernetics is much more closely associated with the mathematics of discrete functions than it is with the mathematics of continuous functions which has provided the backbone of the modern development of mathematical physics. As far as discrete mathematics is concerned, one should think in terms of set theory, mathematical logic, recursive functions, groups, stochastic and Markov processes, and so on and so forth. This indeed is placing emphasis on another aspect of mathematical development which is important in the evolution of modern mathematics.

The theories of Gödel (1931), Church (1936) and Turing (1937) are connected with any symbolic or linguistic system whatever, and with any axiomatic system. These theorems are important landmarks in the history of mathematical logic and the foundations of mathematics. They assert that no theory language (i.e. any sufficiently rich language that is used descriptively in science) can show its own consistency within itself.

The theorems also deal with *decision procedures*, or algorithms or mechanical methods of finding proofs of mathematical statements, and Church was able to show that, for a system rich enough to include classical mathematics, no mechanical method was possible for discovering whether every statement in such a calculus was a theorem of that calculus or not. By calculus, we shall mean a particular postulational system, such as Euclidean geometry of the plane, or what we may call a 'model'. It was Turing who gave the most suitable expression to the point in developing his theoretical computer, the Turing machine, which we shall describe more fully in Chapter 3. These are, or should be, matters of considerable importance to those experimental psychologists and biologists who are interested in cybernetics, because it tells them something of the nature of machinery, as defined in terms of simple operations, and the power of precise linguistic forms. These theorems have also been the foundations of some measure of misunderstanding, because the word 'machinelike', although suggesting what is obviously mechanical, does not exhaust all possible machines.

Mathematically, the above theorems were formulated in pursuit of the goal suggested by Hilbert (1922), that all mathematics was a formal system of symbols (abstract marks or sounds) that were manipulable according to a set of rules, and that there was a sense in which mathematics should be capable of being shown to be *complete*. This is now known to be impossible; the sense of completeness involved, although capable of various precise definitions, is roughly the sense in which we would expect a self-contained system to fit together coherently. This means that every statement made within the system should be capable either of being shown to be a theorem of the system or not, and all the true theorems being shown to be true, and those only. It is this which is not possible.

The importance of axiomatic systems to the development both of cybernetics and mathematics is considerable. The point about axiomatic systems is that they are akin to the process of formalization and provide a precise framework in which precise questions can be asked and precise answers given. Axiomatic systems can take various forms, they all depend on some statements being assumed to be true and some of those being used in the meta-language as rules of inference from which theorems can be derived by methods of proof and in some cases by the use of an automatic procedure or algorithm. In all cases of axiomatic systems, one is concerned with the properties of consistency and completeness. In other words, it is essential that, within the axiomatic system, it is not possible to prove a statement, proposition or predicate to be true or valid and at the same time prove that its negation is also true or valid.

Similarly one is concerned that the axiomatic system is complete in the sense that it does demonstrate all that was intended by its original construction, no more and no less. In fact, of course, the setting up of axiomatic systems shows clearly that the consequences that follow from the formalization were not necessarily foreseen by the original process of formalizing. Thus in the propositional calculus, the consequences of the use of 'if... then—' in the form of the horseshoe symbol are far greater than was originally envisaged by people who intended the interpretation to be 'if... then—'. This is the inevitable consequence of any sort of formalization, it either strips away many of the different meanings intended or actually adds other meanings that were not intended and yet follow from the formalizing process. Thus it is that axiomatic systems, apart from being blueprints for machines, in the cybernetic context, are also means for precise communication. In both roles they have great cybernetic importance.

There are in the main three different schools of thought with regard to the nature and foundations of mathematics. They are: The Logistic school of Whitehead and Russell (1910, 1912, 1913), Peano (1894) and Frege (1893, 1903), which argues that mathematics is a part of logic; the Intuitionistic school of Brouwer (1924) and Heyting (1934), which argues that mathematics is independent of logic, and comes from a direct appreciation of numbers; and the Formalist school founded by Hilbert, who believe that mathematics is a formal game with symbols. These three schools have carried on continued arguments regarding the foundations of mathematics, and it is perhaps fair to say that the bulk of current opinion favours the first view; that mathematics is founded upon logic; but the whole question is a very complicated one, and it is not obvious that the various views expressed are really at variance with each other. However, this is not a matter of primary interest to biologists and psychologists, and it will not be pursued here.

Independently, but still within mathematics, there has been the development of computing machinery, and although the motive force was quite different, the results had a great deal in common with the foundation studies. At the same time, what was to be regarded as an effective procedure or a mechanical procedure, sometimes called 'decision procedure' or algorithm in the sense of Turing, easily covered what a computer was thought to be capable of performing, since computers, in their early days at any rate, were thought of merely as adding and subtracting machines of an automatic kind. It was only later that they were to be thought of as having far greater generality, and capable of being driven by electronic rather than by purely mechanical means. Even now, few people have come to think of a computer as anything but a deductive type of system, and it is the inductive use of the computer which is the one that is of primary cybernetic interest; this, indeed, is one of the main themes of this book, and of cybernetics.

To return to the mathematical foundation of computers, we find that the first calculator that was used for any widespread computations was one designed by Pascal and used for insurance purposes in France, and this same computer was improved by extension from addition and subtraction to multiplication and division by no less a personage than Leibniz. Also in France, it was Colmar who has generally been credited with producing the first commercial computer. But the father of the large-scale *automatic* computer in its modern form is most certainly Charles Babbage.

In his work Charles Babbage anticipated virtually all that is characteristic of the modern computing machine, and during his lifetime he also used the technique of punched cards as a classification system, a method that was rediscovered in America, some years later, by Hollerith.

We shall be discussing the general form that the modern computer has taken in the next section but one of this chapter; at the moment we should notice simply that the concept of a computer, although dependent upon the work of engineers of every kind, was primarily a mathematical project.

Cybernetics also has roots in applied mathematics, in particular in the statistical mechanics of Willard Gibbs, and the general development of statistical thermodynamics and the gas laws. The common ground here lies in the fact that information, in the technical sense of information theory, and the distribution of gas particles have a common descriptive law. Recently a fresh analysis has been undertaken by Wilson (1965) who has tried to show more clearly the relationship between information and entropy.

In analytical mathematics, a considerable contribution was made to the theoretical background of cybernetics (though he was quite unconscious of the connection) by Albert Lebesgue with his special form of definition of an integral. The development of abstract algebra, and in particular the theory of groups, has also contributed to the general theory. The purely mathematical background of cybernetics will not be developed here except in so far as it is necessary to an understanding of the behavioural and biological applications.

Historical

The sudden relatively recent rise to prominence of cybernetics was due, immediately, to World War II. There existed then a series of problems which had not previously been met. The main one was that of range-finding for anti-aircraft guns in high-speed aerial warfare. The older systems involved human computers and these, with manually controlled locators, were wholly inadequate for the job in hand. The essence of the process involved was to track and predict the direction, velocity, and height of enemy aircraft. The human being's part in the operation was much too slow and inaccurate, and there were people available with machines already developed to do the job adequately; these machines were, of course, computing machines.

These computing machines had already been designed, and some built, by Vannevar Bush, Norbert Wiener, and others, and were almost ready-made for the job. These scientists, as well as others such as von Neumann, Shannon, and Bigelow, were in a position to see that machines of an electronic kind were ideally suited to carry out the whole of the operations of range-finding and location without any human intervention whatever.

These electronic computing machines were already developed to a very high degree of efficiency for the solution of mathematical equations, and some technical difficulties had led to the suggestion that a process of scanning, similar to that used in television, might be incorporated into the computer. Another innovation was the use of binary notation rather than decimal notation as in the early Harvard Mark I computer.

The problem of tracking, however, called for the mimicking of another characteristically human type of activity in the form of 'feedback'.

Feedback is what differentiates the machines that we are primarily interested in from the popular docile machine such as an aircraft or a motor car, or even the most obviously docile machines of all such as spoons, forks and levers.

Feedback involves some part of a machine's output being isolated, to be fed back into the machine as part of its input—a controlling part of the input. Man obviously operates on a gross feedback system in so far as he must have knowledge of the results of the actions that he performs in order that he may continue to act sensibly in his environment. A man playing darts will not improve unless he can see the results of his actions. More generally, a man who cannot see his results in a learning task will not improve, i.e. he will not learn; this fact has been well understood in experimental psychology.

A fairly well-known machine that exhibits feedback is a *thermostat* for controlling the temperature of domestic water supplies. A lower and an upper limit of temperature is set, and when the water which is being heated gets to the upper limit a mechanical device cuts out the heat source. The water then starts to cool, and when the temperature reaches the lower limit the device operates again, but in the opposite way, and the heat goes on. The temperature of the water oscillates between the two limits, which may be as high or as low as we please. The important thing is that it is the temperature that itself controls the change of temperature. This is precisely what is meant by a self-controlling machine.

Self-controlled steering mechanisms, such as are used in ships and aircraft, also operate on a principle of feedback, and most human muscular systems work on the same principle. A man cycling, or a driver driving a car, makes small correcting adjustments in his muscular movements so that small errors in directions or balance are corrected. The process is one of error-correction by a series of compensations.

All the instances that we have described are examples of what is called *negative* feedback, wherein a part of the response to some stimulus is used to operate against the direction of the original stimulus. Positive feedback involves the same compensatory or self-controlling aspects, but in this case the energy side-tracked for control purposes operates in the same direction as the principle energy rather than against it, and thus creates unstable, or 'runaway' conditions. In general, cybernetics has been concerned with the negative feedback type of arrangement.

Self-controlling machines, or 'artefacts' as they are sometimes called, have been classified according to the following general characteristics according to Mackay (1951):

(1) The receiving, selecting, storing and sending of information.
(2) Reacting to changes in the universe, including messages referring to the state of the artefact itself.
(3) Reasoning deductively from sets of assumptions or postulates, and learning. Here, learning includes observing and controlling its own purposive or goal-seeking behaviour.

We should add a fourth point to this:

(4) We would point out that learning is for us as it was for Peirce (1931–5) a form of induction. It is this which makes inductive reasoning and inductive logic play such a key part in the development of cybernetics.

It is these characteristics that include artefacts within the definition of the organism. Indeed, as we have seen, the basic assumption of cybernetics is that the human organism definitely comes within the framework of our definition, and it follows that the human operator is (in an obvious sense) a machine.

Computers

The computer, particularly that of the digital type, is of the greatest importance to cybernetics. Such machines are now constructed for a variety of different purposes. As well as solving mathematical equations, which was their original purpose, they are, of course, capable of adding up numbers, sorting and classifying information, making predictions that are based on forms of induction, and performing at least all the operations which are capable of being stated in precise language. The theoretical possibilities inherent in such systems are almost without limit, although in practice there may be serious limits of a definite kind.

It is not always easy for the technician to achieve results in practice which appear to be perfectly possible in principle. This is one reason why the technique of machine-construction and organization has developed far faster in blueprint than it has in hardware. It costs large sums of money to build computing machines and, after they are built, further large sums to keep them working; it is well, therefore, for those who are interested especially in the potentialities of machines, that it is sufficient to develop an effective technique for discovering the capabilities of a machine without going to the enormous expense, in terms both of money and time, of building it. This subject, and the sort of blueprint techniques practised, with their close relation to mathematics, is of the first importance to our subject.

Computers have advanced mainly with the advances in technological methods, especially of the electrical and electronic techniques which are closely bound up with the realization in hardware of machine theories. This process of realization demands a whole technology involving the design and manufacture of resistances, relays, transistors and micro-miniaturized circuitry, that will function with a certain degree of efficiency under specified conditions.

It is clear that the building-in of a maintenance and repair system will be quite vital if the computer needs to be permanently running. It has been suggested by von Neumann (1952) in this context that we might use a duplicating technique in construction which von Neumann called 'multiplexing'.

The general form of a digital computer

The digital computer is, to put it quite generally, composed of an input and an output system, a control and a storage system. The storage may take many forms but the central store uses what is called core store and is very fast in its operation and is supplemented by tape and discs which are rather slower but have a very large capacity. The present third-generation computers are built on a 'family basis'. Thus it is that the central processor can take so many peripherals in the form of tape or disc units and punched card input and punched paper output and then if a bigger computer is wanted a new central processor can be installed which will take the same peripherals but more of them. This is the general plan whereby the computer does not have to be exchanged for a new computer to expand its size but certain component parts can be changed and the whole thing can be made, as it were, 'to grow'.

The process of operation of the computer could be typically described as that of accepting instruction in the form of coded words, which it stores and then uses to operate on the data which is put into the computer usually in the form of punched tape or punched cards. The storing of the instructions makes the main difference in principle between a calculating machine and a computer, since the inclusion of the instructions in store means that it can run automatically and continuously from the beginning of a program to its end without external interference.

Each instruction and each piece of data in store has to be given a suitable address and the instructions themselves refer to the data to be operated on by virtue of their address. Instruction words can be one-address, two-address, three-address or n-address and there is perhaps a recent tendency to use one-address instructions, i.e. dealing with only one number or piece of data at a time. The speeds of modern computers are thousands of times faster than the early first-generation computers and the size too has gone up by factors of ten. Today's computers work at what is by comparison with human data processing astronomical speeds.

The language of computers

Much more important from our point of view than the physical construction of the computer is the process by which it handles the software. In the first instance we have languages for programming the computer and the basic language which each computer has is called its machine code language. Sometimes, however, the programmer will use a higher-level language such as ALGOL, COBOL, FORTRAN and the like which are then translated in the computer into the machine code language, where it must always finish up so that specific addresses are referred to inside the computer storage.

The advantage of high-level language is, of course, that you do not need to know the precise location of a piece of data in store and its address in using them. You merely need to know it is somewhere there, and then the translation procedure inside the computer will automatically translate the code word used into a specific address. The fact that computers were originally nearly all binary coded was one of the factors which drew attention to the similarity between computers and the human nervous system. In fact, more and more computers are decimal and it is quite clear that the binary nature of the machine code language is incidental to the construction of the computer.

In fact, today there are a large number of different languages used, often in the same computer. Languages such as octal, duodecimal, hexadecimal, 'excess three' and others, are all used for different purposes on different computers at different times. Thus it is that we should not really place heavy emphasis on the binary coded nature of computer codes.

We have used the word 'code' and also the word 'language' and they differ only in degree. The code is literally the alphabet and the syntactical rules which allow you to make up words, and we often refer to the basic language as a machine code which reminds you that language is in codes that differ only by degrees. We nearly always refer to ALGOL or COBOL as languages rather than codes, on the other hand.

One very important point about computer languages is the flexibility with which the programs can be achieved. So often, particularly when we are trying to simulate human intelligence in some form, we need to have a highly flexible storage system. This is achieved by particular types of languages. The best-known type of such a flexible language is called List

Processing. This was developed by Newell (1961) and others (McCarthy, 1961) in America, and various versions of List Processing have been built up for other computer languages. They are all really variants on the same basic theme which allows you to link items and classes together in a convenient cross-classified manner.

Whilst it might be considered that the computer is independent of cybernetic modelling, or even any other kind of scientific modelling, and thus the technicalities of computer science are not the direct concern of cyberneticians, this cannot be entirely true, especially for cyberneticians, because the division between software and hardware is fairly arbitrary and the division between models and the software representation of these models is also largely arbitrary. In other words, one tends to be influenced by the means of constructing models on a computer by the facilities so offered. The development of List Processing is a good example of such a process and one might expect to see in the future software techniques being developed to fit around the type of models being produced, such as those of artificial intelligence.

A good example of the need to consider the computer end of the organization is in theory proving and natural language programming. In both cases, as in the case of data retrieval, the careful organization of information in store is a prerequisite to the success of the undertaking. This does not necessarily, of course, only apply to the suitability of the language chosen but the way in which the information is being organized within store. We should perhaps add that none of these considerations are logically necessary to the modelling capacity of cybernetics but they are empirically of considerable importance.

Systems analysis and programming

In approaching a particular program it is clearly important to spell out the system. It is essential that the system to be programmed is thoroughly understood and it is assumed, of course, that in any particular context the undertaking is both feasible and worth while.

Having understood sufficiently the system, it is a simple matter to construct a model of it in terms of flow charts. From these flow charts or their equivalent in the form of decision tables, a fairly detailed specification is needed of the input and output as well as the particular form of the output and its format. When all these sort of decisions have been taken and when it has been decided what file of information should be kept in what sort of store, then and only then are we in a position to actually encode the system in the form of the program.

The encoding procedure is what is usually referred to as programming and is done relatively easily in a particular language once the system has been defined with great precision in terms of flow charts or decision tables or both.

Digital and analog systems

All that has been said here so far has been about digital systems. There are also analog systems and analog computers. The difference between digital and analog methods is essentially the same as between discontinuous or discrete and continuous functions in mathematics.

We shall not be much concerned with analog systems, but we shall just say a few words about them. They represent numbers and other physical conditions by physical variables (e.g. voltages and currents) rather than by digital numerical means. They are in widespread use as calculators, and also as simulators of various physical states. One example is to be found in the various flight conditions encountered by an aircraft, which can be wholly or partially simulated in a computing machine. It is clear that biologists and psychologists are, in a sense, seeking to simulate human behavioural conditions in their theories and models, and they too may have occasion to use analog methods.

We should mention in the context of analog systems the fact that many of them have grown up in the background of servomechanisms, which we shall be discussing later on. The notion of a servosystem is one of automatic control and one thinks in terms of servos which are used to act in automatic pilots or in automatic location of enemy aircraft or in automatic sighting and firing of guns, etc. In every case the servo control is one based on a notion of 'error'. Therefore if the rudder or elevators of an aircraft are set in the prescribed position for, say, straight and level flight at a particular airspeed, then if, due to turbulence, etc., the angle of the rudder or elevator is changed slightly, this is the 'error' which automatically precipitates adjustments against the direction of error to bring the aerofoil back to its prescribed position. This is a typical analog system.

If we want to generally characterize the difference between digital and analog systems we could do no better than illustrate it by saying that a piano is essentially digital and a violin is essentially analog. This serves to emphasize the point about discontinuous and continuous scales or functions which we referred to above. Analog systems have played a very much smaller part on the whole in the development of cybernetics than digital systems. This is largely because they are much smaller and much less well developed and much less convenient for the programming of things like artificial intelligence. This is not to say that the brain is essentially digital and many people believe that it is a mixture of both digital and analog systems, but this is neither here nor there as far as the simulation of the brain's activities is concerned. It is the convenience of the computer rather than its structure which is so important.

Neurophysiology and psychology

Following up a discussion of digital and analog computers, we must consider the more general questions of automata, artefacts, and machines.

If machines can perform mathematical operations with such success, what else can they do in the same way as human beings, always assuming that they do perform mathematical operations in a manner which is at least somewhat similar to humans? This is probably not always true, but doubtless *can* be so, as we shall see when we later discuss theorem proving in logic.

Psychology and physiology in particular, and the biological sciences in general, have taken notice of the revolution in machine design in order to investigate human behaviour and general physiological function from the machine point of view. We have already suggested that the similarity between machines and organisms is so great that the specifications for one appear to be capable of including the specifications for the other, and we should be able to make use of this fact in our attempts to understand human behaviour, build simulators for it, and so on.

This has led, in turn, to the construction of various machines in blueprint form, and special techniques for their design and construction; indeed, some of them have been constructed. These can be described, preliminarily, as mimicking some aspects of human behaviour. They are models, and they generally mirror *some* aspects of human behaviour, but not all of it. Not that it will always necessarily be impossible to build a complete human machine, but there are various reasons why it will not be useful to do so. The models will endeavour to mimic some of the aspects of behaviour rather as a putting green mimics some aspects of golf, or a wind-tunnel model of an aircraft mirrors the aerodynamic aspects of aircraft.

It is clear that electronic devices which mirror some sides of behaviour will not mirror, for example, the biochemical side, since the biochemical side is peculiar to the use of protoplasmic materials which are those materials used in the construction of *living* organisms, in its usual sense. But the fact of using different materials is no barrier to the use of machine artefacts for understanding behaviour, although the extent to which such considerations do matter must be given some thought.

What is of obvious interest to the behavioural scientist is the fact that machines are said to *think*, and this, too, is why logic is brought into the picture, since it is logic that helps humans to think, in so far as they do think efficiently.

It is believed that the whole development of machines that can *learn* and *think* is a vital product of the general theory of cybernetics, and, of course, first cousin to the process of automation. These models, coupled with methods used in modern psychology, will occupy most of our attention in the later chapters.

'Can we sensibly and seriously say that machines can think?' 'Is it true that humans are, in some sense, just machines?' These are matters of philosophical and psychological interest.

The answer the cybernetician is inclined to give to these questions takes one of two forms: (1) Machines do think, and machines could be made to think just as humans think, or (2) In so far as we can only deal with the machine side of humans, we can behave as if (1) above were true, even if in fact it is not.

We are concerned with a behaviouristic viewpoint, and whether or not the word 'thinking' is appropriate, and philosophers will often object to its use here, the processes inside humans and those inside *possible* machines are capable of being made the same.

It must be emphasized that cybernetics as a scientific discipline is essentially consistent with behaviourism, and is indeed in part a direct offshoot from it. Behaviourists, in essence, are people who have always treated organisms as if they were machines.

Communication theory

We have already seen that the control and the communication of information are completely bound up with each other in a computer, as indeed they are in a human. These two closely related subjects are the focal point of all knowledge. They are most certainly the central theme of cybernetics.

The theory of communication, or 'information theory', as it is sometimes called, is a very general and rigorously derived branch of modern mathematics; a branch of probability theory. The theory introduces the notion of an information source and a message which is transmitted, by any of the many possible means, to a receiver that picks up the message. There may also be an interference source that interrupts or otherwise disturbs the transmission of the message along the communication channel, and this is called a noise source; this very general situation may be represented diagrammatically.

The message may be coded, or it may be sent in a language that itself requires to be interpreted with respect to its meaning. Codes and languages are much the same, and ordinary languages are really codes for our 'ideas' or concepts. The fact of coding or encoding messages naturally

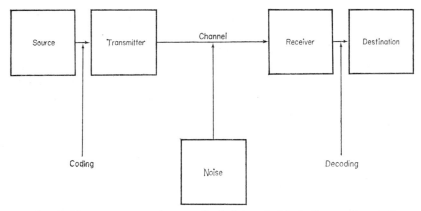

Fig. 1. COMMUNICATION. A generalized picture, in block diagram form, of the communication situation on a noisy channel. The coding and decoding may be repeated any number of times and a filter may be utilized in the channel to regain information lost through noise.

implies the process, at the receiving end, of decoding or interpreting the same message.

The amount of information that passes along some channel can be measured, as can the capacity of the communication channel; this leads us into some mathematical technicalities which we will take up in the next section of this chapter, but in the meantime there are one or two other points which must now be mentioned.

In the first place, languages have certain properties of a statistical or probabilistic character. In particular, certain letters and certain words occur more frequently than others, both in English and any other language. There is a definite probability that can be associated with the occurrence of any particular letter, which means that the notion of information is closely associated with probability. Information is measured by the probability of occurrence of the particular message passed.

The sequences of symbols that characterize any sort of language, or any set of events, have certain statistical properties; indeed, our ability to decipher languages or language-codes depends upon its repetitiveness: what statisticians call its statistical homogeneity.

Generally, we say that any sequence of symbols which has a probability associated with each symbol, is a 'stochastic process'. Now a particular class of stochastic processes, called 'Markov processes', has the extra condition that the probability of any event is dependent on a finite number of past events; often the name Markov process has been restricted to a conditional probability on one past event, but we can think of it as operating over any finite number of events. If the Markov process also has the property of statistical homogeneity, it is called an 'ergodic process'. These names will be already familiar to psychologists, as they represent closely allied ways of regarding human behaviour (Bush and Mosteller, 1956). We shall return to this aspect of the subject later.

Let us consider a very simple language, with an alphabet of only the four letters A, B, C and D. If the occurrence of each of these letters is equiprobable, we might expect a typical series, or a string, of letters in a message such as ABBACDABDDCDABDBCABDCACC, and so on, where all the leters occur equally often. If, however, A is three times as likely to occur as B, and B twice as likely as either C or D, then we might get AABBAAAAABCAADAACDBBABABAACDBBAAAAA CDBAAAAAACAD. We can make the matter more complicated by saying that if we get A then there is twice as much chance of B following it as there is of C; D is never followed by A, and so on. We can then build up closer and closer approximations to any ordinary language whatsoever by using words (collections of letters) and by considering their frequency of occurrence and their order. Such a rule as: U always or almost always follows Q, for example, would be true of English. These will be probability statements, it must be remembered, and therefore there may be exceptions to the rule.

Let us—following Shannon and Weaver (1949)—use the words

0·10 A	0·16 BEBE	0·11 CABED	0·04 DEB
0·04 ADEB	0·04 BED	0·05 CEED	0·15 DEED
0·06 ADEE	0·02 BEED	0·08 DAB	0·01 EAB
0·01 BADD	0·05 CA	0·04 DAD	0·05 EE

with the associated probabilities of occurrence next to each word. This stochastic process, composed of the five letters A, B, C, D and E with the words listed above, gives a typical message such as: DAB EE A BEBE DEED DEB ABEE ADEE EE DEB BEBE BEBE ADEE BED DEED DEED CEED ADEE A DEED and so on.

In the same manner as this we can approximate to any ordinary language whatsoever. Thus a zero-order approximation is one in which the symbols are independent and equi-probable. First-order approximations have independent symbols, but the same frequency of letters as in the language. The following is an estimate of the frequency of letters in English per 1000 letters (Goldman, 1953).

E	131	D	38	W	15
T	105	L	34	B	14
A	86	F	29	V	9·2
O	80	C	28	K	4·2
N	71	M	25	X	1·7
R	68	U	25	J	1·3
I	63	G	20	Q	1·2
S	61	Y	20	Z	0·77
H	53	P	20		

A second-order approximation has what is called a 'digram' frequency; this connects two successive letters in terms of probabilities, as in our conditional probability case mentioned above. A probability influence that spreads over three successive letters is called a 'trigram' frequency, and this, for English, is a third-order approximation; and so we go on until the second-order word approximation is obtained.

The bulk of the mathematical aspects of the theory had been developed quite independently of the theory of communication, since it is a branch of probability theory. The importance of the direct relation between the information flow and the change of the state of the particles of the world and their distribution is still problematic. Entropy, which is the measure of disorganization, is said, in statistical thermodynamics, to be increasing, and has an analog in the passing of information. It is a strange picture, but in terms of the world, control systems are seen as little pockets of negative entropy that are running against the main flow of the tide of disintegration (Wilson, 1965).

The full significance of the relation between entropy and information is by no means wholly clear, but it has the ring of fundamental importance.

The idea of a statistical distribution of particles can be made clearer if we consider the distribution of particles of air in the ordinary room. Unless conditions are unusual—such as the window being open and causing the door to slam with a gust of wind—we may expect the particles to be, roughly speaking, equally distributed through the room. Gases, like air, are known to fill their containers completely and arrange their density according to the space available. The Clerk Maxwell demons, those fictional twin characters—who, had they existed, would have made perpetual motion possible—are to be pictured as standing at each of two doors which lead away from the room to a heat engine and back into the room again. The demons open and close the doors according to the velocity of the particles which approach them. The first exit is opened only for the high speed particles, and the second is opened only for low speed particles, thus creating a temperature gradient which can be made to do mechanical work and therefore permitting the possibility of perpetual motion. This keeps the energy in the system constant, but does not allow for the increase of entropy, against which the demons would be fighting a losing battle.

The most important feature of communication theory is perhaps that, considered as feedback control systems, machines and organisms are essentially the same, and therefore have the same problems of communication.

The theory of communication can be regarded from at least three different levels. In the first place, there is the technical problem of transmitting accurately the symbols used in communication. It is fairly obvious that telecommunications should be of interest here, and the problem is primarily syntactical. We mean 'syntactical' to suggest the organization of the basic symbols according to rules, in a sense to be discussed later.

The second level problem can be called the semantic problem, and deals with the *meaning* that the symbols are said to carry. Thirdly, we want to know whether, or to what extent, the meaningful communications affect behaviour. This last might be called the 'pragmatic' problem. Some attempts have been made to develop the semantic theory of information, but little has been done at the pragmatic level. This is, again, precisely the domain of cybernetics.

All that has been said so far in this section has been about the syntactical problem at the technical level, and has been largely concerned with pointing out that a technical problem of communication exists. The problem is primarily electronic, at least for those who are concerned with the development of the theory, and their interest, and indeed the theory generally, has been directed towards the more technological forms of communication such as radio-telegraphy, radio-telephony, radio, television, and a wide variety of methods of signalling. This involved Morse code and teleprinters and, with it, the essentially mathematical process of making and breaking codes. It is of immediate interest that the theory in fact covers much more than these technical problems—technical, that is, in a narrow sense—for in particular it covers the ordinary, though vital, problem of communication between people, both as individuals and groups.

The technical aspect of communication

Communication theory really represents the attempts of the communication engineer to understand what he himself is doing.

It should be said, in passing, that *information* as used by the technologists has a slightly limited usage (which is characteristic of any term that has been given a precise meaning), and refers to all the messages that *are capable of* being sent, rather than to any sentence that has already conveyed meaning. The actual measure of information is given by

$$H = -\sum p_i \log_2 p_i$$

where p_i is a Laplacian probability and such that $0 \leqslant p_i \leqslant 1$.

A simple example will make the position clear. If the well-known choice in the *Merchant of Venice* had been extended from 3 caskets, as in the play, to 16 caskets, and a message had been passed to the suitor telling him which casket contained 'fair Portia's counterfeit', he would have been given just 4 bits of information. This can be seen from the general formula, or it can be thought of as the number of times that we have to divide 2 into the number of alternatives before we reduce them to 1. If there were 4 caskets, then a message indicating which casket contained the portrait would have just 2 bits of information. The word 'bit' is a contraction of 'binary digit', and the significance of this unit is that a message containing 2 bits of information needs 2 binary digits to communicate all the possibilities defined by the situation. The case of the 4 caskets demands the need for 4 messages for all possible outcomes, hence these can be coded as 00, 01, 10 and 11, thus requiring only 2 binary digits (bits).

Many other technical facts have been discovered, such as the Hartley Law which relates bandwidth to frequency of information. This makes it clear that any signal, being ergodic, will be a continuous periodic function, and thus will be characterized as a wave function, having frequency, wavelength, bandwidth and so on. Similarly, there are problems of noise. A practical example is that of the needle-hiss on a gramophone record. There is a well-known theory of filtering, due to Wiener (1949), that is intended to reduce the noise-to-signal ratio to a minimum. The procedure is, in essence, a statistical one, and can be thought of as picking one's way through the noise to minimize its effect. A channel with noise is a function of two stochastic processes, one for the message and one for the noise. This is closely connected with the familiar processes of frequency, amplitude, and other forms of modulation.

Hartley himself developed a theory of information similar to the one now widely accepted, wherein the concept of meaning was rejected, and the process of selecting from a set of signs organized as a language, with an alphabet, characterized the central notion of 'information'. The concept of bandwidth is quite fundamental to all communication, and Hartley's Law can be broadly interpreted for all such systems as meaning that the more elements of a message that we can send simultaneously, the shorter is the time required for their transmission. Some applications of these ideas to psychological data will be discussed in later chapters, although our primary emphasis in this book will not be on the application of information theory, but on the application of finite automata.

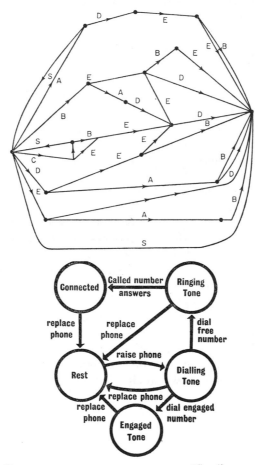

FIG. 2. TRANSITIONAL PROBABILITY DIAGRAMS. The diagram shows the transitional steps from state to state in terms of the artificial language described in the text. The second diagram shows the same thing for a simple telephone system.

Let us now return to a consideration of some further aspects of the technical definition of communication. We can graph stochastic processes in a manner that brings out the importance of the constraints that are enacted on any code that may be used.

The graph in Fig. 2 illustrates the states and the transition probabilities that will affect the artificial language of our example with the words A, ADEB, ADEE, etc. The dots represent states of a kind, and the lines represent the transitions from state to state, with the associated probabilities marked against them.

The constraints on language are illustrated by this graph. If we consider a language like Morse code it is clear that, having just transmitted a dot or a dash, anything can follow; whereas if there has just been a letter space or a word space only a dot or a dash can follow. If, for example, we did not have a letter space between Morse letters, it would be quite impossible to tell whether four successive dots was meant to be four successive E's, or H; such examples abound. In a sense this is part of the syntax of any language, and directly affects the technical problem of transmission.

One further example of a technical problem, code capacity, will be noticed before we leave the technical and syntactical problems of communication theory.

The code capacity of a channel has to be appropriate to the passing of a code, and the code capacity in the simple case, where all the symbols used are of the same length, has a simple form. If we have an alphabet with 16 symbols, each of the same duration, and thus each carrying 4 bits of information, the capacity of the channel is $4n$ bits per second, where the channel is capable of transmitting n symbols per second.

The subject of coding and transmission of codes, as well as the problems of decoding and breaking codes, is an extensive one. We shall return to it briefly later when we consider problems of the modelling of behaviour.

Language, syntax, semantics and pragmatics

The distinction between syntax, semantics and pragmatics is fundamentally a logical one, and has here been borrowed to apply to the general theory of communication. It is a distinction due largely to Carnap.

The idea is that *syntax* is a formal set of signs that have certain grammatical properties; they follow rules which allow certain combinations to occur and not others (in theory construction we shall think of these as being like models). Mathematics is purely syntactical until we say that the signs that mathematics uses: 0, 1, 2, 3, +, −, and so on are: nought, the positive integral numbers one, two, three, and the operations of addition and subtraction, and so on. Similarly, the x, y and z of elementary algebra can stand for fish, people or anything at all that follows the same rules; and when the correlation or association is performed, we have a descriptive language or theory.

As soon as we say that the symbols in our syntactical model *refer* to or *name* certain objects or relations, then we have added rules of meaning, and we are in the province of *semantics*; and if we then add the reactions of the person talking and the person spoken to, we are in *pragmatics* which deals with the behavioural effects of language.

In many ways it is true to say that syntax is mathematical logic, semantics is philosophy or philosophy of science, and pragmatics is psychology, but these fields are not really all distinct. The relation between syntax, semantics and pragmatics, and the desire to extend their integration at certain levels of description, is a motive power involved in the present book, and one that is perhaps not *logically* necessary to a cybernetic standpoint; nevertheless it is taken as a justification for the examination, cursory as it is, of logic and philosophy in the next chapter. We shall, therefore, be talking in terms of these distinctions in other chapters when we are dealing with logic, language, mathematics, as well as general problems of communication. The closeness of all these to communication theory will be quite apparent.

Servosystems

Another pillar of cybernetics appears in the development of that branch of engineering concerned with servosystems. As with computers, this is a specialized field, and there are many textbooks available for a suitably detailed study should the reader feel this to be necessary to his purpose. Here, we shall only outline the general principles of servosystems.

A servosystem is a closed loop control of a source of power; it is usually an error-actuated control mechanism operating on the principle of negative feedback. A servomechanism is a servosystem with a mechanical output such as a displacement or a rotation, although the closed loop of control could be used to model a far broader range of outputs.

Servosystems themselves can be divided into those that are continuous (these are the most usual), and those that deal with error or whatever is the controlling factor, in terms of discontinuities, such as step functions, where the variable makes sudden jumps from one value to another. They can also be divided into manually and automatically controlled systems, where we think of such characteristic activities as temperature regulators, process controllers, and remote position controllers.

The power source and the amplification and transmission of signals in servosystems may take many forms, although the electronic and electrical are by far the most popular. We should, however, mention hydraulic and pneumatic methods as alternatives to electrical ones.

Servosystems are self-controlling systems, and of course in this, again, they bear some resemblance to human beings.

They are capable of being represented by differential equations. Linear differential equations represent linear servosystems, and non-linear differential equations represent non-linear servosystems. Here again, a great deal of mathematics could be generated, but this would not be of direct interest to the cybernetician. The mathematical development is in the form of differential equations and functions of a continuous variable, or variables, and there is an analog of this in theories of learning (London, 1950, 1951; Estes, 1950, and many others) where differential equations are used as defining certain crude molar changes in learning, remembering and other cognitive acts.

To put it briefly, a servosystem is a standard engineering method for producing automatic control in actual hardware components; it is used as part of most automatic control systems. The computer-controlled machine tool cutter is an example of a servo-controlled system. The actual positioning and moving of the cutter, relative to the piece to be cut, depends on the transmission of information to the control by virtue of servomechanisms. In this case, one servomechanism was needed for each dimension of movement.

Similarly, in such devices as automatic pilots we have the basic manipulations of the control surfaces of the aircraft depending on servomechanisms. Characteristically, we have the input signal made up of a desired position signal, and the error—or departure from the desired position—which derives from the output, involving a comparison between the actual and the desired state of affairs, and then a compensating message being sent by the control to the item controlled, effecting whatever changes are necessary.

There are many physiological processes that appear to operate as closed-loop systems, and this idea is supported by the appearance of the general principle of *homeostasis* that has been closely associated with behavioural descriptions of organisms.

Finite automata

One most important concept within cybernetics is that of finite automata and, rather especially, their representation as logical nets. It is, in fact, so important as to receive explicit and detailed description in Chapters 4 and 5. Here, as a brief introduction, we should say that it was an insight of McCulloch and Pitts (1943) to see that Boolean algebra (discussed more fully in the next chapter) could be directly applied to the description of something very much like idealized nervous systems.

The essential link was, of course, the fact that—as we have already mentioned—computers could be described in Boolean terms, on the one hand, and nervous systems seemed like two-way switching devices, on the other.

This book is going to be concerned primarily with the development of the theory of logical nets, or 'Automata theory', as it is sometimes called. We hope to show how certain finite automata can be constructed in a manner similar to organisms, and thereby to offer an alternative approach to modelling behaviour mechanism.

Universal Turing machines (to be discussed in Chapter 3) are infinite automata to be analysed briefly as important to possible limitations on machines, and we shall further distinguish between the theory and the syntheses of finite automata, by which we mean simply the difference between paper and hardware machines.

Logical nets are themselves dependent on mathematics, computer design and communication theory, and represent the syntheses that are most immediately applicable to biological ends.

Cybernetics has, we shall argue, not only helped the telephone engineer, and those concerned with the technological problem of communication, by making their problems explicit, but also—and even more obviously—helped the biologist and the psychologist. For example, for many years the neurophysiologist has been guided by the idea of a reflex arc, like a telephone switchboard system, but he is now graduating to the idea of controlling systems of a homeostatic type. This advance not only broadens our understanding of biological function, but it also makes way for the application of mathematics, and the generally increased precision of prediction.

Summary

In this chapter we have summarized the principal constituent parts of cybernetics, and some parts of its central feature, that of artificial intelligence. The principal constituents are: (1) Mathematics, (2) Computers, (3) Communication theory, (4) Servosystems, and (5) Finite Automata. The last of these is rather more in the nature of a development than a foundation constituent part.

These subsections of cybernetics are, of course, subjects in their own rights. Here we are concerned with experimental psychology and biology, and have only summarized as much of the above as seems necessary to our proposed development of cybernetics for those purposes.

We could think conveniently of 'pure' cybernetics as mainly concerned with artificial intelligence, and the 'applied' branches as being Biocybernetics, Behavioural Cybernetics, Mathematical Cybernetics, Educational Cybernetics and so on.

Cybernetics in general is defined as the study, in theory and in practice of control and communication systems. Its relation to language, by virtue of its communication interest, ensures a vital link with logic, and also encourages the study of language which, in turn, inevitably touches the domain of philosophy. It also involves us closely in the study of heuristics.

CHAPTER 3

PHILOSOPHY, METHODOLOGY AND CYBERNETICS

UP TO now we have concentrated our attention upon cybernetics which is a new science and which has an important role as an integrating science. Now it is impossible to carry out a plan which involves the application of new methods in science without considering the philosophical or theoretical consequences, and this is especially so in cybernetics, which is so closely connected to logic, mathematics and scientific method; such considerations are the main reason for the inclusion of the present chapter.

The great importance of the contribution made by cybernetics to biology is that, under certain circumstances, it can formalize theories and make them precise. This same contribution is often claimed for mathematical logic, and it is relevant to quote Carnap (1958) on this point:

> If certain scientific elements—concepts, theories, assertions, derivations, and the like—are to be analyzed logically, often the best procedure is to translate them into the symbolic language. In this language, in contrast to ordinary word language, we have signs that are unambiguous and formulations that are exact; in this language, therefore, the purity and correctness of a derivation can be tested with greater ease and accuracy... A further advantage of using artificial symbols in place of words lies in the brevity and perspicuity of the symbolic formulas.

Much more could be said about formalization, but at the least we may claim the above advantages for cybernetics, with the additional advantage that our logical model is *effectively constructable*, and is therefore operationally effective. Indeed, as we have seen, actual hardware constructions are often desirable.

Another side to this matter, which seems to be closely related, is the philosophic (almost antiphilosophic) movement of *pragmaticism*, and this at least includes the general belief that science can contribute to the solution of philosophical problems, and, by dropping the classical search for universality and certainty, can solve its own theoretical problems (George, 1956a, 1957b; Crawshay-Williams, 1946, 1957; Pasch, 1958). This whole matter will be discussed to some extent in this chapter, but it is in fact a subject which calls for far more detailed treatment, with its specialized philosophical interests, than it can be given here. However, we hope we have already said enough to convince the experimental biologist and psychologist of the necessity for a theoretical analysis of his own activities, assuming that he was not already convinced.

Naïve Realism is probably a good starting point for scientific endeavour, but it is difficult not to believe that there are times when a more critical appraisal of one's starting point becomes necessary. Not, we would emphasize, that we wish to become involved in ontological or epistemological disputes but we should at least be fully aware of our own logical and philosophical commitments.

We must be prepared to revise our scientific theories continuously, and this means that we are committed to an understanding of our methods for constructing theories in the first place.

There is one possible misunderstanding about this sort of work that should be cleared up right at the start. The kind of therapeutic linguistic analysis and criticism that is to be considered in this chapter is at least as much meta-theoretical as theoretical. Let us put it this way: scientists indulge roughly in the following activities: making ordinary day-to-day observations, carrying out controlled observations, making observation-statements which purport to state what is observed and no more, generalizing about these observation-statements in the form of hypotheses, theories, etc., and finally, criticizing their findings, both the practical and the theoretical. Criticism is what is meant here by meta-theory, as against theory which is *inside* the science itself, as it were.

It is a commonplace that virtually anything can be a model of anything else, and that description and explanation depend on this fact. Similarly, any theory or language can be described in another theory or language, which we call a meta-theory or meta-language. In turn, the meta-theory can be the subject of a meta-meta-theory, and so on.

In psychology certainly, theory and meta-theory are often confused. The tough-minded experimentalist asks how a piece of linguistic analysis can help him in his work, and looks for theoretical help when he is being offered meta-theoretical help. The idea of methodological analysis is to help clarify the viewpoint of the scientist about his theories, point out his logical and linguistic confusions whenever possible, and help to orientate him in an *explicit* point of view. Science is, more than anything else, an attitude, and the object of our methods is to try to inculcate a clear-headed attitude. This whole purpose is to be distinguished from theoretical science which constitutes, broadly speaking, the generalizations within the subject and remains, in the form of cybernetics, our principal topic.

We should mention that the term 'psychology' will be used throughout this chapter in the broadest sense, to cover all and any parts, of the science of behaviour. Thus, physiology may, for convenience, be subsumed under the same term, as may any other part of biological science.

A particular problem that arises is the relation of psychology to philosophy. This is a vexed question in the eyes of philosophers, and it is noticeable that there is all too often an attitude of armed neutrality between the two camps which leads to the detriment of both. The writer takes the view that the distinction between science and philosophy is essentially one of degree, rather than a division marked by a sudden gulf, as is suggested by the sharp distinction sometimes made between the analytic and the synthetic, or between formal and factual sciences (Quine, 1953; George, 1956a).

We are not concerned here with discussing possible distinctions between the pragmatists and the formal semanticists, the logician and the experimentalist. A useful distinction certainly *can* be drawn between the logical and the empirical, and at a certain level it is possible to distinguish *formal* from *factual* commitments, without pressing the matter too far. The reason this is important to the scientist is because he must decide what end his generalizations are to serve. In this chapter we shall explicitly state the theory-construction methods that are to be adopted in the application of cybernetics to psychology and say something of the relation of philosophy to cognition. One reason for this is that psychologists should be familiar with the work of the philosophers, as has been suggested already, and in this pursuit the whole question of the relation between the two approaches is brought into relief.

It is not our intention to claim that a methodological analysis of learning or perception is an alternative to a scientific theory of learning or perception; indeed, we believe that the scientific theory is the proper aim of the psychologist, and the methodological analysis is primarily a preliminary which helps to clear the way. We believe that much that has been said by philosophers about perception is either misleading or wrong, and indeed it must be so in the eyes of scientists when philosophers write in terms of their own 'casual' observations of themselves and others.

An important reason for encouraging the psychologist to read at least an outline of philosophical problems is to make him more sophisticated about language and its use, since one distinction that generally seems to hold is that philosophers are far more perceptive of linguistic difficulties than are their psychological counterparts, although in fact the psychologist needs this sophistication just as much. He has recently been blinded in these matters by his overwhelming faith in experiment, and while experiment is vital to science, so also is theory, and the need to avoid conceptual confusion. Wittgenstein (1953) has said:

> The confusion and barrenness of psychology is not to be explained by calling it a 'young science' ... for in psychology there are experimental methods and *conceptual confusion*... The existence of experimental methods makes us think we have the means of solving the problems which trouble us; though problems and methods pass one another by.

There has been some doubt as to what Wittgenstein meant by this passage, and it is possible that he meant one or other of at least two different things. Certainly it is true that psychology has sometimes foundered on methodological rocks, in that some of the workers in the field appear to think that experimental methods of the 'molar' kind can be used to solve problems of thinking, imagination, and the like, *in a manner* in which behaviouristic and molar techniques could not possibly succeed. Thus it sometimes appears that the essence of the problem is often missed by a particular experimental approach. This usually means that the problem demands methodological rather than experimental techniques, or waits on the advance of neurophysiology ('Molecular' experimental methods), or both. We shall continue throughout the book to use the words 'molar' and 'molecular' as relative to each other, and meaning 'with respect to large scale variables' and 'with respect to small scale variables', respectively.

In a sense, pragmatics and cybernetics together attempt to give an answer to Wittgenstein that might have satisfied him. The choice of the sensory, perceptual and learning fields arises only because, needing a particular and central problem on which to exercise the techniques, they appear to be the most central ones for behavioural studies.

Our approach to cybernetics is through a methodological or analytic approach to psychological problems. Our interest, then, is no longer in the problems that can, in any narrow sense, be made to follow from certain assumptions; we are now interested in the development of a scientific theory, the second half of Braithwaite's 'zip-fastener' theory. In other words, we may start by appeal to marks on paper and give an interpretation to these in developing descriptive statements, on the one hand. On the other hand we can turn to what is the more important business for scientists, the making of inductive generalizations based on a series of observations. Philosophers are really concerned with what it means to talk of making observations, and so really only one part of the formal half of the zip-fastener theory is touched upon in their domain, the other formal part and the factual part being utilized in the field of science. Our main interest here is in trying to make a Braithwaitean type of approach more realistic in meeting scientific needs.

Implicit in this whole work is the feeling already alluded to, that the division between philosophical and descriptive sciences is artificial and, at most, one of degree; thus, when words like 'factual' and 'formal' are used, they are used on the understanding that they are rough classifications employed merely for convenience, and in no sense fundamental. This approach has an explicit attitude to the mind–body problem which, from the scientific point of view, is not a problem at all, and from the philosophic viewpoint is capable of a new interpretation (Pap, 1949; Sellars, 1947; Quine, 1953; George, 1956a; Morris, 1946) Descriptive pragmatics, in which the observer and the speaker both occur (as well as the signs they use), are regarded as wholly continuous with semantics or pure pragmatics, and no sort of gulf or sudden discontinuity is thought to arise between them.

Cybernetics and philosophy

Philosophical or linguistic analysis may be regarded, then, as being *preliminary* to any sort of scientific process, and we are in fact limiting our science to cybernetics. In other words, our explanations are intended to be in the form of blueprints for machines that will *behave* in the manner made necessary by the observable facts.

There is some evidence that all scientific explanations take this form, or should take this form if they are to be effective. The same sort of insistence on the empirical reference of scientific theories is seen in so-called *operational definitions* (Bridgman, 1927).

It seems worth repeating that cybernetics, which is only incidentally concerned with the actual construction in hardware of machine manifestations of its theories, is consistent with behaviourism. It takes behaviourism further along its path in making it *effective*, without destroying any of the increasing sophistication that behaviourism has recently acquired.

Our next task is to outline, for the non-philosopher, the various philosophic categorizations and classifications. This must necessarily be brief and couched in general terms.

Viewpoints in philosophy

In trying to draw up brief and yet coherent classifications of different philosophical viewpoints, one is confronted with a certain measure of difficulty and ambiguity. This is, of course, true of most classifications, and stems from the fact that there are virtually as many different philosophical views as there are philosophers. Furthermore, all the different philosophical categories cannot be placed in a single dimension; indeed, apparent inconsistencies in terminology would quickly arise if such were attempted.

Bearing in mind these basic difficulties, an attempt will be made to give a brief account of the principal philosophical views, with the idea of providing an orientating background to the analysis of cognition from a philosophic and ultimately cybernetic viewpoint. Since such an analysis must necessarily be brief, it will not serve every purpose, and it is *only* intended here to be sufficient for an understanding of the various philosophical approaches to knowledge and perception. It may be thought of as an attempt to classify on the philosophical level what psychologists have called learning and perception, although it really involves all of cognition.

Convenient classifications

As a basis for discussion it will be useful to consider the categories suggested by Feigl (1950) as being roughly appropriate for the study of methodology and epistemology. Feigl lists the following nine views:

1. Naïve (physical) realism.
2. (Fictionalistic agnosticism) fictionalism.
3. Probabilistic realism.
4. Naïve (conventionalistic) phenomenalism.
5. Critical phenomenalism (operationism, positivism).
6. Formalistic (syntactic) positivism.
7. Contextual phenomenalism.
8. Explanatory (hypothetico-deductive) realism.
9. Semantic (empirical) realism.

(These views will be referred to hereafter *without* use of that part of the title which is placed in parentheses.)

We consider these nine possible philosophical viewpoints sufficient for our initial classifications. The issue could be narrowed by overlooking even more of the differences between the various views held, and combining 1, 3, 8 and 9 under the heading of Realism, and combining 2, 4, 5 and 6 under Phenomenalism, and leaving 7 as a sort of half-way house between the two. Thus, in one dimension our main distinction is to be between some form of Realism and some form of Phenomenalism. We might when thinking of Realism, however, still maintain a distinction between Naïve and Critical Realism. Any attempt at a final integration, which may leave many particular questions undecided, would probably say that Critical Realism and Critical Phenomenalism (if in each case they are sufficiently critical) would differ very little, and yet there would still be *internal* differences with respect to questions of cognition.

Language

Cutting across almost all that has been said is the question of language and its use, and the more general problem of communication. There are at least two apparently different views about the nature of the linguistic problem. We may on one hand take up G. E. Moore's view that natural language is the proper and sufficient description of the real world, and that the problem of the philosopher and of the scientist is to see that he uses natural language in its correct way. This view of language could be maintained independently of an epistemological or ontological commitment. It would hold, roughly speaking, that to say as the fictionalists do that 'atoms do not really exist' is to misuse the term 'exist', for whatever one conceives to be the *sense* of existence, the fact that atoms exist is certainly true. In a sense the problem here has been to push language away from the ideas underlying it. We can interpret what you say according to common usage, but its underlying sense may not be so obvious.

In fact, we shall not accept this viewpoint, but shall try to be aware of the ways—two at the very least—in which realistic philosophers such as Moore regard language. Realists holding the second view, while trying to keep as near as possible to natural language, would feel free to lay down conventions and rules about language, although these constructed languages would ultimately be within the structure of a natural language. This does not necessarily mean that what the constructed languages say can be wholly reduced to natural language without the vagueness that attends the use of simile and metaphor, since the whole point of such constructed languages is to avoid such vagueness. What, on the other hand, we cannot do is to explicate 'truth' or 'meaning', or any other problem term of natural language, within a constructed language and hope to explicate its natural use, which may of course be vague, and whose meaning depends, as they do with so many such terms, on their context. A formalized system lays down rules by which such vagueness may be ruled out, but it does not by virtue of this *explain* the *meanings* of the basic terms. This, we personally conceive, is closely related to the study of signs from a pragmatic viewpoint.

It is along these lines of providing appropriate contexts that we believe that science can be as vital to philosophy as philosophy is to science.

Scientific theory construction

Now we shall turn to the explicit process by which we shall construct theories of science, and by which we believe they should normally be constructed. This is the theme of the remaining section of this chapter.

Again, as in the case of philosophical analysis, we believe—and for the same reasons—that an explicit statement of methods is necessary. Psychology, biology and the social, behavioural and information sciences, have continually suffered from verbal and methodological muddles, and this at least might be avoided with a little care.

First of all we shall illustrate our conception of the nature of the scientific procedure in a simple, anecdotal manner, showing its close and crucial relationship to the role which cybernetics plays in the scientific process. This relationship will be clarified at the end of the present chapter.

The nature of science in general

In order to relate our intuitive ideas of logic to the general process of communication and to the very basic ideas of science, let us suppose that an observer has just arrived at a town in Erewhon, where he is to study the behaviour of shopkeepers. For the sake of the example we will assume that he does not know the language of the country, and that in any case he is too shy to ask questions (physicists cannot ask questions of particles with any hope of an answer). His mission is to construct a scientific theory that describes the shopkeeping behaviour of the Erewhonians.

He starts by observing the behaviour of shopkeepers on the first day, a Monday, and he finds that they work from nine until five. On Tuesday he finds that the same times are observed, and he is now in a position to make his first inductive inference, to the effect that they work every day from nine until five. The next day, Wednesday, confirms this hypothesis, but his observations on Thursday show that his first hypothesis is inadequate, since on this day the shops are closed at one o'clock. Friday brings working hours of nine until five again, and Saturday is the same, but on Sunday the shops do not open at all. This upsets completely any second hypothesis which he might reasonably have formulated on the evidence up to that point, and it will be some weeks before our observer begins to see the repetitive nature of the facts.

After a few months the observer may be reasonably sure that he now has a hypothesis that adequately covers all the facts, and it will not be shown to be inadequate until the occurrence of a national holiday or its equivalent. It is probable that he will never be able to understand completely the variation of certain national holidays, such as Easter, and even if he does learn the rule which governs this particular holiday, it is quite certain that he will never be able to understand what rule governs the occurrence of certain other holidays which are given merely to celebrate some unique event, and *never* recur.

In the above analogy the rules will never be quite sufficient to make a completely watertight theory, but the method will be sufficient for most purposes, and this is all science is ever concerned with: a theory and a model *for some purpose.*

For similar reasons we can never have more than probability laws in science, since we can never be sure that they will not subsequently be in need of revision.

There are other aspects of the analogy that also hold good. If we had employed only one observer to discover the shopkeeping laws of Erewhon, he would have been in the akward position of having to decide at which particular point he should set up his observation post. We should be interested to know whether what our observer saw was typical of the behaviour of all the shopkeepers, or not. Suppose our town was such that different rules applied to other shopkeepers that he did not see; how would he know how to answer such an implied criticism? All he could say would be that he tried to take a fair sample of the population. The efficiency with which he carried out his sampling is a measure of the accuracy of the results. This is really a matter of individual differences, and is treated in experimental psychology by statistical methods.

This story has represented roughly what scientists are doing, and we can now discuss the problems of the psychologist in particular, bearing in mind that our illustration still needs to be explicitly linked to the cybernetic approach.

PRINCIPLES OF THEORY CONSTRUCTION

Psychological theory

The psychologist has to construct theories of behaviour: learning, perception, etc., that satisfy some logical standards, quite apart from incorporating our knowledge of behaviour, neurophysiology, and what is intuitively accepted in behavioural terms. Indeed, the process of producing any theory of behaviour requires the production of *effective pro-*

cedures for determining the application of the theory at a variety of different descriptive levels. This of course is already widely accepted in the physical sciences.

The essential steps that need to be outlined are: (1) that any particular scientist must go through the process of making observations, as already illustrated; (2) he must generalize upon these observations, and (3) will eventually produce scientific theories which are initially hypotheses, and become 'laws' when they are highly confirmed. Now it is not important whether what is being described or constructed is mathematics or a science such as physics or psychology. Whatever it is that is under discussion or investigation at any particular time is what we will call the *object-language*, and we must discuss it in some other language, a *meta-language*. This meta-language may be itself an object-language for some other investigation, but this is of no importance at the time.

We are also vitally concerned with the construction of object-languages, and these can be represented as models of whatever the non-linguistic entities are that need to be modelled.

Scientists are forced to start from assumptions, which represent their prior agreements with themselves for the sake of a particular investigation. The assumptions are represented by only partially analysed statements; the notion of partly analysed terms is secondary to this, and will represent an internal analysis of sentences into their parts. Language and that is what a scientific theory is, in a sense, part of—has the sentence as its natural unit. The syntax of the propositional calculus or any systematic marks on paper, any structure such as a lattice, blueprint, or map, is capable of being used as a model for a scientific theory, and here we accept the essential distinction, made by Braithwaite (1953), between a model for a theory and the theory itself. The model will be *explained* in the theory. All this is couched in the natural or symbolic *language* that is used for descriptive purposes by particular scientists.

It may be necessary to add certain pragmatic devices to any scientific explanation, in the form of ostensive rules or definitions, operational definitions, and the like. These may serve to sharpen the meaning of the language used for the theory, or the meta-theory, for even here we soon find that only very few and very limited investigations can be restricted to one clearcut theory language. We must therefore be prepared to think in interconnected chains of such theory languages, which will give repeated descriptions of different facts of nature on different levels and in different ways. It is, in a sense, the particular investigation that is the scientist's working unit. The whole of science or any of its divisions can thus be reconstructed in any number of ways.

For the psychologist, working beyond a narrow behaviourism and yet determined to avoid that which cannot be treated on a basis of public observation alone, the problem is to find more and more models and interpretations, as well as theory languages, for the coherent description of his vast collection of empirical facts.

The result of an uncertainty about the correct progress of theory and explanation in science has sometimes led to models being used descriptively, whereas in fact what needs to be developed is a model with a theory that has a controlled vagueness: that of the *surplus meaning* of its theoretical terms. This lack of specificity, this possibility of many interpretations of the same model, rather than the attempt to construct a model which fits in detail one possibly non-representative piece of the whole set of observations to be explained, is necessary to the fruitfulness of science.

The scientist will be concerned with the following procedures that may be listed in the order they usually occur:

(1) Learning by description the existing information (George, 1959a) on a branch of the subject we will call *A*. Testing this information for consistency (internally and externally) and finding it wanting in certain respects either in generality or consistency.

(2) The stating of simple, observational facts collectively with inductive generalizations originally called *A*, and now *A'* (if different from *A*). This requires a language the foundations of which are to be agreed upon; it will not necessarily be the same as in (1) but will necessarily be capable of being interpretable in the same language, at some level, as (1), or alternatively (1) in (2).

(3) The generalization process which is based inductively on a certain number of instances is always subject to revision.

(4) A model for *A*, essentially deductive, which is utilized in terms of the inductive parts of the theory. It may be pictorial, symbolic, or anything at all that is capable of interpretation in terms of the language of either (1) or (2).

(5) If we use a merely descriptive language for the generalizations, we must be prepared to show the nature of the underlying structural model,

since a description of empirical facts is really a description of structural relations. This process is called the *formalizing* of a theory.

(6) This whole process is sufficient for any science.

(7) This process may go on without end, with continual checking, criticism and analysis, which may take any part of the whole (or the whole) of science as the object of its investigation.

So much then for the initial complications, wherein theories are particular (or particularized) languages, or parts of independently formulated languages, ultimately capable of interpretation in natural language (or a slightly more rigorous equivalent). Thus, if we use the word 'language' for the interpretation of a system of marks, we are already committed to a certain theoretical structure. This is why a scientific theory and a language are interdependent, and *may* be one.

Models

We are concerned with cybernetics and therefore with logic and, what is essentially the same, logical nets as models of behaviour (see Chapters 4 and 5). We do not intend, here, to describe in any detail the whole of the possible range of models that *can* be used in the processes of scientific theory construction. The most obvious of those that have already been used are the syntax of the propositional calculus, the functional calculus, and the various existing calculi that are intended to be given an intepretation as propositions and functions, and have thus been widely used by philosophers and mathematicians. These are open to use in science and will, if the logistic foundation of mathematics is to be accepted, lead to the whole of mathematics. Mathematical structures such as lattices, abstract algebras and other symbolic models or structures may also serve as such models. From the viewpoint of cybernetics, these systems may be constructed in hardware; indeed, any symbolic model can be regarded as a physical system and produced in hardware.

The model that we have been mainly using—one that can be seen to be closely related to other models and theories that we have mentioned—is that of a *finite automaton* which, for all practical purposes, is an idealized organism.

At first our aim here was certainly not strictly neurological, but rather, while using a model that can also be used for neurology, to seek to develop a theory that has usefulness, precision, and the possibility of predictability at every level.

The logical nets which we are to discuss are roughly isomorphic with a part of logic, that part called the propositional calculus coupled with a part of the lower functional calculus, all suffixed for time. The word 'roughly' occurs above because in fact the logic concerned is actually *supplemented by* a time-delay operator. There is a relationship between the nets that can be drawn, and the formulae that can be written which is closely analogous to the relationship between geometry and algebra.

Logic and cybernetics

We have already said something about logic and its relation to logical nets; now, we must try to be more specific, and describe at least as much of logic as is necessary to an understanding of cybernetics and of our theory of logical nets.

In the first place, logic arises because logic seems to represent the process of ideal reasoning, and it is reasoning that the machines in which we are interested can do. They have to be able to perform the operations of a deductive and inductive character if they are to be of cybernetic interest. Such machines have sometimes been directly described in logical terms; in fact there has been a general theory of machines, of the control and communication type, that draws on mathematical logic in its description. We shall now describe something of the development of modern logic and decision processes in paper machines.

Logic in ordinary language

In an historically given or natural language such as English it is not always possible to draw strict inferences, because of the vagueness and ambiguity of some of the words we ordinarily use. We sometimes mean something special by a word, but there is no complete and definite set of rules for what words should mean, and vagueness is therefore inevitable, for inferences depend on meanings, and meanings in natural language are vague. But in spite of this there are many obvious examples of the use of logic. Thus, when I say 'Jack is a man', I do not need to know any more facts about Jack to know that he is also a featherless biped, since all men are featherless bipeds. This simple inference follows from the meanings of the words 'man' and 'featherless biped', and I am assuming that there is little chance of these words being misunderstood; but there are very many sentences which refer to classes, events and relations which are very far from clear.

For a long time philosophers have analysed language with the object of trying to sort out logical puzzles, but in the meantime mathematicians have developed a mathematical theory.

Since mathematics has to be definite in a way that ordinary language does not, we should expect to find, and do find, that mathematical logic is a perfectly precise arrangement of symbols, like ordinary algebra wherein instead of saying that x stands for anything at all, we say that x stands for a class of objects: x is all featherless bipeds, or all automobiles, or all of anything at all. Now the most interesting sort of relations are those of class-inclusion and class-exclusion. All red shoes, for example, are included in the class of all red objects, and excluded from the class of all green objects. Of course, difficulties can arise, because it can be argued that red shoes are perhaps not all-red, or that green shoes may not be all-green, and that both are a mixture of different colours. The answer to this is that the algebra of classes, or Boolean Algebra as it is often called, only holds for objects which are capable of being classified as a member of some class. More complicated algebras have been developed, and some mention of these will be made later in this chapter.

One particular interpretation of the Boolean algebra of classes is of special interest. This involves the assumption that all the classes are to be understood as propositions or sentences. Thus, if we say in the algebra, where the dot '.' between x and y is taken to be 'and', that $x.y$ is the class of all objects that are (say) red *and* round, then, following the convention of changing x and y to p and q, we can say that $p.q$ is the conjunction of two statements, say, 'Jack is a man' and 'All men are featherless bipeds'.

The mathematician, having said that he means his variables p, q, r, . . . to be understood as sentences, then constructs relations between his symbols that seem to be in keeping with the way we use logical inference in ordinary language. In fact he will preserve the intuitive meanings of 'and' and 'or' (for which he uses 'v', and which he means to be an inclusive

'or', meaning p or q or both); he will also have a symbol for 'not', i.e.
'$\sim$', and from these he builds up a whole system of mathematics.

We shall just repeat here, using the ordinary calculus of classes, the
essential relations from which, by use of careful rules, the whole system
is built up.

$$X.Y \text{ means } X \text{ and } Y$$

$$XvY \text{ means } X \text{ or } Y$$

$$\sim X \text{ means not-}X$$

The diagrams show clearly the significance of these simple relations.
Let the square stand for the whole possible universe under consideration
and be symbolized by 1, then the opposite, or nothing, is symbolized by 0.

It will be easily seen that simple reasoning can be carried out in this
system. Let us use the symbol '$\subset$' for 'is contained in', '$\rightarrow$' for 'implies',
and '$=$' for an equivalence relation, then,

$$A.B = A \rightarrow A \subset B$$

The syllogism about Jack and featherless bipeds can now be written

$$A \subset B.B \subset C \rightarrow A \subset C$$

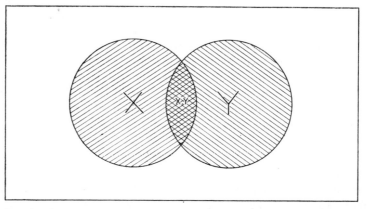

FIG. 3A. AND. $X.Y$ is short for X and Y and is represented by the area of
the overlap of X and Y, where X may represent all red objects say, and Y
all round objects, then X and Y represent all red *and* round objects.

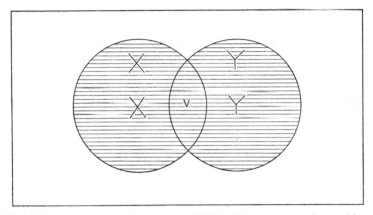

Fig. 3B. Or. *Xv Y* is short for *X* or *Y* in the inclusive sense of or and is represented by the whole area of *X* and *Y* taken together.

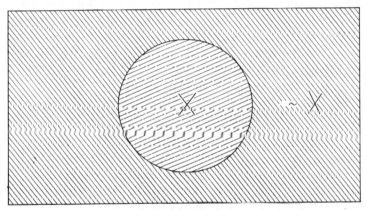

Fig. 3c. Not. Everything not within the circle of *X*, is not-*X*. If *X* represents all green objects, then all objects of other colours lie outside the circle because they are not green.

With these simple examples we shall leave Boolean algebra and turn to the propositional calculus, which interprets the variables of Boolean algebra as propositions.

Before stating the formal requirements of the Propositional Calculus as an axiomatic system we would explain that we are now explicitly stating, in a meta-language, the symbols to be used in the object-language (here, the propositional calculus), and the way they can be formed into acceptable units, like words, sentences, or formulae. In English, for example, the word 'word' is well-formed and the word 'xxyyzz' is not. This reminds us that all combinations of symbols do not satisfy our formation rules. We set down, then, certain well-formed formulae (wff) called axioms, and use another wff as a rule of inference to generate further well-formed formulae which have the additional property of being true in the system, i.e. theorems.

THE PROPOSITIONAL CALCULUS

The propositional calculus is said to formalize the connectives *and*, *or*, *not*, and *if—then*.... There are many different systems and various notations for the propositional calculus. The formulation (called $\bar{P}$) which we shall give is one of those used by Church (1944). $\bar{P}$ is composed of:

(1) *Primitive symbols:* [,], $\supset$, $\sim$, and an infinite list of propositional variables for which the letters p, q, r, s, u, v, w (with or without numerical subscripts) may be used.

(2) *Formation rules:*

(A) Any variable alone is well formed (wf).

(B) If A and B are well formed, so are $\sim A$ and $A \supset B$. Where A and B are syntactical variables (variables in the syntax language) which designate formulae of the calculus (in this case $\bar{P}$).

(3) *Rules of inference:*

(A) From A and $A \supset B$ to infer B *(modus ponens)*.

(B) From A to infer $S_{B'}^{A'} A \mid$ where $S_{B'}^{A'} A \mid$ means the result of substituting B' for A' in all its occurrences in A.

(4) *Axioms:*

(A) $p \supset [q \supset r] \supset .p \supset q \supset .p \supset r$

(B) $p \supset .q \supset p$

(C) $\sim p \supset \sim q \supset .q \supset p$

It should be explained that the dots (.) in these axioms take the place of brackets, and that the general rule is one of association to the left. Thus $p \supset q \supset p$ could be regarded as ambiguous as it stands, and could mean either $(p \supset q) \supset p$ or $p \supset (q \supset p)$; if no dot occurred, then it should be taken to be the former, but the dot in axiom B implies the latter. Similarly, axiom C with brackets reads:

$$\sim p \supset \sim q \supset (q \supset p)$$

As a result of these axioms and the rules of inference we can define a theorem. A theorem is a well-formed formula (wff) which is obtainable from the axioms by a finite number of applications of the rules of inference. We could, it should be noticed, reduce the list of rules of inference to only one by the omission of substitution and the use of an infinite list of axioms.

We are not, of course, concerned with what might be called the technicalities of logic, so we shall not discuss the deduction theorem, regular formulae, completeness, duality, independence, etc. However, it is worth mentioning that the decision problem (the effective procedure or algorithm for discovering whether any wff is a theorem) has been solved for the propositional calculus, and it says that every tautology is a theorem and every theorem is a tautology. By a tautology we mean a wff of the propositional calculus which has the truth value t (see below) for all possible combinations t and f (to be interpreted as 'truth' and 'falsehood') replacing the propositional variables in the wff. The decision problem for the lower functional calculus, and therefore all higher functional calculi, has been shown to be unsolvable. In the network models of Chapter 3 we shall use '$\equiv$' rather than '$\supset$', where '$\equiv$' means 'if and only if' rather than the one-way relation 'if—then ...'.

We shall also mention the Sheffer stroke (used by von Neumann in his logical nets), which is another constant in the propositional calculus. It is written $---|\cdots$ and is defined $a \mid b = $ df. $\sim av \sim b$, where 'df.' means 'is defined as'. There is also a conjunction stroke symbol $\downarrow$ which is defined by $a \downarrow b = $ df. $\sim a. \sim b$. It was of interest that the propositional calculus can be constructed in terms of the one single primitive constant term, the Sheffer stroke, and this is the reason for von Neumann's choice of basic logical net elements.

We should remind the reader at this point that we are thinking in terms of formal or axiomatic systems which start from axioms and use rules of inference to generate theorems. One of the first things we look for in an axiomatic system is a decision procedure or algorithm which will shortcut the procedures of proof which otherwise would be lengthy and unwieldy;

we also look for the consistency and the completeness of the axiomatic system. There are other features of axiomatic systems which we should mention but not discuss further and these include the development of theorems in the meta-language which is where all the rules formalizing the system in the object-language are couched. This often means the development of theorems which considerably simplify proofs in the actual object-language.

THE FUNCTIONAL CALCULI

To go from $\bar{P}$ to F^1 (the functional calculus of the first order) we need to add individual variables: x, y, z, x_1, y_1, z_1..., and functional variables F^1, G^1, H^1, F^1_1, G^1_1, H^1_1, ... F^2, G^2, H^2, F^2_1, G^2_1, H^2_1, ... F^n, G^n, H^n, F^n_1, G^n_1, H^n_1, ... these being singularly, binary ... n-ary functional variables.

The functional calculi permit the analysis of predicates and functions, and we shall wish to make assertions such as 'for all x, $F^1(x)$' and 'there exists at least one x, such that $F^1(x)$', and we shall thus need to add the Universal and Existential quantifiers, respectively, to our notation; they are (x) and (Ex) respectively, which makes the above two sentences:

$$(Ax)F^1(x) \text{ and } (Ex)F^1(x) \text{ respectively.}$$

We shall need, also, to construct new formation rules, rules of inference and axioms to meet the needs of our new primitive symbols which will include, as part of it, the whole propositional calculus.

It is, of course, possible to generalize further to the functional calculus of order 2, (F^2),—there are many different kinds of such functional calculi—and so on up to F^n.

We shall now add a word on truth-tables. We cannot discuss the Matrix method, as the tabular method is called, in detail here, but it is sufficient for a two-valued interpretation where t and f are used (these may be thought of as 'truth' and 'falsehood', or as 'firing' and 'not firing' in the logical networks) if we ascribe t and f exhaustively to all the variables in our formulae. Thus, to take a simple formula of $\bar{P}$ such as $\sim p$, its truth-table is:

p	$\sim p$
t	f
f	t

and *pvq* (where '*v*' may be read as 'inclusive or', i.e. *p* or *q* or both) has truth-table:

p	*q*	*pvq*
t	*t*	*t*
t	*f*	*t*
f	*t*	*t*
f	*f*	*f*

then $p \supset q$, which can be translated as $\sim pvq$, has truth-table arrived at by combining the above two truth-tables; it is as follows:

p	*q*	$p \supset q$
t	*t*	*t*
t	*f*	*f*
f	*t*	*t*
f	*f*	*t*

For the functional calculus the truth conditions on the existential and universal operator demand that one or all values of *x* satisfy the respectively given formulae:

$$(Ex)\, F^1(x) \text{ and } (Ax)\, F^1(x).$$

As far as the functional calculi are concerned, there is a whole set of such calculi and it has been shown that whereas a lower functional calculus has the property of completeness and consistency, there is no decision procedure for it, and furthermore with the higher functional calculi we get to the point where we cannot even show consistency and completeness at the same time within the system. This is part of what is entailed by Gödel's incompleteness theorem.

The development of the functional calculi and the associated Theory of Types which distinguishes sets from sets of subsets from sets about sets about sets and, in other words, distinguishes different levels of propositions in the system to avoid the well-known paradoxes, is that it depends on functions and variables and the question arises as to whether the dependence on functions and variables is absolutely necessary. The answer has been shown by Rosser and by Church (1944) that you can develop a formal language or calculus sufficiently rich to provide virtually all that is required by classical mathematics, certainly by way of constructive theorems, by use of constants alone. This has been done by what is known as combinatorial logic or, in the case of Church, the calculus of lambda conversion.

We shall not pursue a detailed examination of these systems here, but merely note they exist because there are times when the elimination of functions from the argument facilitates particularly the computerization of the system. Against this facilitation of the computerization remains the difficulty that substitution seems to be a natural operation of mathematics and translating it into combinatorial terms merely makes the equivalent of substitution that much more complicated. As usual, what we gain on the swings, we tend to lose on the roundabouts.

It is easy to see how it may be possible to extend the notion of truth-tables to 1, 2, . . ., n truth-values (Rosser and Turquette, 1952). Thus a truth-table for 'v' in a three-valued logic could be written.

p	q	pvq
1	1	1
2	1	1
3	1	1
1	2	1
2	2	2
3	2	2
1	3	1
2	3	2
3	3	3

Much thought and effort have gone into the construction of many-valued and modal logics (Rosser and Turquette, 1952), and we can do no more here than summarize the general scheme of things, while suggesting a little of their possible value for cybernetics.

It is clear that just as we can generalize geometry from the best known two- and three-dimensional cases to any number of dimensions, so we can for logic. We can simply say that we do not wish to limit our interpretation to 1 and 0 as 'truth' and 'falsehood'; we can have n truth values whether we give the other n-2 values an interpretation or not. We shall say something later of the significance of this matter for switching systems, but straightaway we can see that the law of the excluded middle, which says that everything is either a or not-a, may be discarded if this sort of logic is to be used descriptively. Indeed, intuitionistic logics have long denied the law (Heyting, 1934). However, we can regard our many-valued logics as satisfying this law by retaining some corresponding law of the excluded $(n+1)$th. Intuitionistic logics and many-valued logics, it should be noted, are not necessarily the same.

The modal logics give a specific interpretation to the truth values beyond true and false. Reichenbach, for example, has attempted to analyse the foundations of Quantum Mechanics in terms of a three-valued logic wherein the third truth-value had the interpretation of 'undecidable'. Other qualifying modalities can be introduced as interpretations, such as Necessarily true, Contingently true, Possibly true, Impossible, etc., and modal operators such as Np, Cp, Pp, Ip, etc., have been introduced into the literature.

There has been much discussion as to the possible usefulness of many-valued logics, and it seems that on most occasions when it might be useful, the descriptions are usually capable of being reduced to the usual two-valued terms. Yet again there are many sorts of situations, both with regard to truth and in ordinary empirical descriptions, where things are not conveniently regarded as being either a or not-a. This, of course, involves matters of probability, and is the reason for our later discussion of what have been sometimes called empirical logics.

The horseshoe sign $\supset$ that we have used for material implication in the propositional and functional calculi is by no means the only sort of implication sign that might have been introduced into our formal logical scheme of things, and much argument has surrounded the interpretation of this symbol as 'material implication'. C. I. Lewis (1932) has developed a logic based on strict implication which he believes comes nearer to what we normally mean by 'implication' in ordinary language. He takes '$\Diamond p$' to mean 'p is possible', and 'o' as meaning 'is consistent with', and this leads to the possibility of p being given a definition in terms of the self-consistency of p:

$$\Diamond p = p \, o \, p$$

Similarly for two variables p and q, we have

$$\Diamond pq = p \, o \, q$$

and implication, which is symbolized by ... $\prec$, is defined

$$p \prec q = \sim (p \sim q)$$

which, on application of the above, leads to

$$p \prec q = \sim (p \, o \sim q)$$

This sort of logic is more important in the analysis of language than in logical networks, nevertheless in the study of networks the various possible logics and the evident infinity of possible logical calculi should be borne in mind.

To take our artificial languages or calculi one step further we should introduce predicates P, Q, R, ... which can be associated with particular 'argument expressions' a, b, c, ... so that by $P(a)$, $Q(b)$, $R(c)$ is meant 'a has the property P', etc., or to take a particular example, 'Napoleon was a Corsican'.

It is now possible to construct calculi (and therefore models) of enormous complexity and richness, many of which are directly important to cybernetics. In this context special notice should be taken of the artificial languages of Woodger (1952); unfortunately we lack the space to illustrate his work here (see page 66 et seq.).

Generally, we shall remember as much as we can about logic for three reasons: (1) Logical calculi can be used as models and be reproduced in hardware. (2) Logical calculi can be given explicit interpretations for descriptive purposes in scientific theories. (3) Logical calculi and their interpretations are, like scientific theories, examples of some of the most complex and sophisticated human behaviour, and are thus of considerable psychological interest.

We shall be discussing in a later chapter the question of drawing inferences in computer programs. At least here for the record we should mention that a lot of work has recently been done on theorem proving by computer. There have been two different motives involved. On the one hand (Newell, Shaw and Simon, 1963) there has been a search to prove logical theorems in the manner that humans use, by heuristic methods, and on the other hand there has been an attempt (Wang, 1960) simply to try to make mathematics, or the derivation of proofs in mathematics, possible on the computer. Inevitably the second method tends to be more nearly algorithmic and follows processes such as that of pattern recognition which are far more effective in producing theorems at a great rate.

This is the purpose of the operation and one that is basically different from that of the heuristic approach which is concerned with showing how human beings do it. Inevitably, the heuristic approach to theorem proving by virtue of its goal is slower and different in its construction. It is very much the same as the difference between proof the long way by a sequence of steps, in, say, the propositional calculus and proof by using a decision procedure.

Paper and pencil machines

Our next subject for discussion concerns what are sometimes called Paper Machines (specialized automata). The aspect which has our particular interest springs directly from the decision procedure considerations described earlier. The idea is, as has been said before, that there are some aspects of mathematics that are machine-like in their characteristics and, once the directions are laid down, even a stupid person could follow them and eventually find an answer to whatever problem is posed. What is so important about this is the fact that we have a ready-made method for laying down a blueprint, or a theory, that we shall know is effectively constructible, without the need for actual construction to take place. It means that we can build paper machines without going to the expense of finding out *in practice* whether the blueprint will work or not.

But before pursuing this notion further, a little more must be said on that vitally important matter, the postulational or axiomatic method. This involves making a set of basic statements usually taken to represent facts or hypotheses that we are going to assume. The process is then to have some rule of inference, such as the one used in the last section for the syllogism, whereby we can deduce theorems from the postulates. It is the complementary process to that gone through by our Erewhonian observer, and is dependent upon it.

The most widely known examples of postulate systems are those of geometry, such as Euclidean geometry in two or three dimensions, and group theory, which is a part of modern abstract algebra. There the problem of proving theorems was one of showing that the statement in the theorem was reducible to the statement of the postulates; if this could be shown, then the theorem was true or, as mathematicians sometimes say, provable.

We should remind ourselves that mathematics, in view of its incompleteness, is not quite the cut-and-dried system we once thought it to be, though some of its partial systems, like geometry, are sufficiently precise and complete. Geometry is a symbolic system, like all other constructed languages, that contains general concepts which are themselves an offshoot of behaviour.

There is one point, before we return to 'paper machines', that we must make quite clear: we *could* produce in hardware all the machines we have in blueprint, given the time and the money, and provided our blueprint methods have a decision procedure, and they could also be of immeasurably greater complication than anything that actually exists. In the meantime we have these *effective theories*, and indeed many of our most exciting discoveries have been theoretical. The problem now arises, in view of a certain widespread distrust of theory, as to how we can convince the world at large that the theories work, without actually building the machine in hardware, and it is here that 'paper machines' become important.

The words 'paper machine' were used, probably for the first time, by Turing in an unpublished paper on 'Intelligent Machinery', and we can describe a paper machine as the process of writing down a set of instructions or rules, and a procedure that could be carried out by a man who was quite ignorant of the purpose of the rules or the procedure. This has already been discussed, and now we must explain the position a little further.

Consider, for example, a problem demanding such a machine-like procedure. One might ask a child to look through all the integers between one and one thousand to see if any one or two or more of the numbers have some special property. To take a trivial example, are there two such integers whose product is 827? And if so, how many such pairs are there? Granted that the child knows how to multiply integers together, and has the most ordinary intelligence, he could give a definite answer to the question. We have already seen how this works for the propositional calculus in discovering whether any wff is a theorem or not.

Now this sort of 'blind' procedure of following rules when given them, and using paper and pencil for the process, is in effect a computing machine. It is now a reasonable question to ask what sorts of problems can be solved by such procedures. The use of a man, a pencil, a piece of paper and a rubber, is what we call a 'paper machine', and what we now have to face in programming the man are some of the most important problems in modern science. It is one obvious approach to the subject of the theory of machines.

Let us look at this matter in a more historical context. The notion of an effective procedure, or a decision procedure, has its place in mathematics and logic, and we will consider some of the simpler cases.

There are various examples in mathematics of the search for such decision procedures or methods. For example, there is an algorithm called Euclid's algorithm which will tell us whether or not, in the elementary theory of integers, two numbers are relatively prime. If we are presented with a statement to the effect that any two numbers p and q are relatively prime—two numbers are said to be relatively prime if they have no factor in common except unity—then the algorithm will tell us whether this is so or not, i.e. whether the statement for any particular values is true or false. Thus the whole set of such statements can be divided into two groups, those that are true and those that are false, and no such statement is undecidable. This process has been described as machine-like.

The point that is of special interest is that undecidable formulae do occur in any system sufficient to generate all we now refer to as classical mathematics, and although it does not follow on this account that there is no decision procedure for all of classical mathematics, this nevertheless is also a fact, a fact that has been shown to be the case by Church (1936).

Church's theorem, as we have called it, shows that if there are no undecidable formulae in a formalized system, then it must have a decision procedure. These are matters of paper machines that are vital to a consideration of what can and what cannot be built, from a theoretical point of view. Let us now consider the problems outlined in this paragraph from another aspect, that developed by Turing under the title of Turing machines.

Turing machines

A Turing machine consists of a length of tape which may be as long as we please, and therefore potentially infinite. The tape is marked out into squares on each of which a symbol can be printed. The body of the machine is a scanner that scans, one at a time, squares which each contain one symbol. The machine can alter the symbol on the scanned square, move to the right one square, move to the left one square, or stop. The symbol actually scanned, the internal configuration of the machine at the moment of scanning, decide which actual operation will next be performed. The machine indeed is *not* one that needs to be built; it is a paper machine, and is mainly of interest to consider precisely what machines are capable of *in principle*.

Turing was able to show that there existed a Universal machine that was capable of doing anything that any other machine whatsoever was capable of doing, provided a description of the other machine was forthcoming, i.e. if the details of any machine whatsoever are printed on the tape of a Turing machine, then it will be able to carry out the operations of the machine so described. This means, of course, that all machines are, in a sense, reducible to a Universal Turing machine.

A Turing machine is completely defined by a set of quadruples (set of four symbols) which act as the orders that determine the behaviour of the machine and its process of calculation.

We shall now define, by way of illustration, a simple Turing machine, and show how it operates (see Fig. 4).

A simple Turing machine is defined by three types of quadruple, using symbols q_1, q_2, ... q_n to indicate the state of the machine, and

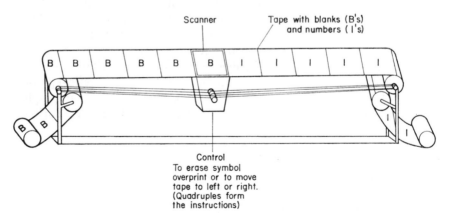

FIG. 4. TURING MACHINE. A Turing machine is composed of a tape ruled into squares, a scanner and a set of instructions that moves the tape to the left or right one square at a time, or allows the symbol on the square to be overprinted.

S_0, S_1, ... S_m to indicate the symbols on the tape. The three types of quadruple are:

$$q_i S_j S_k q_l$$
$$q_i S_j \rightarrow q_l$$
$$q_i S_j \leftarrow q_l$$

The first two symbols of each quadruple give the present states of the machine and the symbols scanned, whereas the next two symbols of the quadruple tell us the next act of the machine and its subsequent state. For example, the quadruple

$$q_1 S_2 \leftarrow q_4$$

says that the machine, when in the state q_1, scanning the symbol S_2, will move one square to the left and go into state q_4.

Two particular symbols S_0 and S_1, written B and 1, have special significance, in that overprinting with a B amounts to erasure of a symbol on the tape, and S_1 will be used to represent 1's which are of special importance, since we wish to represent decimal numbers by collections of 1's.

We will now observe a Turing machine performing a very simple operation, that of addition. Our numbers are to be represented on the tape by one more 1 than actually occurs in the number, which means that 2 is written 111, 4 is written 11111, and so on. If we wish to add 2 to 4, or indeed any two numbers m_1 and m_2, say, we proceed in the following way.

Let f be the function $f(x, y) = x+y$ which represents addition; in our case we are interested initially in m_1+m_2. Z is a Turing machine which will compute this function. Let Z consist of the following quadruples:

$$q_1 \ 1 \ B \ q_1$$
$$q_1 \ B \ \rightarrow \ q_2$$
$$q_2 \ 1 \ B \ q_3$$
$$q_2 \ B \ \rightarrow \ q_2$$

Now if A_1 is the initial instantaneous description, where by instantaneous description we mean an expression containing only one q-symbol and containing otherwise only S-symbols, without $\leftarrow$ or $\rightarrow$, which means

6*

that it is of the form

$$Pq_iS_jQ$$
$$Pq_iS_jS_kQ$$
$$Pq_iS_j$$
$$PS_kq_iS_jQ$$

or $$q_iS_jQ$$

where P and Q are expressions possibly empty, that is, involving no symbols whatever, then here

$$A_1 = q_1\,(\bar{m}_1,\,\bar{m}_2) = q_1m_1Bm_2$$

where A_1 is simply a way of writing the two numbers to be added in l's, remembering that there is one more 1 in this rendering of A_1 than in the number itself. We may incidently write m 1's as 1^m. The B separating the m_1 and m_2 is effectively a comma. If we suppose initially that $m_1 = 0$, then $\bar{m}_1 = 1$, since it has one more 1 than the number represented, and

$$A_1 = q_1\,1\,B\,1^{m_2+1} = q_1\,1\,B\,11^{m_2}$$

Therefore $A_1 \to q_1\,B\,B\,1\,1^{m_2} \to B\,q_2\,B\,1\,1^{m_2} \to B\,B\,q_2\,1\,1^{m_2} \to B\,B\,q_3\,B\,1^{m_2}$, and this last is terminal ($\to$ means 'yields' here), since of course there is no quadruple starting q_3B, and therefore no instructions on which to proceed further.

Therefore the computation yields an answer as above in the terminal instantaneous description, and this expression contains 1^{m_2}, or m_2 1's, and this means (by convention) that the answer is m_2, where at the end of the computation the number of 1's in a number correctly represents that number. The result of our addition is thus seen to be $0+m_2$, on the assumption of $m_1 = 0$.

If we had supposed $m_1 \neq 0$, then $A_1 = q_2\,111^{m_1-1}\,B1^{m_2+1} \to q_1\,B\,1\,1^{m_1-1}\,B\,1^{m_2+1} \to Bq_2\,1\,1^{m_1-1}\,B\,1^{m_2+1}\,B\,q_3\,B\,1^{m_1-1}B\,1^{m_2+1}$ which is terminal.

This gives m_1+m_2 as answer, and of course if we had made $m_1 = 2$, and $m_2 = 4$, and written them in as 111 and 11111 respectively, we would have found the tape containing six 1's at the end of the computation.

This example has been, of course, of a simple Turing machine, and shows it performing merely a simple operation; more complicated Turing machines can be constructed, using more quadruples and even more than one tape, and with such machines we would of course be able to deal with more complicated functions. This would have led us in time to a consideration of recursive function theory and its identification with effective computability, but that is a pathway we shall not tread here, since it is primarily of mathematical interest, and the general results have already been mentioned. However, perhaps this much should be said by way of elucidation: the idea of a recursive function is important because, as we shall see in computer programming, it represents a general method for manifesting the totality of mathematical operations—or virtually so.

Before we leave Turing machines, we should include a note on what has already been mentioned with regard to Turing machines which have been developed with more than one tape, and also with more than one row of symbols on a single tape. Sometimes the tapes all run together synchronously and other times they run independently, and furthermore, work on Turing machines (de Leeuw, 1956) has shown that computations can also be performed by probabilistic Turing machines as well as deterministic Turing machines. The interesting result mathematically is that whatever the method the range of computation seemed not to be effected. From the cybernetic point of view this might be of considerable importance because although the computation is of interest, the method from the cybernetician's point of view is of even greater interest than the end obtained.

One thing that should be made quite clear is that although a Turing machine can make any machinelike computation whatsoever, it will take a long time to do the more complicated operations, and so will often be extremely wasteful of time. This, of course, is not a practical difficulty, since we are here only interested in what a machine is capable of, *in principle*.

We do not wish to push the matter of mathematics and logic any further. What seems to be of vital importance for the theory of machines is this: whatever can be done by humans can be done by machines. This is, of course, contrary to many opinions which have resulted mainly from misunderstanding the processes of these paper machines, but there is in fact no obvious reason to doubt that a machine could be built to do what a human being could do in *all* cases, provided that an adequate description is available of what the system to be mirrored actually does.

The fact that there exists no decision procedure for mathematics as a whole does not mean that there are parts of mathematics that are not investigatable by machines. It does mean, however, that the methods to be employed are beyond the reach of what has been called a decision procedure. Other methods are needed, of a more random character, such as cannot be put in a manner that could be followed by an unintelligent helpmate. Let us try to throw a little more light on this point.

The theorems of Gödel, Church and Turing are not a barrier to what machines can do, any more than they are a barrier to using an unintelligent helpmate. If we can tolerate an occasional wrong result—such as human computers sometimes produce—then we can use machines that can be constructed to pursue the further mathematical inquiries just as humans pursue them. This point can hardly be overemphasized, since it has sometimes been used as an argument against cybernetic development, which of course it is not. We can now discuss these same methods of paper machines from a more positive standpoint.

Machines and biology

Although nearly all of the discussion in this chapter has been concerned with the development of logic, it is not here that our primary interest lies. Mathematics is a convenient place to try out such machine theories of logic, and it is an historical fact that it is mathematicians who have so tried them out, but the machines with which this book is primarily concerned are of other kinds.

Learning machines of various sorts have been built, and these are of great psychological and behavioural interest. What are the problems here? The main point is that it is not possible to build all the machines we would like. But we can and do build the blueprints, and by such decision procedures we can discover what is and what is not possible.

It is certainly the case—and this is exhibited by the development of computing machinery—that we can construct an analog that could do anything that can be described sufficiently definitely by biologists. This, perhaps, may not appear helpful, and indeed it is certainly not the reason for studying 'thinking machines', but the fact is that such a criterion may be taken in a sense as a measure of the meaningfulness of a biological statement. 'Is it effectively constructible or reconstructible?' might be the form of such a test. If not, then it seems that the mechanism has been insufficiently described.

There are, of course, technical difficulties. We do not as yet know sufficient of colloidal chemistry to construct systems of the same colloidal materials of which humans are built; but though we cannot at present construct the analog of human behaviour in hardware, these purely technical difficulties are irrelevant to matters *in principle*.

The general argument about paper machines and their implications in the general field of biology may seem trivial, but it is being emphasized for the reason that it is not widely recognized by biologists and psychologists that there is a field of mathematics and mathematical logic that has a direct relevance to their own fields of interest. The fact is that paper machines tell us a great deal about the nature of machine construction, and which thinking operations are possible, and about the possible construction of nervous and other biological systems, and their possibilities. Their main use—and it is indeed a very valuable one for most scientists—may be to suggest experiments, but such investigations have an even greater value than this in that they suggest theories, not only of particular branches of knowledge but also about the nature of reality.

Now we must return to our discussion of scientific theories and their evolution.

The evolution of scientific theories

The next stage in our analysis of the theoretical problems for psychologists is to enlarge on the methods of the earlier sections of this chapter at the most general level, and consider the possible modes of development of scientific theories. In particular, we shall continue to consider, but more explicitly, the case of experimental psychology.

The existing state of experimental psychology is perhaps at the transition from the 'taxonomic' stage (collecting data) to the theoretical stage. The second stage of a theory is marked by the fact of having a theoretical language that allows the role of the experiment to become primarily that of a test for theoretical predictions. This clearly expresses the need for theory, and it also re-emphasizes the need for carefully considered experiment. So much of psychological theory is limited in value by the fact that most writers in the field use imprecise, discursive methods, and so many of the experiments carried out are ill-conceived. It is surely obvious that while not all the questions involved in scientific theory construction are merely linguistic, a great many of them are; and even those which are not merely linguistic are coloured by linguistic considerations. What is needed in psychology, apart from rare skill in experimental techniques, is some of the linguistic skill of the methodologist and the logician.

We will now turn to a more explicit consideration of the work of Braithwaite, in which the relation of models to theories has been analysed.

Braithwaite (1953) has pointed out the relation between models and scientific theories with great clarity. His view is that there is a sort of parallel between the development of scientific theories from observation statements, on one hand, and the reconstruction of empirical data from a model, on the other. These are two parallel zip-fasteners, as it were, the theoretical-zip being tied to observations at the bottom, and the model-zip being tied to observations at the top. In this chapter we have discussed some of the problems, and the structure, of the formal languages and the cybernetic models, which start from sets of marks on paper and proceed by rules to generate further sets of marks or strings. These sets of marks are models, and are then open to interpretation as languages which may be used for any purpose whatsoever that is consistent with the interpretation placed on the marks. It is rather as if, to speak metaphorically, the collection of marks (called calculi) have certain structural properties like maps of anywhere at all, and the problem is to select a map that fits the country in which the scientist is interested at any particular time. Braithwaite's analogy of a zip-fastener depends on the fact that the model at the lowest level and the theory-language at the highest level are both attached to reality, and we can go up and down the levels (meta-levels) in between, in either direction. We are using hierarchies of languages as the bases of the themes.

It is generally believed—as our earlier anecdote illustrated—that we can proceed from a set of statements of direct observation to generalizations by inductive inference, and from the generalizations back to the testable particulars by deduction. This is the theory; the model is in essence the skeleton logical structure of this theory, and it is therefore clear that there is the closest relation between theory and model.

Before proceeding to make any comment on this view of Braithwaite's, it is important for theoretical psychologists to note that he has also given considerable support to a view held by F. P. Ramsey (1951) that the theoretical terms that occur in scientific theories are not merely logical constructs. This means that the theoretical terms cannot be defined solely in terms of observed entities if we wish our theory to be capable of expansion to incorporate new information as it arises, and this of course we surely do ultimately need.

Let us now consider the broader nature of psychological theories. We shall start with natural language and its use as descriptive of particular occurrences and generalized hypotheses, and we shall try to refine its statements by setting up glossary (George, 1953a, 1953b) definitions for our principal logical constructions and observable variables. This involves the necessity of adding refining contextual definitions to all except the explicitly primitive terms of the system. We could, on a more precise level, do the same thing by using either reduction-sentences, or by reformulating from time to time our sets of explicit (eliminable) definitions. Rules of inference are not usually explicitly formulated at the natural language end of our continuum, but are so formulated, of course, as and when we proceed to the use of formalized languages. Indeed, we regard the important sense of the word 'formalization' as that of 'making rigorous', and making the rules of use for a set of symbols explicit. We should proceed from the observables on the *molar* levels of observation and, by use of theoretical terms (inferred entities, logical constructs, or intervening variables, are points on a continuum of the Realist-Nominalist kind by which we may mean that they stand for actual physical systems in one extreme or mere functional connections without any implied physical existence at the other) to build a psychological *qua* psychological theory. From this as our datum, the process of levels of language allows us to expand the system in many different (as it were) dimensions. The most obvious extension that seems to be necessary is to descriptions of a neurophysiological kind. Thus, the constructions on the 'molar' level should be capable of redefinition in the language of neurophysiology. There is, however, an important sense in which this procedure of redefinition on any level of description has been confused with a different thesis known as 'reductionism', but what is intended here is only the ability to translate from the language of one level of description to the language of another level; indeed such translation should be possible between different linguistic frameworks on the same level of description.

There is no obvious way, on a purely molar level, of granting priority to one linguistic system, with a certain choice of terms and categorizations rather than to another, except by the tests of a pragmatic kind that can be carried out at all levels of description. Actually, any particular molar theory must be *tested* by seeing whether it uniquely defines, in certain test cases, such as under classical or instrumental conditioning, a definite operator such as those that have been suggested by Estes (1950) or Bush and Mosteller (1951a). They may be further tested, of course, by any logical nets that may be derived from them. Theories that are so vague that *any* mathematical operators or logical nets can be derived from them are insufficiently precise, and can only be tested on molar-pragmatic grounds as to alternative interpretations of the same precise operations. The psychological theorist is therefore under obligation to show the breadth of utility of his theory, and its plasticity in allowing precise rules, etc., to be derived from it whenever the need arises.

The above statement argues that a theory must at least satisfy the following conditions: It must have certain molar explanatory properties that place it in advance of any existing theory; it must therefore have some, even if crude, explanatory powers in a language that has been made sufficiently precise for its use. It will be realized parenthetically that the precision of the questions to be answered will decide the precision of the theory to be used. Then the molar theory must be flexible enough to allow implicit redefinition of its primitives and theoretical terms at any other level of description (either more or less molar than the datum-language). We should then be able to translate it into a molecular language that permits of being made precise at any moment, and from which logical nets and mathematical models are capable of being derived. It is extremely important that a theory be tested in this ramified way since, at the purely molar level, it appears that we cannot always adequately distinguish the predictive value of the different theories offered. It may, of course, *turn out* that there is an important sense in which the purely molar theories are little more than scaffolding for the presentation of the important questions which are concerned with, say, the relations of logical nets with each other; or the more general problem of producing a blueprint for the relation of the internal parts (variables) of the human machine.

We should notice the difficulty that the work of Braithwaite has made for the view that logical constructs are definable in terms of observable entities. This becomes more acute as we approach a more formalized level of language. However, Braithwaite's own suggestion that such theoretical terms should be reserved for the high level statements, and can only be implicitly defined, is certainly acceptable. The writer has drawn attention to the use of logical constructs in psychological theory before (George, 1953a), and has pointed out that it is precisely the vagueness attendant on the surplus meaning of such logical constructs that gives them both their power and their vagueness. The difficulties of theoretical terms in more formal languages still demand some further research; indeed, this problem appears already to have reared its head in the attempts that have been made to apply mathematics to psychology.

There are two further matters that now demand comment, the first being a sort of criticism of Braithwaite, in that there is something of a gap between the way science actually works and the cut and dried systems he suggests. It is as if he were giving a prescription for the ideal state of an ideal science, whereas we have tried to talk realistically in terms of the actual situation with which the experimental psychologist is faced. He starts with a great mass of data, based mostly on observation, upon which generalization is to be made; the nature of the generalization will depend upon intuitive and anecdotal notions. Thus, although one may start in principle from a model and give interpretations of that model, one may also formalize a theory, i.e. one may proceed from a set of scientific generalizations to the logical core of those generalizations. In fact, the original generalizations will be partially confused with a model as often as not, and the explicit stages of Braithwaite only arise, if at all, after much work has been done on the confused mass of empirical data that represents the normal growth of a science.

The second point takes us outside the theory-construction to the directives and foundation principles upon which the theory is to be built. Here, the cleavage is along the lines of behaviourism and introspection, and it is a dispute characterized at some level by the 'Mind–Body problem'. At the working level of the scientist there are still problems of what behaviourism implies, i.e. how broadly or how narrowly the behaviouristic notion is to be employed, and if taken too narrowly, how much of a science of psychology is lost, if anything.

The answers to these last questions can be given here only briefly. Some form of behaviourism, involving at least the study of that which is obviously public, is quite vital. A science of behaviour so based should include all the data that the introspectionist deals with, but it will not use the same language. Indeed, self-observation is essentially part of the subject matter of behaviouristic psychology, but necessarily approached in a public manner. Self-observation statements are therefore indispensably involved in a behavioural science, and such statements are continuous with (ordinary) observation statements. There should be no confusion here at the level of the absolute behaviouristic science, but in fact confusion does sometimes arise, since we do not always see where the observer enters into the apparently public scientific system. In the practice of psychology we have to combine, for many purposes, information from introspective and behaviouristic sources, and we are forced into a degree of eclecticism. It is to the behaviouristic approach that our processes of formalization, the applications of logic, and all the matters discussed in this chapter, are applied. Failure to recognize the nature of the complicated problems of constructing scientific theories has vitiated a great deal of the work of psychologists; recognition of this should lead to improved scientific standards.

One last, clarifying word should be said on the matter of behaviourism. What it is hoped to avoid in modern psychology is on the one hand, the narrowness of early behaviourism, which simply ignored problems which did not fit into its over-simplified notions. On the other hand, it is equally vital not to become embroiled in a morass of ontological and epistemological disputes. We are concerned with the systematic construction of scientific theories, meta-theories, and criticisms of both; and with the nature of the actual assumptions, and the interbehavioural interpretation that is both possible and desirable for psychology, and indeed for the whole of science.

Explanation

We have seen that explanations may take more than one form. The reduction-sentence methods of Carnap are made necessary by the notion of 'dispositional properties'. The notion of *causal consequence* certainly presents a difficulty for logic, i.e. in the logical model, but for science it is not a genuine *problem*. We simply act in accordance with what we believe would happen if some action were performed. This is, in fact, induction at work, and no scientist is worried by the knowledge that he cannot be *certain* of what would have happened if he had done something that he did not actually do. The general form of the Hempel–Oppenheim (1953) theory looks something like what is needed as a form of scientific explanation. The conditions they set down are certainly too strong, but the general form comes nearer to what scientists actually do. Let us consider this matter a little further.

Hempel and Oppenheim's theory can be stated (oversimply) as that of finding true sentences C_1, C_2 ..., C_r which are antecedent conditions, and L_1, L_2, ..., L_k which are general laws together forming the *explanans* for the *explicandum* (E), which is made up of statements which are the description of empirical phenomena: that particular phenomenon (or phenomena) that is to be 'explained'. Their method deals with what they call *causal* (as opposed to statistical) explanations, and demands many special properties of the explanans. The sentences of the explanans, which are the general laws, are to be true (they will not accept 'confirmed to some degree' with respect to certain evidence); they must also be 'familiar' in a certain sense, and testable. The language they would use to formulate a model theory would be that of the lower functional calculus without the identity relation. There are many more complicating conditions which cannot be discussed here, and with which the writer would generally agree, but the total sum of their plan—while it should be familiar to every psychologist—is in fact too strict to be followed by every scientific theory.

The same criticism of over-strictness is applicable to Carnap's conditions as laid down in 'Testability and Meaning' (1937), which expresses the process of reduction (to be distinguished from definition) of sentences to observation sentences.

Most of the predicates of science being dispositional predicates, everyone knows of the non-eliminability of such predicates as 'soluble', the ordinary word used for the property of being capable of being dissolved in water. This led Carnap to the process of reduction sentences of the form: If x is immersed in water then, if and only if x is soluble in water, x will dissolve. This is of the logical form

$$(x)[P(x) \supset Q(x) \equiv R(x)]$$

The process of reduction of the dispositional predicate by reduction-pairs may finish in non-dispositional predicates, referring to a test-operation. A weaker test, involving unilateral reduction-pairs, is usually used in experimental situations. (A brief account of this process can be found in Pap (1949, chapter 12), and, again, should be familiar to every psychologist.) This process of 'reductionism' is an alternative to explicit definition, and has some advantages.

The psychological theories of Hull use the traditional theory-construction method of psychology; it is hypothetico-deductive, a postulational method (with complications) which uses 'logical constructs', and derives consequences. Operationism is not excluded from such a system, and the more nearly operational such definitions, etc., can be, the better for most purposes. This is not to be taken as an indication of a final answer to the most suitable method of constructing even the molar sort of behaviour theory. Investigation of theory-construction in science *is as much a subject in evolution* as science itself.

What is needed by the psychologist is a systematic method for translating statements of observation into generalized laws or hypotheses, without hopeless vagueness. This demands that the meta-language assumed, and the language refined for the actual statement in the theory, are sufficiently clear. For this, *definition* is probably vital; there is certainly no point in introducing false rigour, but for the more rigorous part of psychology, where disputes are mostly about terminology, the calculus of empirical classes and relations is perhaps the ideal form of description. Here, the terms and their relations are relative to the context of inquiry; they do not insist on rigid class membership, but permit a degree of vagueness that heralds the use of probabilities. Here, as in all formalized systems, the theory and the model are closely and explicitly related. Such a formal, yet elastic, language also goes a long way to avoid the hazards of talking of 'things having properties', etc.

The use of natural language, languages, and scientific theories, has one further complication. A precise, descriptive language (including an explicit or implicit model) is a scientific theory. The marks on paper (or sounds in the air) which have no meaning (interpretation) are not, of course, a language. The point is that our precise, descriptive language should be capable of interpretation in natural language, but that the precise relations themselves are not necessarily capable of being precisely produced in the natural language, other than by analogy. To believe that natural language (a theory of the world on a crude level) is sufficient for science simply because the final interpretations of precise language have to be in natural language, is surely a mistake.

What is vital for the psychologist to notice is that logic (all systematic languages) has two different roles to perform for him: (1) in clarifying their existing statements and theories, and (2) as a precise, descriptive language itself. Both roles are vital, and it is vital to distinguish them.

We shall now leave philosophy of science and return to the closely related matters of logic.

Empirical logics

We have referred to empirical logics and their use to behaviouristic-cybernetic methodology, and we shall now say something more about them.

It has generally been thought that the logics of the type of the propositional and functional calculus are too precise to deal with the vagueness in most of the ordinary situations that we wish to describe. This has suggested to many people that more realistic descriptive languages could be found by using probabilistic logics, and we shall see later that the use of probabilistic logics has a direct application to logical networks, which are at the very heart of cybernetics. However, the main idea is to avoid vagueness in description and still retain enough rigour to avoid the pitfalls of ordinary language. These methods may be thought of as analytic tools, or as descriptive methods for a science (Kaplan and Schott, 1951; Woodger, 1937, 1939, 1952; Körner, 1951). We shall here merely outline what we believe is likely to prove a very powerful linguistic tool in both experimental and social psychology. Its importance lies partly at least in its close link with logical nets, because these logics can, like the logical nets, be given an interpretation at any level of investigation, making it easy to pass from a description at one level of generality to another.

To put the matter simply, the idea is to map the calculi of classes, relations and predicates on to the calculus of probability. This means that we talk of class membership, or of relations between classes, we talk rather of the probabilities that exist between these items or classes. In other words, instead of saying 'Jack is a man', we shall simply say that 'Jack is probably a man', where we mean, of course, to imply an incomplete description of Jack which leaves us in doubt and implies that the probability falls short of 1. This example may at first sound over-simplified, but on the basis of a perfunctory description one might be unsure as to whether the person referred to as 'Jack' was a human; even if human, 'Jack' could be a woman disguised, and so on.

If we bear in mind that in logic we are concerned with giving an interpretation to a system of formal symbols, then we will realize that an alternative interpretation of such empirical logics would be to say that

'Jack is a man *to some extent*'. This may seem a less plausible interpretation, but it could at least apply to those unfortunate cases of endocrine disorders where change of sex is involved. If we use the example 'Jack is to some extent a neurotic', we can clearly see the point of substituting a probability in place of a certainty with respect to class membership.

It is not being suggested that imprecise description is to be preferred to precise description, but rather that where the facts described are imprecise (our own knowledge of them is incomplete) it is better to have a precise description of their imprecision. Mathematics is a language with which you can actually carry out the measurements, and there is some point in saying—by analogy with well-known methods in statistics—that empirical logics are non-parametric mathematical descriptions.

It is clear that a description of any situation can be couched in terms of a probabilistic language of this sort, where the interpretation on the variables may be anything we like. The probabilities may be computed on the basis either of *a priori* probabilities or of empirical probabilities. Let us briefly illustrate the method in one of its many forms.

Suppose that a set of variables of a physiological kind are associated with a certain piece of molar behaviour, then, if we can obtain a set of measures for a certain range of behaviour, we can describe the total behaviour pattern as a relation. Let us say *Rab* is such a relation, where a and b are two states of the organism and R is to be interpreted as 'probably follows in time'. A definite value may be calculated from the cases measured.

R itself is made up of the measurable variables $A, B, \ldots, N$. Then we may measure these variables, and although they may not constitute a complete basis for describing R, we can discover which are the best indices for R. Then we might also consider relations between the variables and so on, so that, given any subset of the variables, on some future occasion we can ascribe a probability to the relation

Rab

Alternatively, we can interpret the logic as we did above with respect to an utterance such as 'Jack is married to Jill', also of the form

Rab

If we assume we do not know all the facts but know certain indices of marriage, such as 'they live in the same house', 'they appear to be affectionate towards each other', and so on, then we can ascribe *a priori* probabilities to these subrelations r, s, ..., t which are a basis for the relation R. The more we know of the subrelations the more completely can we ascribe a probability to R. Obviously, we may weight the subrelations so that they do not necessarily contribute equally to the total probability ascribed at any particular time.

As far as the notation is concerned we need not bother about that here (see Chapter 5), except to notice that we can easily think of a, b, ..., n as either items or classes, to be distinguished where necessary, and R, S, ..., T as relations which may be monadic, diadic, etc., having subrelations r, s, ..., t and so on, with sub-subrelations for as many levels as we want. Then the $X.Y$, XvY, $\sim X$ of Boolean algebra become two diadic and one monadic relation:

$$Rab, \ Sab, \ Na$$

where it will doubtless be wise to retain particular letters for particular relations, as in the Lukasiewicz type of notation where the relational operator is written first to save the bother of manipulating brackets. Here, of course, the relational operators conceal a probability, and to make this explicit we could write

$$Rab_p \quad \text{or} \quad Rab(p)$$

say, to remind the reader that a probability p will be ascribed to the relation under description.

It should be added that Woodger, in his biological language previously mentioned, uses explicit predicates of a biological kind, over and above the symbols of the propositional and functional calculus. He introduces such predicates as

$$Tr \ (x, y)$$

which is read as 'x is before y in time'; and

$$Sli \ (x, y)$$

meaning 'x is a slice of the thing y'; and then again

$$Org \ (x)$$

meaning 'x is an organic unit', which can be put into an axiomatic form:

$$Org(x) \supset Th(x)$$

which means to say that 'each organic unit is a thing'.

TBC 7

We shall be discussing this matter again later but the obvious development of empirical or applied logic is in the direction of describing total systems. Such systems can be likened in some respects to empirical games, where the purpose of the system is clearcut, even if not precise, in other words it is a goal-directed type of activity with a precise solution (possibly requiring an optimization procedure) which is needed. The use of heuristic methods, which frequently in practical situations would lead up to accept a quasi-optimum solution and adaptively improve the standard of the quasi-optimum solution possibly reaching an optimum in the course of experience if experience is possible. If experience is not possible the same process of improvement must be attained through simulation.

This is a core notion in the development of cybernetics and one which will be discussed explicitly later on in the chapter on artificial intelligence, but the main point to appreciate fully at this stage is that logic for the cybernetician plays two roles; on one hand it plays the conventional analytic role and theorems about it tell you something of the limitations which are imposed on any sort of system. This work culminates in the work of Gödel and Church and Turing, but on the other hand, and on balance this is probably the more important, logic is also used as a descriptive language. This is so even though in some cases the description may be extremely complicated as it certainly becomes in the case of neural nets (which have an equivalent logical description) where the nets are sufficiently complicated to be interesting. When they are that complicated the fact that they can be put on to a computer makes them nevertheless tractable.

These simple beginnings in Woodger's language are soon made quite complicated, and a precise biological description is built up and used to describe processes of genetics and cell division. Although these descriptive languages may sometimes seem to state the obvious with unnecessary precision, it must nevertheless be admitted that this is a beginning of a somewhat different, yet similar, descriptive language which, with the help of the computer, may become of great importance.

Now if the members of Y are organic units

$$[Yxy \supset Org\ (x) \cdot Org\ (y)]$$

Now if we suppose Yxy, and that u is the end slice x and v is the first slice of y, then u is either a part of v or v is a part of u,

i.e. $\qquad [Yxy \cdot ESli\ (u, x) \cdot ISli\ (v, y) \supset (u \neq v) \cdot (Puv\ V\ Pvu)]$

Given that *Mom* (x) means that spatio-temporal area is only momentary, we have

$$Mom(x) \; (u) \; (v) \; (Pux \cdot Pvx \supset \; \sim Tr \; (u, v))$$

where *Tr* is the asymmetric time relation

$$Tr \; (x, y) \supset \; \sim Tr \; (y, x)$$

We shall not pursue this matter any further here, but should notice the link with empirical games in Chapter 6 and with empirical axiomatic systems in Chapter 14.

Stochastic processes

In discussing logical net models we have frequently mentioned the important part played by stochastic processes, and the fact that they had been used in cybernetics. They have at least been used in attempts to apply the mathematical descriptions to psychological phenomena, and this is part of cybernetics.

The work of Bush and Mosteller (1951, 1955) comes to mind in a consideration of Stochastic Processes. They have tried to apply the mathematical paraphernalia of certain types of stochastic process to behavioural problems, and in particular, to the analysis of particular experiments.

It will be remembered that a stochastic process is a sequence of symbols that implies a temporal order and yet is itself random. A particular stochastic process, of importance in behavioural analysis, was called a Markov net, in which the steps of the sequence are related by definite probabilities. Furthermore, if nature is something like an *ergodic source* we may expect that the Markov processes, with which behavioural descriptions are going to be concerned, will be of the statistically homogeneous kind.

For Bush and Mosteller the process starts with a stochastic model, and proceeds through statistical methods to the mathematical model for some aspect of behaviour. This is all meant to apply to molar behaviour activities. They are thus concerned with operators, especially matrix operators, and the statistical description of behaviour in terms of these operators, which represent the response tendencies implicit in a class of events as described by probability variables.

We shall later show briefly some of the close connections that exist between the work of Bush and Mosteller and the work of logical nets. We can straight away say that both conceive of molar behaviour as capable of a statistical description and indeed as being essentially a Markov process. The methods actually used differ largely in that logical nets are concerned in deriving a description of molecular behaviour *as well as* molar behaviour, and so have involved themselves more deeply in descriptions of the organisms.

The end of the anecdote

We should now add an epilogue to the anecdote which we related earlier. The cycle of events involving assumptions, tests and generalizations is claimed to be typical of science, but what we should now notice is that it is typical of human behaviour. The processes of deduction and induction may be irrational and private in man, but the essentials are identical.

Cybernetics is concerned with showing that the inductive as well as the deductive part of the Erewhonian observer's behaviour could be carried out by a machine.

The whole field of methodology in science is vast, and the subject matter could be extended to many volumes. However, what is perhaps most obvious is that logic and language can be applied to all sorts of problems. The method is to construct artificial languages and then place the appropriate interpretation upon them. From one point of view, cybernetics can be regarded as being precisely a branch of this general field of applied logic.

It should be emphasized that linguistic problems will occur in science, even in the realm of applied logic. As long as this is remembered, then such matters can usually be cleared up in the contexts in which they occur.

Summary

This chapter has outlined a many-levelled method of modelling human behaviour by the use of empirical descriptive methods and of theoretical terms that are capable of redefinition on other levels of description.

A particular view of science is delineated by which the scientific process is seen as the collecting of data and the making of inductive generalizations from those data, and then the drawing of deductive inferences from the generalizations. This, it is claimed by many of those interested in cybernetics, is a process that can be achieved by machines as well as organisms.

Logical systems which are to be used as models for our cybernetics theories are summarized briefly, and some mention is made of the more obscure logical calculi.

Effective procedures are seen to be paper computers, and are of the utmost value in a discussion of what is possible for hardware construction. This is one of the firmest links between mathematics, computer design and the construction of effective theories of behaviour.

Some further discussion has also taken place with respect to the evolution of scientific theories, and some of the difficulties met in constructing such theories. Finally, a point of view of relevance to philosophy has been implied, although the program of pragmatics suggested has not been carried through. The emphasis is on methodological rather than philosophical forms of analysis, since from this aspect classical philosophical analysis seems to have a limited contact with the needs of modern science, which is concerned not with absolutes but with limited contexts of meanings

CHAPTER 4

FINITE AUTOMATA

A FINITE automaton, in the sense of McCulloch and Pitts (1943), is a stimulus–response system which could involve representations of the previous stimulus states of the system. From this model we must go on to inquire, with Kleene (1951), about the general nature of finite automata, and what kinds of events can be represented by them.

We shall first set out the McCulloch–Pitts definition of a finite automaton, and we shall call our particular automata 'neural nets', initially, thus preserving the original title of the founders. We shall, however, change the title to 'logical nets' in the next chapter (and from then on), when we outline the particular finite automata that this book will use fo its analysis and synthesis of psychological problems. The reason for this change of name is largely to preserve the distinction Braithwaite (1953s makes between a model and a theory, and in this way to make it clear that a finite automaton is not in any way *committed* to being a model for a theory of the central nervous system.

Automata theory

Before we commit ourselves to discussing automata that are of special interest to cyberneticians and people working in the field of cognition, we should say something about the general development of automata theory. The very first thing to say is that automata theory is a development, primarily mathematical, in its own right and does not depend on the interpretation that could be placed on the various types of automata, such as in the form of digital computers or, as we have already said, central nervous systems. The theory stands in its own right regardless of the interpretation placed on it in the Braithwaitean sense.

A very general definition of an automaton (McNaughton, 1961) is: 'An automaton is a device of finite size at any time with certain parts specified, with inputs and outputs, such that what happens at the outputs at any time is determined by what has happened to the inputs.' This definition is admittedly somewhat vague, but can be made as precise as we wish for any particular purpose. This raises the point that there are at least three different interests in automata theory, one from the world of computers, one from the worlds of mathematics with which automata theory is primarily concerned, and one from our own point of view, that of cybernetics. It is important to establish these different interests otherwise we may look at automata developed for cybernetic purposes and question whether the results are of mathematical interest. We might equally look at automata theory developed as part of mathematics and ask whether it has any relevance whatever to cybernetics. The short answer to this, and part of this we have seen already in the previous chapter, is that automata theory does tell us something about the limitations on what is possible cybernetically, and often helps to provide clues of one kind or another as to how the actual model construction may be carried out. On the other hand, theorems which are developed as a normal process of the development of a mathematical subject are not of special interest to cybernetics. Cyberneticians will use automata theory, as they use the rest of mathematics, as a means to abbreviate or simplify or conceptually clarify their own particular interests, which are of course in the modelling, both synthesizing and simulating, of various systems mostly of a self-adapting or feedback kind.

The main point about automata theory, certainly in its tape-and-scanner forms such as in the case of the Turing machine, is that it is primarily concerned with what is mathematically possible and not with the other forms of modelling. For example, it is important that we should know that there are no computations that can be performed with a multi-tape to a Turing machine that cannot be performed by a simple-tape Turing machine. This is not, however, of the same interest to cyberneticians, who are less interested, while still being interested to some extent, in what the class of computations are that can be performed by any particular automaton as the manner in which they are performed.

We are concerned primarily with two different things, one the search for suitable algorithms, and this is typical of the mathematical search, and also the search for heuristics, and this is the process that must necessarily take over when the algorithmic methods come to a halt. This does not mean that heuristics will not often be used where algorithms are possible, since this is just another aspect of the cybernetic 'facts of life'. Let us follow McNaughton (1961) in his summary of the theory of automata.

He makes a number of distinctions which are extremely useful. *Growth automata* are automata that can become arbitrarily large in size and therefore the potentially infinite Turing machine is clearly capable of being interpreted as a growth automaton. Some *partial growth automata* are limited in the upper limit to which they can grow and precisely because of this limitation it can be said that they are no more powerful than fixed automata. This is so because the upper limit placed on the part of growth systems is wholly equivalent to the upper limit placed on the size of the fixed automaton and clearly they can be made coextensive.

Automata can also be *synchronous* or *non-synchronous*, they can be *deterministic* or *probabilistic*, they may have an initial state or they may not be said to have an initial state. An example of the latter kind of automata would be those of Edward F. Moore (1956, 1964). One further distinction that we should make in possible classification of automata is that between *continuous* and *discrete*. This is the same sort of distinction as is made in classical mathematics and applies whether or not there are continua of values for each input and output or only a discrete set, whether potentially infinite or not. This in turn leads to a consideration of other forms of automata such as a switching circuit which could be interpreted as a fixed discrete automaton whereas a classical electrical circuit in its abstract aspects is a continuous automaton. However, all these classifications, as always, are arbitrary and many of these systems can be viewed in many different ways.

If we now turn to more precise efforts to define automata we look first at Rabin and Scott (1959) who suggest the following definition:

A finite automaton over a finite alphabet E is a system R equals (S, M, s^0, F) where S is a finite set (the internal states of R), M is the function of E multiplied by S with values in S (the table of moods of R), s^0 is an element of S (the internal state of R) and S is a subset of S (the designated final state of R).

And a rather similar definition has been offered by McNaughton (1961).

A finite automaton is an ordered principle (S, I, U, f, g) where $S, I,$ and U are elements, f is a function mapping S multiplied by I into S, and g is a function mapping S multiplied by I into U. Then for every element of f in S and i in I, $f(s, i)$ is an element of S and $g(f, i)$ is an element of U.

In the case of the second definition in a manner which is very similar to that of the first definition S, I, U, f and g are a set of states, set of input values, set of output values and the transition function and the output function respectively.

We should add at this point that all the many different types of automata we have mentioned the ones which most often we have in mind when we use the phrase 'finite automata' are those which are fully described as fixed, discrete, synchronous, deterministic finite state automata. So we can assume that that is what we shall always mean by the phrase 'finite automata'. And this is certainly covered by the two more precise definitions just applied.

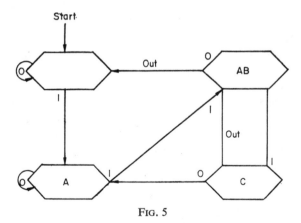

Fig. 5

We should emphasize here the use of state graphs which are often used to represent automata. The graph shown in Fig. 5 represents a binary scalar. The odd numbered 1's are dealt with at C where the arrow from state C to state A represents the transition from C to A. The input symbol here is 0 and the result of 0 as an input is to change the state from C to A. If the input at C is 1 the state is changed at AB, and so on. The binary scalar is a simple counting device which counts up to 2. We can also draw these state graphs as logical nets.

One especially important distinction, from the cybernetic point of view, is that between deterministic and probabilistic automata. One example at least of a probabilistic approach (de Leeuw *et al.*, 1956) was to compare probabilistic and deterministic Turing machines, and they were able to show that there was nothing a probabilistic machine could do that a deterministic one could not. However, once more we should be careful about such results since they involve only one interpretation of a probabilistic automata, and they refer to the class of events which could be processed by the automata and not by the methods used, and from our point of view it may be the methods that are more important than the class of problems soluble by such methods.

In talking of von Neumann's automata later in this chapter we shall see that a probabilistic approach has certain important criteria from the point of view of brain models.

McCulloch–Pitts neural net

A neuron is a cell body whose nerve fibres lead to one or more endbulbs, where we can think of an endbulb *with respect to one element* as being simply the next element in the net. A nerve net is an arrangement of a finite number of neurons in which each endbulb of any one neuron impinges on the cell body of not more than one other neuron. A special case arises where a cell body is its own endbulb. The separating gap between cells is a synapse, and an endbulb may be one of two kinds, excitatory or inhibitory, but not both. The neurons are called *input neurons* where no endbulbs impinge, and otherwise, *inner neurons*. The conditions on the firing of input neurons are determined by conditions outside the net, while for inner neurons a threshold number h must be exceeded, or at least equalled by the balance of excitatory over inhibitory inputs, firing the instant before the time t (say) under consideration.

The conventions on which the networks are drawn are as follows: A circle represents an element (or neuron) which is in one of two states at any instant t, it is either *live* or *dead*. If live, then its output fibre will be sending out an impulse at the instant it is live. The output fibre must be in one state at any instant, and an *instant* is assumed to be the firing time of all the elements. The output may bifurcate as often as is needed, but it can only be in one state for all its bifurcations. There can be as many inputs as we like, and these inputs can be divisible into two classes, excitatory and inhibitory. The excitatory ending is represented by a filled-in triangle, and the inhibitory by an open circle. A heavy dot is used to indicate that wires crossing over are also having contact, except that when three wires are involved, since no loose endings will occur apart from the input and output elements, there will be no ambiguity in omitting the heavy dot. This replaces the $+$ notation sometimes used in electrical circuits. The number h in the circle is the threshold number which is such that, if e be the number of excitatory fibres live at any instant and i the number of inhibitors live at any instant, then the condition for the element to fire is that $e \geqslant i+h$. The neural net of Fig. 6 illustrates some of the principles so far described.

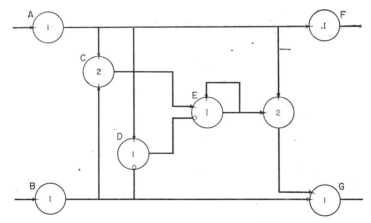

FIG. 6. A LOGICAL NET FOR SIGNS. The logical net is one that could be taken to represent a sign. If A and B fire together this fact is 'remembered' by the loop element E, and if then A fires alone G fires as if B had fired; A is 'a sign for' B.

If we assume that a nerve net has k input neurons N_1, N_2, ..., N_k for positive k, then for any period of instants, reading back from the present p (say r instants), we can represent the total activity of the automaton by a k by r matrix. The matrix will be made up of 0's and 1's according to whether the particular input neuron fired at a particular instant or not.

A typical matrix for $k = 2$, $r = 3$ is:

$$\begin{bmatrix} 1 & 1 \\ 1 & 0 \\ 0 & 1 \end{bmatrix}$$

for columns N_1 and N_2 and rows p, $p-1$, $p-2$.

Such a matrix represents, or could be taken to represent, the whole history of the input, and in terms of this we define an *event* as a property of the input of an automaton. An *event* is any subclass of the class of all possible matrices describing the inputs over all the past time right up to the present. Such matrices will be called *input matrices*.

An example of an event in terms of the above matrix would be the firing of N_1 at $p-1$ and the non-firing of N_2 at the same time. This event would be one of the events represented by the above matrix.

We must now, following Kleene (1951), narrow our definition of an event. First we shall define a *definite event* as an event that took place within a fixed period of the past, and that the relevant matrix is said to cover definite events of duration r.

It will be noticed that there are kr entries in a kr matrix which covers k neurons over a period of duration r. This means that there are 2^{kr} possible matrices, since they can be made up of all possible combinations of 0 and 1, and there will be $2^{2^{kr}}$ definite events represented by such a set of matrices. A *positive* definite event is one in which at least one input neuron fires during the duration of the event.

Now we must briefly consider the representation of definite events, since we must be sure that when we use neural nets for our behavioural purpose, they are within the safe ground of logical consistency; they are, in fact, taken to represent *regular events*, for which we must seek a definition. In this respect Kleene has proved many theorems which are primarily of mathematical interest, and those interested in the mathematical theory of finite automata should consult his work.

One of the important consequences of Kleene's theorems should be stated immediately. He has shown that almost any event which is likely to be of biological or psychological interest can be constructed in neural nets; he has even shown an effective procedure for the construction of the necessary net.

An *indefinite* event is one that cannot be described by precise reference to a past firing of an input element. Figure 7 shows a simple example of an indefinite event. It uses the notation of the lower functional calculus as well as that of the propositional calculus suffixed for time.

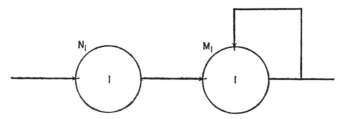

FIG. 7. A LOOP ELEMENT. If N_1 fires, it fires M_1, and then M_1 continues to fire itself indefinitely. M_1 is called a loop or looped element.

Figure 7 can be represented by the logical formula

$$(Et)_{t \, > \, p} N_p \supset M_{p+1}^1 \tag{1}$$

where (Et) is the existential operator, and means 'there exists a (time) t such that'. Here we use the usual symbol for a material implication.

The element of Fig. 7 could, of course, be characterized in simpler terms. If we label the element M_1 in terms of its input and output (say A and B respectively), we could write either

$$(Et)_{t<p} B_t$$

or we could write

$$B_t \equiv A_{t-1} v A_{t-2} v \ldots v A_{t-n} \tag{2}$$

i.e.

$$B_t \equiv A_{t-1} v B_{t-1}$$

which clearly characterizes the behaviour of the element.

There are many mathematical complications over the 'starting conditions' of automata, and further complications of detail, but our main concern is now over that further class of events called *regular* events. These will be defined.

A *regular* event exists if there is a regular set of input matrices that describe it in the sense that the event either occurs or not according as the input is described by one of the matrices of the set of input matrices or none of them.

A *regular* set of matrices shall be the least class of sets of matrices (including unit all and null sets) which is closed under the operation of passing from E and F to EvF, to EF and to E^*F, where v is the Boolean disjunction, EF means $E.F$ where . is the Boolean conjunction and * is defined by $EE...EF$.

These regular nets (nets that represent regular events) are *primitive recursive* (Kleene, 1951) and realizable, and logical difficulties can be wholly avoided as long as we keep within their domain. This we shall do, and all the logical nets discussed from here on are ones that represent regular events and can be described by a regular set of matrices. This refers to a certain kind of finite automaton within the compass of which our investigations will operate.

We cannot explain the full significance of such terms as 'primitive recursive', but we should state that primitive recursive functions are those defined by Gödel in search of a function that encompassed *all* the familiar mathematical functions. Primitive recursive can be taken to be identified with 'effectively computable'.

Uneconomical finite automata

Most of our later discussion of finite automata will not be concerned primarily with economy of elements used. Culbertson (1950, 1956) has explicitly investigated the properties of uneconomical automata; his work is close to the needs of experimental psychologists who are concerned with the construction of models for molar use, as well as those which are primarily concerned with being interpreted as a 'conceptual nervous system'.

Culbertson (1948), in his earlier work, developed scanning mechanisms and models of visual systems in neural network terms, and these will be discussed later at the appropriate time. The same is true of memory devices and other mechanisms that might help towards the construction of robots, where, by 'robot', we mean a finite automaton reproduced in hardware.

He also devised the outlines of a theory of consciousness, designed to elucidate the mind–body problem by exhibiting the relationship between subjective awareness and the objective activities of the human organism.

A further interesting discussion of memoryless robots has shown that they could exhibit behaviour that might be called intelligent, and this intelligence (or apparent intelligence) can be increased by making the memoryless robot probabilistic rather than deterministic. In the same context, Culbertson has also investigated the possibility that a robot can be constructed satisfying any given probabilistic input–output specifications.

Von Neumann (1952) has investigated the alternative problem of showing how deterministic robots can be constructed in terms of unreliable elements.

Von Neumann's work is of great importance and of great practical value. His paper was significantly entitled *Probabilistic Logics*, and it is concerned primarily with the role of error in logic and, by implication, in finite automata. He constructed his own notation, built like Kleene's in terms of the logical notation of McCulloch and Pitts, and he was able to show that typical syntheses of logical nets are possible by simple and effective devices. Some of these findings have been incorporated into the particular models which we shall be discussing in the next chapter.

The main part of von Neumann's work—and although we shall not be considering this very much further, we must continue to be aware of it—is the manner in which he deals with error. First, to summarize his findings, we shall look at what he calls the 'majority organ', the 'Sheffer stroke' element, and then the 'multiple line trick'.

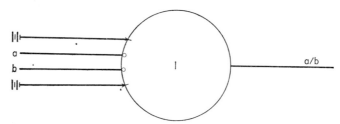

FIG. 8. SHEFFER STROKE. The Sheffer stroke element fires unless both inputs *a* and *b* fire together when the ouput is inhibited.

It is well known that the whole of Boolean algebra can be derived from the one connective called the Sheffer stroke and symbolized |; von Neumann makes this a basic organ of his system. The following figures indicate the nature of the Sheffer stroke in logical net terminology,

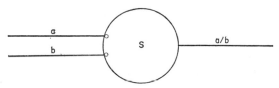

FIG. 9. SHEFFER STROKE. Von Neumann's symbolic representation of the Sheffer stroke element of Fig. 8. The two diagrams are synonymous.

and also the derivation of the other well-known Boolean connectives from it where '⊩' means permanently stimulated. Figure 9 shows the shorthand symbol for the full Sheffer stroke organ of Fig. 8.

Now we can derive 'or', 'and' and 'not' in terms of Sheffer stroke organs as follows:

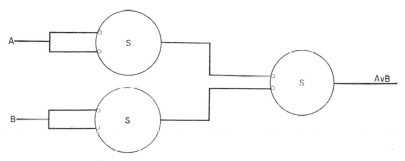

FIG. 10. OR. The inclusive *or* of logic as represented by Sheffer stroke elements.

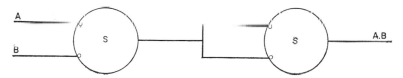

FIG. 11. AND. The *and* of logic as represented by Sheffer stroke elements.

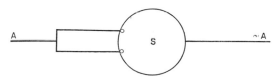

FIG. 12. NOT. The *not* of logic as represented by Sheffer stroke elements.

The other basic organ to be considered is the majority organ, and this can be written

$$m\,(a,\,b,\,c) = (a\,v\,b).(a\,v\,c).(b\,v\,c)$$
$$= (a.b)\,v\,(a.c)\,v\,(b.c)$$

and this can be drawn as in Fig. 13.

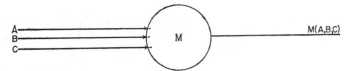

FIG. 13. THE MAJORITY ORGAN. The output fires if a majority of the inputs *A*, *B*, *C* fire.

The operations of conjunction and disjunction can be derived from the majority organ quite easily:

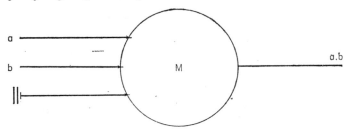

FIG. 14. AND. Representation of logical *and* by the majority organ.

where '∥⊢' means never stimulated, and

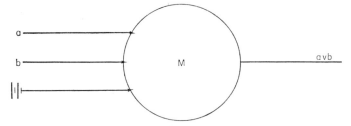

FIG. 15. OR. Representation of logical *or* by the majority organ.

The multiple-line trick

The basic problem that von Neumann sets himself to solve can be stated in the following way. Suppose we construct an automaton, and that we build it in terms of the single organ represented by the Sheffer stroke, and then we represent the probability of the malfunctioning of a particular element by ε ($< \frac{1}{2}$). If we are given a positive number δ, where δ represents the final allowable error in the whole automaton, can a corresponding automaton be constructed from the given organs which will perform the necessary functions while committing an amount of error less than or equal to δ? How small can δ be? Are there many different methods of achieving the same end?

We see straight away, of course, that δ cannot be less than ε, since the reliability of the whole system cannot be greater than that of the final neuron, which may have error ε. This applies to the first question but not to the second.

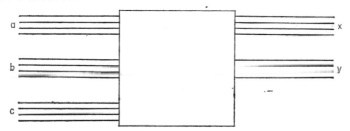

FIG. 16. MULTIPLEXED SYSTEM. With inputs a, b, c and ouputs x, y the system is connected by n lines, represented here by ≡. The probability of ouputs firing for inputs firing can be calculated at different rates of error of connection.

Consider Fig. 16. The multiple line trick, as von Neumann calls it, merely involves carrying messages on multiple lines instead of on single or even double lines.

We first set a fiduciary level to the number of the lines of the bundle that is to be stimulated. Let this level be k. Then for $0 \leqslant k \leqslant \frac{1}{2}$, at least $(1-k) N$ lines of the bundles being stimulated, the bundle is said to be in a positive state; and conversely, when no more than kN are stimulated, it implies a negative state. A system which works in this manner is called *multiplexed*.

8*

Von Neumann next proceeds to examine the notion of error further for a multiplexed automaton.

The rest of this section gives a fairly rigorous example of von Neumann's argument, and this may be omitted by the reader who is not explicitly interested in the mathematical theory. The argument is only a part of the general form by which von Neumann was able to demonstrate the point that reliable automata can be constructed from unreliable components; or, more simply, that error in an automaton can be controlled.

Denote by X the given network (assume two outputs in the specific instance pictured in Fig. 17). Construct X in triplicate, labelling the copies X^1, X^2, X^3 respectively. Consider the system shown in Fig. 17.

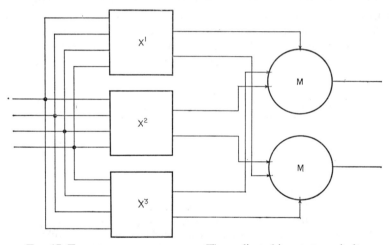

FIG. 17. THE MULTIPLEXED CONTROL. The replicated inputs to majority organs increase the probability of successful transmission of information.

For each of the final majority organs, the conditions of the special case considered above obtain. Consequently, if N is an *upper bound for the probability of error* at any output of the original network X, then

$$N^* = \varepsilon + (1-2\varepsilon)(3N^2 - 2N^3) \equiv f\varepsilon(N) \qquad (3)$$

is an upper bound for the probability of error at any output of the new network X^*. The graph is the curve $N^* = f\varepsilon(N)$, shown in Fig. 18.

Consider the intersections of the curve with the diagonal $N^* = N$. First, $N = \frac{1}{2}$ is at any rate such an intersection. Dividing $N - f\varepsilon(N)$ by

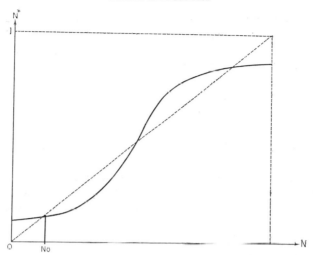

FIG. 18. ERROR CONTROL GRAPH. N is upper bound for the probability of error at any output of an original network (X in Fig. 17), and N^* for the new network derived by multiplexing ε is the error. N_0 is a root of the equation for N^* shown in graph as curved line (see text for explanation).

$N - \frac{1}{2}$ gives $2 ((1-2\varepsilon) N^2 - (1-2\varepsilon) N + \varepsilon)$, hence the other intersections are the roots of $(1-2\varepsilon)N^2 - (1-2\varepsilon) N + \varepsilon = 0$, i.e.

$$N = \frac{1}{2} \left[1 \pm \sqrt{\frac{1-6\varepsilon}{1-2\varepsilon}} \right]$$

i.e. for $\varepsilon = \frac{1}{6}$ they do not exist (being complex (for $\varepsilon > \frac{1}{6}$) or $= \frac{1}{2}$ (for $\varepsilon - \frac{1}{6}$)); while for $\varepsilon < \frac{1}{6}$ they are $N = N_0, 1 - N_0$, where

$$N_0 = \frac{1}{2} \left[1 - \sqrt{\frac{1-6\varepsilon}{1-2\varepsilon}} \right] = \varepsilon + 3\varepsilon^2 + \dots \qquad (4)$$

For $N = 0$; $N^* = \varepsilon > N$. This, the monotonic nature and the continuity of $N^* = f\varepsilon\,(N)$, therefore imply:

First case, $\varepsilon \geqslant \frac{1}{6}$: $0 \leqslant N < \frac{1}{2}$ implies $N < N^* < \frac{1}{2}$; $\frac{1}{2} < N \leqslant 1$ implies $\frac{1}{2} < N^* < N$.

Second case, $\varepsilon < \frac{1}{6}$: $0 \leqslant N < N_0$ implies $N < N^* < N_0$; $N_0 < N < \frac{1}{2}$ implies $N_0 < N^* < N$; $\frac{1}{2} < N < 1 - N_0$ implies $N < N^* < 1 - N_0$; $1 - N_0 < N < 1$ implies $1 - N_0 < N^* < N$.

Now there are numerous successive occurrences of the situation under consideration, if it is to be used as a basic procedure, hence the iterative behaviour of the operation $N \to N^* = f\varepsilon\,(N)$ is relevant. Now it is clear from the above that, in the first case, the successive iterates of the process in question always converge to $\frac{1}{2}$, no matter what the original N; while in the second case these iterates converge to N_0 if the original $N < \frac{1}{2}$, and to $1 - N_0$ if the original $N < \frac{1}{2}$.

To put the matter another way, in the first case no error level other than $N \sim \frac{1}{2}$ can maintain itself in the long run, where $\sim$ means 'approximately the same as', or 'the same in the limit', i.e. the process asymptotically degenerates to total irrelevance. In the second case the error-levels $N \sim N_0$ and $N \sim 1 - N_0$ will not only maintain themselves in the long run, but they represent the asymptotic behaviour for any original $N < \frac{1}{2}$ or $N > \frac{1}{2}$, respectively.

These arguments make it clear that the second case alone can be used for the desired error-level control, i.e. we must require $\varepsilon < \frac{1}{6}$, i.e. the error-level for a single basic organ function must be less than ~ 16 per cent. The stable, ultimate error-level should then be N_0 (we postulate that a start be made with an error-level $N < \frac{1}{2}$). N_0 is small if ε is, hence ε must be small, and so

$$N_0 = \varepsilon + 3\varepsilon^2 + \ldots$$

This would therefore imply an ultimate error-level of about 10 per cent (i.e. $N \sim 0{\cdot}1$). (For a single basic organ function error-level of ~ 8 per cent (i.e. $0{\cdot}08$).)

This argument is taken a great deal further, and made very much more rigorous, and von Neumann introduces the concept of a 'restoring organ' which helps to control the error. He hazards the guess that 'neuron pools' in the human nervous system may work on such a procedure as he outlines.

It is probable that von Neumann's principial contribution to the behavioural theory of neural nets lies in his demonstration that error in the components at least will not be a reason for believing that very large switching devices would be hopelessly inadequate because of the multiplication of error. There are, of course, many other ideas that spring from his work, and which we should bear in mind in our search for suitable behavioural models.

The syntheses of finite automata

We next turn to the subject of the actual hardware machines that have been built as syntheses of the general theory of finite automata. We shall exclude some machines from this discussion and leave them until the end of the next chapter, where they may be better understood after the discussion of the particular set of finite automata there described.

There are many difficulties confronting a discussion of the syntheses of finite automata, and we can but summarize some of the better known of these models. We shall subsequently make some generalizations about the nature of the syntheses.

We should bear in mind that we have already outlined the structure of digital computers, and these are the most obvious of all examples of such syntheses that are of interest to us in the behavioural sciences. We shall say no more about them at the moment, although their special use when programmed as learning machines should be borne in mind.

Grey Walter's models

Grey Walter (1953) has produced two syntheses of finite automata. The simpler one is called Cora, a conditioned reflex analog, and its general structure and function are briefly noted in the following description.

Cora's response to changed conditions is indicated by a short discharge in a neon glow tube, seen as a flash of pink light, which is the response to a particular stimulus. With such a system, a sound such as a whistle can be made a sign of a forthcoming light stimulus. In other words, it is a simple association system, and it will be seen later that this is the basic idea underlying our logical networks of the next chapter.

Machina speculatrix (popularly known as 'the tortoise') is somewhat more complicated. It has two sensory elements in the form of a simple contact receptor and a photoelectric cell. The tortoise is mobile, being driven by an electric motor, and it carries an accumulator, two valves, registers, condensers, and a pilot light (Appendices B and C, Walter, 1953).

Technical description of *M. speculatrix*

M. speculatrix is intended as a model of elementary reflex behaviour, and contains only two functional elements: two receptors, two nerve cells, two effectors. The first receptor is a photoelectric cell, mounted on the spindle of the steering column always facing the same direction as the single front driving wheel, which is one effector. In the dark the steering is continuously rotated by the steering motor (the other effector) so that the photo-cell scans steadily. The scanning rotation is stopped when moderate light enters the photo-cell, but starts again at half speed when the light intensity is greater—the dazzle state. The driving motor operates at half speed when scanning in the dark, and at full speed in moderate or intense light. The other receptor is a ring-and-stick limit switch attached to the shell, which is rubber-suspended. When the shell touches something, or when a gradient is encountered, its displacement closes the limit switch. This connects the output of the 'central nervous' amplifier back to its input through a capacitor so that it is turned into a multivibrator. The oscillations produced by the multivibrator stop the circuit from acting as an amplifier, so that simple sensitivity to light is lost; instead, the connections alternate between the 'dark' and 'dazzle' states. The steering-scanning motor is alternately on full- and half-power, and the driving motor, at the same time, on half- and full-power, the effect of which is to produce a turn-and-push manoeuvre. The time-constant of the feedback circuit is selected to give about one-third of the time on 'steer-hard-push-gently', and two-thirds on 'push-hard-steer-gently'. This gives a prompt response to the first contact with an obstacle. Though there is no direct attraction to light the obstacle-avoiding state, the feedback time-constant is shorter when the photo-cell is illuminated, so that when an obstacle is met in the dark, the avoidance drill is done in a leisurely fashion, but when there is an attractive light nearby, the movements are more hasty.

The electrical circuit is shown in Fig. 19. This is only one of many possible arrangements, but it is probably the simplest in components and wiring. The photo-cell is a gas-filled type, and generally needs no optical system, a single light-louvre giving sufficient directionality. It is convenient to connect the tube between the grid of the first amplifier tube and the negative side of the 6-V accumulator needed to run the motors. The grid of the input tube is connected to the positive side of the 6-V battery through a 10-megohm resistor; illumination of the photo-cell can therefore only change the bias on the input tube from zero to about 4 V negative. In the dark the first tube, having zero bias, passes its full current,

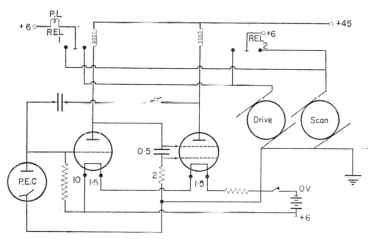

FIG. 19. CIRCUIT OF *M. speculatrix*. This figure shows the circuit of *M. speculatrix* (after Grey Walter).

and the relay in its anode is 'on'. This tube is a triode, or a triode-connected pentode. The relay should have a resistance of about 10,000 Ω, or rather less than the anode impedance of the tube, and a single pole change-over contact. The resistance of this relay and the anode impedance of the first tube form a potentiometer which fixes the screen voltage of the second tube. The anode of the first tube is thus connected directly to the screen of the second and also, through a 0·5-mF capacitor, to its grid. This provides a relatively high gain for changes in illumination and steady-state amplification when the input is larger. The effect of this coupling is to permit transient interruption of the scanning motion when a faint light enters the photo-cell, thus gradually bringing the model on to the beam at a distance, then a steady inhibition of scanning when the light is brighter or nearer. The relay in the anode of the second tube is of the same type as the first, but the moving contact goes straight to the positive terminal of the 6-V battery, instead of through the pilot light. The stationary contacts are connected in the same way, 'on' to the driving motor, 'off' to the scanning motor, in both relays. In faint light, relay 2 is closed momentarily; in moderate light it is held closed, and in bright light it remains closed but relay 1 opens, thus providing for swerving away from a bright light.

The pilot light, which is in series with the moving contact of relay 1, is short-circuited when relay 2 closes, and is therefore extinguished when the driving motor is turned to full power and the scanning movement is arrested by light. When the light from the pilot bulb is reflected by a mirror into the photo-cell, it is extinguished, but the disappearance of this light restores relay 2 to 'off', and the light appears again.

Grey Walter tried the interesting experiment of connecting Cora to the obstacle-avoiding device in the tortoise and, as a result of associating touch with the onset of trouble, it was found that the whole model would retreat when touched. The education process involved, in Grey Walter's own words, 'blowing the whistle and kicking the shell a few times'. This simple sort of associative learning is of the greatest interest from the point of view of learning theory.

One special point of interest arises with the combined model, and it is one of those which justify the construction of hardware models. After the defensive backing reflex had been conditioned the whistle was blown and, without reinforcement by kicking, the flash of light that indicated the activation of the memory circuit occurred without an explicit eliciting stimulus. This meant that every time the dodging operation occurred the pink light flashed, and although this *could* have been predicted from the blueprint, the prediction was not in fact made.

But we must curtail discussion of these machines and carry on to the next model. As in all these cases, the original references should be used when the full detail is required.

Ross Ashby's model

Apart from Ashby's lengthy justification of the principle of ultra-stability in the design of human brains (Ashby, 1952), he has produced the well-known 'Homeostat'. This models the process of ultrastability, and is of special interest to psychologists.

The Homeostat is an analog computer, and consists of four boxes with a magnetic needle pivoted on top of each. The magnets can be deflected from their neutral positions from which they will return to a position of equilibrium, although the return is not always by precisely the same method. The magnets are connected to water potentiometers, and the four boxes are interconnected with each other.

The Homeostat is thus composed of four main units, and the angular deviation of each magnet constitutes the variables in the situation. Each of the four units emits a d.c. output proportional to the deviation of its magnet from the neutral. In front of each magnet is a trough of water, and electrodes there provide a potential gradient. The magnets carry wires which dip into this water and pick up a potential difference that depends on the position of the magnet, sending it to the grid of the

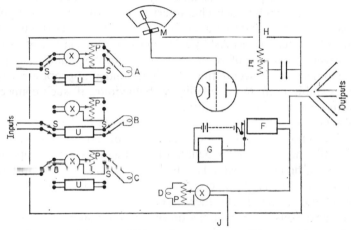

Fig. 20. Тhe homeostat. Wiring diagram of one unit. *J* provides anode potential at 150 V, while *H* is at 180 V, so *E* carries a constant current. *M* is the magnet. *A*, *B* and *C* are coils. *X* is a commutator, *P* a potentiometer, *S* a switch, *U* a uniselector, *G* a coil of a uniselector and *F* is a relay.

triode (see Fig. 20). *J* provides the anode potential at 150 V, while *H* is at 180 V, so *E* carries a constant current. If the grid-potential allows just this current to pass through the valve, then no current will flow through the output; whereas if the valve passes more or less than this amount of current, the output circuit will carry the difference in one direction or another. So, having been fixed, the output is proportional to *M*'s deviation.

The next stage involves the interconnecting of the units so that each sends its output to the other three. This leads to the torque on all of the magnets being proportional to the sum of the currents in coils A, B and C (see Fig. 20). There is also an effect from D itself as a self-feedback. Each input passes through a commutator X and a potentiometer P before it reaches the coil, and these determine the polarity of entry, and the fraction of input to reach the coil.

This system, so Ashby claims, exhibits the important characteristic of *purposiveness*, and he believes that the variations in the manner of achieving ultrastability are a characteristic not normally seen in machines, but usually seen in living organisms. The point is well made that organisms show this purposiveness, and any machines that purport to be humanlike must exhibit such characteristics. In the logical nets of the next chapter we shall find that a motivational system will exhibit some of the same characteristics as Ashby's Homeostat. One cannot but wonder at the possible outcome of connecting the Cora–*Speculatrix* compound to the Homeostat; it seems that it might, under appropriate circumstances, exhibit even more intelligent behaviour, if such connections proved to be a practical possibility.

Ashby (1956a, 1956b) has set out a large-scale design for a brain in terms of step functions and the characteristic of ultrastability and, more recently still, has argued on behalf of set theory for the appropriate description of finite automata. This is, in fact, a form of description that is implicit in our own logical nets. A more recent set-theoretic description by Beer (1960) is also of relevance here.

Let us next consider Shannon's maze-running machine.

Shannon's model

Figure 21 shows the Shannon's maze-runner which will be briefly described (1951).

The top panel of the machine shows a maze derived from a 5×5 array of squares. There is a sensing finger which has contact by touch with the walls of the maze, and the finger is driven by two motors which orient it in a north–south and an east–west direction. The finger now has to feel its way to its goal.

The finger searches each square in turn, and if it reaches a partition it

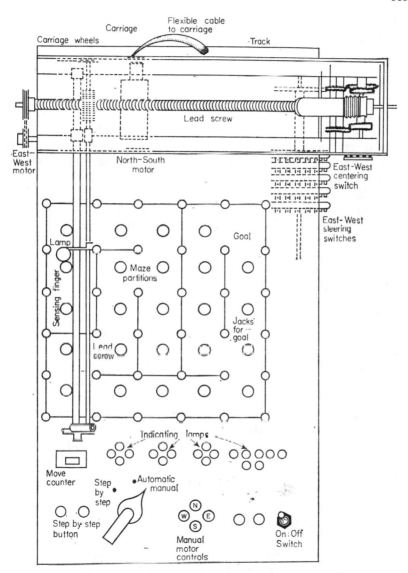

FIG. 21. MAZE-RUNNER. On the panel there is a 5×5 range of squares, these can be rearranged to any desired pattern, thus changing the maze through which the sensing finger must find its way.

goes back to the centre of the square and starts again. The systematic search depends on previous knowledge and certain strategies. It can also get into a sort of 'neurotic' cycle when an old solution becomes a part of another path which leads back into itself.

The strategy involves the use of two relays for each square of the maze, and they can remember any of four possible directions such as north, south, east and west. This means that any square has a special orientation associated with it. Solutions lead to the locking in of relays, and there are also ways in which the machine can forget. If, for example, the goal is not reached in a specific number of moves, then the previous solution is regarded as no longer relevant, the assumption being that the maze-runner has got into a cycle.

Shannon's model shows some of the same characteristics as do the logical nets we are to consider, and it certainly exhibits many of the simple characteristics of learning. It has, indeed, all the essential features of a learning machine in the form of a memory, a receptor system, an output system and is selective in its operation.

Uttley's models

In many ways Uttley's syntheses of finite automata are the most interesting of all, from our point of view, since the essential process of classification and conditional probability are both accepted as necessary parts of the logical net system that we are to use to analyse behaviour.

Uttley's original classification system had the following properties: it was based on the sensory system of an automatic card filer of the Hollerith type. The idea that the human senses worked on a classification principle had previously been suggested by Hayek (1952), and Uttley was able to build a simple classification system in hardware. Its circuit is given in Fig. 22.

The principle is a very simple one, and merely demands that any number of elements can be gathered together into any or all the possible sets of combinations of their elements. We can extend this in both a temporal and a spatial manner by considering the same element an instant or two instants later as being effectively a different element in the sets that one is classifying. Since this is an essential part of our argument on perception and sensory processes, and is going to play a major part in the rest of the book we shall not pursue it at the moment.

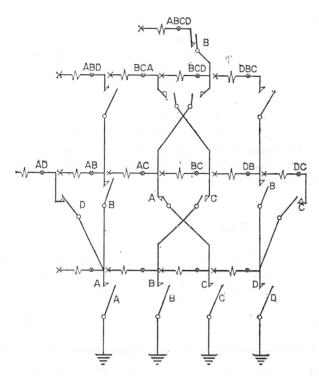

FIG. 22. CLASSIFYING SYSTEM. This is a simple example of a hardware realization of a classifying system, constructed by Uttley, and classifying the inputs, *A*, *B*, *C* and *D* into every possible combination.

Uttley's second machine (1955) is a conditional probability machine. This, again, is a hardware representation of a basic concept that will be taken over into the logical nets. Its essential characteristics are that it is capable of counting different combinations of occurrence, and computing that, given a particular stimulus *a*, then the probability of *b* following is the number of occurrences of *a* in the past when followed by *b*, divided by the total number of occurrences of *a* in the past, regardless of whether or not they have been followed by *b*.

It should be emphasized that in Uttley's system we can regard what he calls the 'tunes' (patterns of occurrences) as being spread out either spatially or temporally.

It is also of interest that Uttley's work, unlike that of Shannon, Walter or Ashby, has been explicitly aimed at the synthesis of the principles on which organisms behave, and less in terms of actually presenting minia-ture organisms.

George (1958) has built models that have the same essential properties as Uttley's two models, but since these were constructed in terms of the theory of nets we shall not discuss them until a later stage in the present work. A model called *Flebus* has been built by Stewart (1959), and a model by Chapman (1959). Chapman's model will be described now, and Stewart's—since it is closely related to logical nets—will be dealt with in the next chapter.

Chapman's self-organizing classification system

The principle of Chapman's classification system differs from that of Uttley's in its demand that any number of elements can be gathered together into several of the possible sets of combinations of their elements, not exceeding an arbitrary number. There is a further condition: that the several combinations of elements which can be gathered together shall be those which occur most frequently together.

At first sight, the limitation on the number of combinations that can be classified appears to be a simplification imposing an unjustifiable con-straint on the system. However, if we consider a situation similar to that of visual perception, where the number of elements is so large that only a tiny fraction of the possible number of combinations occurs, the econ-omy of Chapman's system becomes obvious. The condition of relating priority of classification to frequency inevitably means that the system does not classify elements as soon as it is conceived, and at that stage it is therefore not strictly a classifying system. Its structure is such that, by operating on it with groups of elements, it 'grows', and learns to classify them.

The technique by which this is achieved in the hardware model is one of inhibition. Each of the inputs to the machine representing an element or primitive stimulus is connected to every one of the outputs, repre-senting events, by a number of barely conducting paths, consisting of threads of cotton moistened with lime water. When a group of elements is 'fired' by application of a positive potential to the ends of the cotton threads, the event is registered by the lighting of several of the ouput lamps. For each such event, all conducting links connecting inputs which were not active to outputs which were active, are rendered less conducting by the passage of a large current, and the consequent evaporation of moisture. In addition, the active links are rendered less conducting, at a different rate, unless or until the output on which they terminate only just fires (i.e. its threshold is only just exceeded by a small quantity ε). In general, if a number of different events occur, a tendency is observed for the outputs to distribute themselves among the events, and eventually to represent each event uniquely. However, with suitable adjustment of the rates at which the two sets of conducting paths for each event are modified, it is possible for certain outputs to respond, not to separate events, but to several events all containing a common subset of elements. In a sense the machine has recognized a general characteristic of its environment.

By careful control of the vapour pressure surrounding the cotton threads, the machine can be made to forget events which have not occurred recently, or whose frequency has diminished, and so allow more frequent events to overwrite them. Although a system which allows overwriting would cause confusion if used to store detailed information, it has a very obvious advantage as an early warning system in an organism whose environment is changing, and it seems likely that a system of this type plays an important part in directing attention.

Chapman's machine is significant in itself as a pointer to the way in which economy can be achieved in a large classification system; but what is of more importance is that he, like Pask (1958, 1959), has demonstrated that a very highly organized specific system can grow from a nonspecific medium with a relatively simple structure, obeying generalized rules of growth.

An interesting comparison occurs between Chapman's model and the Mark II cell assembly of Milner, which will be discussed in Chapter 10.

Another approach to the 'growth nets' which are implied by Chapman's model is through matrices. An input matrix has rows which represent input elements, and columns representing the successive states of the input. The initial structure of the net is given by a structure matrix, a square matrix whose elements represent the sensitivity of the various links (cotton threads) between input and output elements. This structure changes as a function of the input matrix, and there is a series of structure

TBC 9

matrices with links whose sensitivities are changing. For example, where the critical threshold is 0·10, the following *structure matrix* defines a simple growth net with three inputs and three outputs (the rows and columns of the structure matrix):

$$S_1 \equiv \begin{pmatrix} 7 & 10 & 5 \\ 6 & 8 & 4 \\ 5 & 4 & 6 \end{pmatrix}$$

Now for input vector $\{1, 1, 0\}$ the resultant output is $\{1, 1, 0\}$. The result is that a new structure matrix is formed, and the elements of S_1 are all diminished, the links which are fired being diminished less than those not fired.

This whole problem of matrix description of growth nets is now undergoing a careful analysis, and will be discussed no further here.

General synthesis

Obviously if one asks general questions about syntheses of theories, one is immediately transported back to those theories from which the syntheses emanated. We should say, though, that a very important account of the synthesis of two-terminal switching circuits has been written by Shannon (1949), and this deals with questions as to which logical theories can be translated into hardware, and it deals especially with questions about the simplest form that such syntheses should take. This matter is rather concerned with mathematical and electrical engineering aspects of switching circuits, and will hold no immediate and direct interest for the behavioural scientist.

Except to say that there have been many other models built apart from those here briefly discussed, we shall be content at this point to leave the question of the synthesis of automata, and return to it much later after we have seen more clearly what sort of systems we might next try to convert into hardware models. It should perhaps be said, from the behavioural point of view, that the sorts of models that are likely to be most useful are liable to be a very great deal more complicated than anything that has so far been built.

An alternative method of approaching the same problem (George, 1957d) is to consider the possibility of programming a general purpose digital computer with a full description of the automaton we are interested in, and then feed the inputs into the automaton that is now inside the computer. The difficulty here is the inadequate size of memory stores in any of the existing general purpose digital computers. However, it might be possible to use this idea in one of two ways, (1) either by enlarging existing memory stores, or (2) by giving a most abbreviated description of the automaton. This last suggestion might reduce to a simple form of mathematical operator, in the same way as when we approximate to a description of a molecular model by a molar description, and in turn to a mere mathematical operator or set of operators. This again suggests the possible usefulness of the work of Bush and Mosteller (1955).

By use of the same molar theoretic ideas as mentioned above, we might hope to be able to reproduce, in the future, many of the best understood psychological variables in an analog computer, and study their relations there under various sets of conditions. This is something that waits primarily on the search for well-defined behavioural variables, and well-defined relations between them.

Summary

This chapter has been concerned with introducing finite automata. It starts by considering the general properties of finite automata as defined by McCulloch and Pitts and followed up by Kleene. The form that these finite automata take is that of logical or neural nets, although of course they could also be regarded as tape automata, with input and output tape, a scanner, and a storage system which is either independent or a part of the input and output tapes.

The next type of automata considered was the net designed by von Neumann, and this led to a brief discussion of his treatment of error and the control of error in automata. Von Neumann's automata had the interesting property of being defined in terms of a single basic element, the Sheffer stroke.

The second half of the chapter deals with the synthesis of automata, and we considered a few well-known and representative hardware models built by Grey Walter, Ashby, Uttley, Shannon and Chapman.

In this chapter the microscope has, as it were, been turned on to that part of cybernetics that is concerned with constructing, in paper and pencil and in hardware, models of behaviour systems. These models are of both conceptual and general methodological interest, and from among the conceptual models we are interested in models which predict behaviour accurately. Ultimately, of course, we are interested in the particular model or set of models that bear *structural* as well as behavioural similarity to the human being.

CHAPTER 5

LOGICAL NETS

WE SHALL now develop a general notation for the use of 'logical nets', as we shall call them from now on. These are essentially the same as the neural nets of the early sections of the previous chapter; they are finite automata, and we are interested in the pursuit of *effective* methods for constructing behavioural theories, rather than in developing a mathematical theory for its own sake, or in the logical or philosophical aspects of the analysis. Using such means, our interest lies in improving their predictive value, as well as in their property of allowing easy revision of existing psychological and biological theories. This can be done by making clear the assumptions and the process of theory construction.

After we have outlined the principles on which the nets are to be constructed, with suitable illustrations, we shall proceed to a preview of the sort of finite automaton we need to reconstruct organisms in terms of the known experimental psychological facts. These are to be thought of, initially, as being broadly descriptive or *molar* only, and not until later chapters shall we start to consider possible neurological interpretations of these models.

We shall not only attempt some sort of preliminary reconstruction, but we shall also consider existing theories of cognition in the light of the models we are using. Such theories of learning as those of Guthrie, Hull and Tolman are typical of those we have in mind to begin with, but the later modifications of Hull by Spence, and the more recent theories of Seward, Deutsch, Broadbent and Uttley must also be considered.

We wish, then, to outline an automaton that mimics human behaviour; to build a machine which is capable of learning, not merely by utilizing what has been *built into* it, but also by acquiring information to which the machine is exposed, and using this information predictively. We must therefore 'build in' the *capacity to learn*, and not the details of the learning itself, as this is essential to adaptive behaviour. However, we shall not pursue this general discussion here, but rather we shall consider how the behavioural theorist may use his information in building up a conceptual nervous system in the form of logical nets.

We must first assume certain properties of a somewhat simplified character about the net we are going to construct, in the same way as did McCulloch and Pitts. We can then develop and test the suitability of the construction principles as we compare the nets with what we know of actual behaviour and neurology. The complications of individual differences can then be introduced.

Just as physics started by considering ideal spheres, or ideal particles, neglecting moments of inertia, and friction, so we must start with some idealizations, as we have already done with neural nets.

Our building bricks we shall call 'elements', rather than neurons. These are intended to be interpreted later as neurons after the principle of Braithwaite, which makes the elements initially formal symbols like those used in symbolic logic. These elements are connected by wires or fibres of two sorts: input fibres and output fibres. Impulses are assumed to run down these fibres in one direction to elements which are strung together in the form of a net.

Briefly, and informally, the principles on which these nets operate are as follows: Each element is assumed to take the same time to fire (an instant), and to be refractory for just that instant of time which is the same for all elements. Each element has a threshold value that has to be overcome before the element will fire. Furthermore, two sorts of inputs can occur: one that will excite and help to fire the element, and one that will inhibit and stop the element firing. These will be called excitatory and inhibitory fibres respectively (represented by closed-in triangles and open circles in the diagrams). If the threshold of an element is only 1, say (see Fig. 23A), then it is excited by the firing of the single excitatory input. If there are more inputs, and the threshold of the element is still 1 (Fig. 23B), then the element will fire if there is one more excitatory input firing than inhibitory inputs.

If the threshold is more than 1, say, 2 or 3, then the condition for the element firing is that the number of excitatory fibres firing at any instant must exceed the number of inhibitory by the amount of the threshold. By this token, Fig. 23c will clearly never fire because there is only one input, and it needs at least two to fire simultaneously to overcome the thresh-

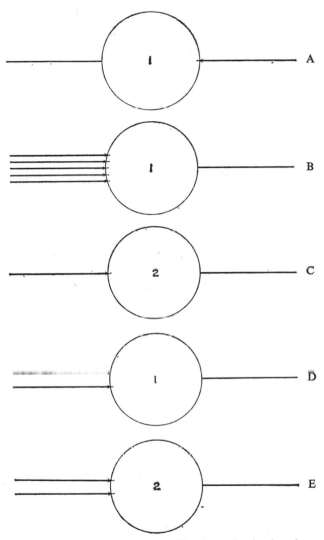

FIG. 23. LOGICAL NET ELEMENTS. Figure 23A shows the simplest element which simply delays an impulse for one instant. 23B shows five excitatory inputs and, like 23A, has a threshold of 1. 23C has a threshold of 2 and since it has only one input it can never fire. 23D fires if either input fires and thus if we label the inputs A and B and the output C, the equation for firing is $C_{t+1} \equiv A_t \, v \, B_t$, where $\equiv$ means 'if and only if' and v is the logical 'or'. 23E shows the logical 'and' with formula. $C_{t+1} = A_t.B_t$.

old. Figure 23D will fire if either one of the inputs fires, whereas Fig. 23E will fire only if both the inputs fire together.

What is interesting about these nets is the fact that they can easily be built using the ordinary relays, or two-way switches, so common in electronic engineering; but they can also be taken to represent the ordinary relations of simple mathematical logic. For example, Fig. 23D fires if either of the inputs (let us call these A and B) fires, and this represents the logical connective 'or'. If we call the output fibre C, we can say that C fires if either A or B fires, and since we mean the 'or' to be 'inclusive', then it will fire if A and B both fire as well as if either A or B fires alone. In symbols,

$$C \equiv AvB \tag{1}$$

where ' $\equiv$ ' means 'if and only if', and 'v' means (inclusive) 'or'.

By exactly the same sort of reasoning Fig. 23E represents 'and'. Thus, using the same lettering as for Fig. 23D, we can say that C fires if and only if both A and B fire together. In symbols,

$$C \equiv A.B \tag{2}$$

where '.' means 'and'.

We can write the formulae for any elements whatsoever in the same logical terms, and could thus replace all our nets by formulae precisely as in the previous chapter, and rather as geometrical figures can be replaced by their equations in Cartesian coordinates. It will be noticed that A and B must fire simultaneously for C to fire, and this can be brought out by using time-suffices in our system. Thus, instead of (2) we could write:

$$C_t = A_{t-1}.B_{t-1} \tag{3}$$

The fact that these nets are correlated with logical notation is, of course, the reason for calling them logical nets, and *later* we shall wish to give an interpretation as nerve cells, axons, dendrites, and the like, and we must even now bear in mind that this is our ultimate aim.

We shall pursue the logical notation to some extent in terms of those branches of logic already described in Chapter 3; it involves no more than the propositional and lower functional calculus. The value of the mathematical logic is that, when the subject becomes very much more complicated, it can be regarded more and more as a branch of mathematics, and we can be led on from mathematical logic to other suitable mathematical techniques. Our discussion here is primarily for those interested in the behaviour of organisms, and it is therefore concerned primarily with the manner of interpretation of such simple nets, both as molar and molecular models.

The elements mentioned above, and their type of connections, are typical of the elements in all the nets in which we are interested. They are all elements which are capable of being in one of two states, that of *excitation* or *inhibition*. They are, as we put it, either *'live'* or *'dead'*. However, we find it convenient to add to our number of elements, or rather, to consider one other kind of connection; this is illustrated in Fig. 24. These are what McCulloch and Pitts called 'circles' (the element M_1), and were illustrated in the formulae of Fig. 24 of Chapter 4, in a discussion of indefinite events.

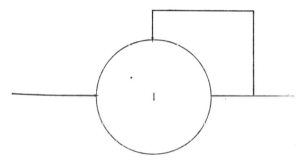

FIG. 24. LOOP ELEMENT. A simple loop element which once fired continues to fire itself indefinitely.

Here the output fibre is also part of the input of the element. This is very important in that it could be interpreted as a primitive form of memory. The element, when fired, will go on firing itself until some inhibitory later stops it firing. If one has such a 'looped' element, or loop element as we shall call them, and that loop element has no inhibitory fibre as part of its input, or if the threshold number is always greater than the number of the inhibitory inputs, then of course the loop, once fired, will never stop. It will not be possible for the element to erase this particular 'memory'. If, however, we added another input fibre capable of inhibiting the loop element, then, of course, the loop element's firing could be stopped. Figure 25 shows this simple element.

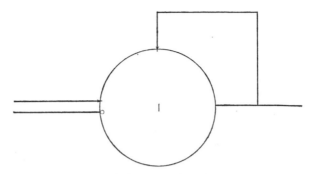

FIG. 25. LOOP ELEMENT. This is the same as Fig. 24, except that we have
added an inhibitor input that can stop the element firing if necessary.

Bearing in mind an ultimate neurological purpose, it is natural that we
should think of a whole network of such elements as being capable of
division into *input elements, inner elements* and *output elements*. It should,
however, be noted that the input elements have output fibres and input
fibres which are free at the other end; output elements have free output
fibres; and of course the inner elements are free at neither end, for they
have both input and output fibres connected to other elements.

Let us next consider one of the simplest significant networks. Figure 26

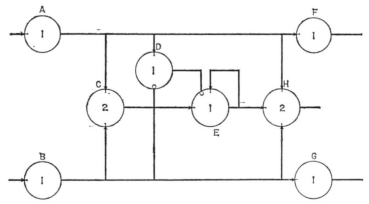

FIG. 26. LOGICAL NETWORK. This is a slightly modified version of Fig. 6
(Chapter 4) and is a 'sign' or 'association' net which associates the firing
of *A* with the firing of *B*.

shows such a simple net which has A and B as input elements, C, D, E as inner elements, and F, G and H as output elements.

First let us see what happens. If A fires alone it fires into F, C, D and H. However, C has a threshold of 2, so it is not activated, or fired, as we shall say. Similarly H, with a threshold of 2, is not fired. So, if A alone fires, it fires F and D only. D fires an ineffective inhibitory into E.

If, however, A and B fire together, then C is fired. D is not fired, as B fires an inhibitory to D. Therefore, the impulse from C does fire E which then goes on firing until A is fired alone again, when the inhibitory fibre from D becomes useful in stopping the firing of E. As long as the loop element of E was firing, it carried the memory of A and B having fired together. The firing of A alone will erase this memory. The importance of this is that if A fires alone after A and B have fired together, then G would have been fired, without the need for B to fire, as the loop element of E also provides one of the necessary two impulses to fire H, and consequently G. This process is a simple analog, or representation, of a conditioned reflex, and is, of course, a logical equivalent to Cora.

Consider A as the unconditioned stimulus and F as the unconditioned response to A, and H as the response which can become conditioned to A. This conditioning will take place when A and B have fired together, so that, in the future, A firing alone will fire H, which it would not have done previously.

Since conditioning experiments will frequently be mentioned, let us say straight away that we are thinking of the typical experiment whereby a flash of light, say, which is to be the conditioned stimulus, is associated with the act of salivating, this itself being the unconditioned response to the unconditioned stimulus of the smell of food. Salivating then will become the conditioned response to the flash of light if light and food occur together for some number of trials. *Extinction* of this association will occur subsequently unless the flash is *reinforced* from time to time by the presence of food.

We would emphasize that the above interpretation is for illustrative purposes. The net of Fig. 26 has, of course, a very short memory, since it forgets as soon as either A or B fires alone. Although the next firing of A alone will elicit H, it will do this once only, which means, of course, that the association is soon extinguished.

As one would expect, more complex nets can and have been constructed, nets that will remember for any number of times we want them to;

such, for example, as will remember either *A* and *B* together or either of them apart. It is possible, also, to construct nets that associate events like *A* and *B* even if they do *not* happen together.

So much for the *basic* informal idea of nets. Not only do they seem to mirror, or be capable of mirroring, some of the properties of nervous tissue, but they can now be used as tools for research.

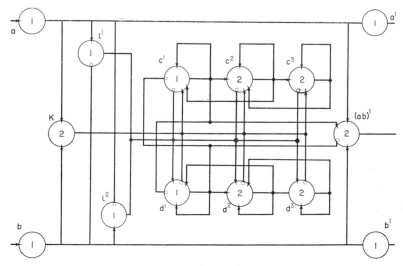

FIG. 27. BELIEF NETWORK. We have referred to this network which is an extension of Fig. 26 (showing more loop elements connected in a particular way) as a Belief-net or *B*-net. In general it associates any number of inputs and counts the degree of association to any extent.

We shall now give a somewhat more rigorous account of the principles upon which these logical nets are to be constructed. Figure 27 illustrates a simple association net based on the same principle as the net of Fig. 26. This is the net we have elsewhere described as a *B*-net (George, 1956a, 1957a, 1957d), and is to be thought of as the basis of the *C*-system. The terms '*B*-net' and '*C*-system' in the model are to be interpreted respectively as belief-unit or *belief* (a theoretical term) and *cognitive system* in the theory.

The equations of the *B*-net element by element, in terms of its firing conditions, are as follows:

$$1_t^1 \equiv a_{t-1}. \sim b_{t-1} \tag{4}$$

$$1_t^2 \equiv \sim a_{t-1}.b_{t-1} \tag{5}$$

$$k_t^1 \equiv a_{t-1}.b_{t-1} \tag{6}$$

$$c_t^1 \equiv (k_{t-1}^1. \sim d_{t-1}^1) \, v(c_{t-1}^2.(Et) \, c_{t-1}^1. \sim (1_{t-1}^1 v 1_{t-1}^2)) \tag{7}$$

In deriving (7), use is made of the obvious simplifying condition:

$$k_t \supset \sim (1_t^1 v \, 1_t^2) \tag{8}$$

Then the generalized equation for any number of c-counters (the name we give to sets of c-elements) is:

$$c_t^n \equiv (k_{t-1}^1 . c_{t-1}^{n+1}.(Et)c_{t-1}^n) \tag{9}$$

(In equations (1) to (6) any delay elements (see Fig. 23A) that may be necessary are ignored.)

The generalized equation here makes use of (8), and of the obvious condition that results from the fact that c^{n+1} fires, then c^n must necessarily be firing. Similar equations can be derived for the d-counters (as we shall call the sets of d-elements), and a final condition on the 'key' element, $(ab)'$ in Fig. 27. The primed notation always indicates an output element, and the combined primed elements are the 'key' elements. These key elements will be composed of every combination of all the primitive inputs $a, b, \ldots, n$ that the system contains. The final condition on the key element $(ab)'$ is:

$$(ab)' = ((a_{t-1}.b_{t-1}.c_{t-1}^1) \ v \ (a_{t-1}.b_{t-1}) \ v \ (a_{t-1}.c_{t-1}^1)$$
$$v \ (b_{t-1}.c_{t-1}^1). \sim d_{t-1}^1) \tag{10}$$

We will next show that our methods of devising these B-nets are *perfectly general*, and that we can cater for any number of input fibres, and can count to any number of combinations whatsoever. The methods for counting can be extended indefinitely; this should be self-evident, for the counters are essentially linearly connected, and any number can be added to either the c- or d-chains. By 'chain' we mean simply a linearly connected set of elements. It is also obvious that we can think of the inputs as any number of the full set of possible combinations of any finite set of inputs, a fact which disposes of the only serious question posed by the need for generalization, that of the counting of any number of inputs.

In considering the net so far described it should be borne in mind that events of duration (or length) 1 are the only ones counted where the distinction is made between $a.b$ and either $\sim a.b$ or $a. \sim b$, and there is no counter system for $\sim a. \sim b$. Elements of threshold 0 could be easily introduced to allow the counting of the last sort of event, and a distinction could easily be drawn between events $a. \sim b$ and $\sim a.b$ if it were necessary; that would simply involve a separate chain of counter elements. Indeed, as we increase the number of inputs in the system, so we shall need new chains of counters. In fact we can radically reduce the number of elements by indulging in a binary counting system which records directly, in numerical form, the number of times a particular event has occurred.

Another distinction we may need later will be that between classification systems which count all events, and those that count only 'positive' events. By 'positive event' we mean an event of which the description does not include any ' $\sim$ ' symbol. Thus we include events of the kind $a.b$, but not of the kind $\sim a.b.c$ which would merely be regarded as $b.c$. For these positive counters the problem of generality is easily solved, since we only need as many k-elements as there are combinations of events, and they can be fed straight into the chain of counters. The first case, where 'negative' events occur, calls for a shade more care since we now have to multiply greatly the number of l-elements. Thus, for three inputs, where all the combinations of events are to be counted, we must have an l-element for the events $a.b \sim c$, $a. \sim b.c$, $\sim a.b.c$, etc., and, given these l-elements, they can now be attached to chains of counters as before.

We might now say a few words about the duration of events. We are normally interested, in behaviour theory, in the relation between events that occur close to each other in time, but not always occurring simultaneously. This suggests that we should be concerned with events of greater length than 1, and it can easily be seen that we can arrange to count events of any duration whatever simply by multiplying the number of inputs for each and every combination that occurs at as many different instants as is necessary. This, of course, would be grossly uneconomical in practice, and we shall be generally concerned with events of relatively short duration and with events occurring at successive intervals of time.

This whole question of temporal order in events becomes extremely complicated, and it will be referred to in more detail from time to time throughout the rest of the book. A consideration of uncompleted tasks and delayed responses, especially in human behaviour, reminds us of the problem, and this immediately raises the question of the relation of the memory store to the classification and control system.

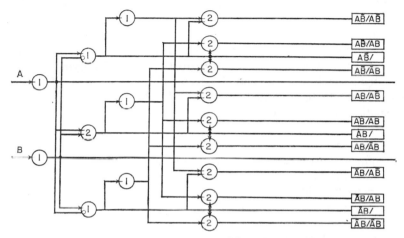

FIG. 28. AN EXTENDED BELIEF NETWORK. This network is a futher extension of Fig. 27 and shows the possible temporal relations between two inputs A and B.

Figure 28 shows the classification of events of length 2, where each event is composed of all combinations of A and B and their negations. In the figure, not-A is indicated by $\bar{A}$. The boxes containing the events such as $A\bar{B}/A\bar{B}$ represent sets of counters arranged as in Fig. 27, or any other of the many possible arrangements.

The basic nets that we have considered, and this particularly refers to the B (6, 2) net of Fig. 27, can be generalized upon almost indefinitely. It is in a sense a paradigm of the whole method. It is easy to show that by the inclusion of delay elements we can get an extended belief network as in Fig. 28 and the belief network can be extended indefinitely to events which immediately follow events or to events which follow events which follow events, etc., thus creating a sort of sequential processor of a Markov net type. Another way in which the $B(6, 2)$ net can be generalized is by talking about any number of inputs, A, B, C, ..., N, not just the two inputs of Fig. 27. Of course this leads to considerable complexity and it leads to an exponential growth of the number of counters needed on the assumption that each particular association and the associations themselves go up exponentially as you include new inputs if the classification is complete; we shall be talking about classifications in the next section which will to some extent bear on the same problem. The thought is, however, that you can have selective classification and the best basic model for representing the human brain is probably an adaptive, partial, partitioned classification system. The argument here being that the classification should be like computer registers and be, up to a point at any rate, capable of taking any information and classifying it rather than being special purpose and classifying only certain types of information. No doubt both special-purpose and general-purpose registers, or association nets, occur in the central nervous systems, but the ones at the highest level are almost certain to be general purpose and therefore we must draw neural nets which show how to cream information off and take information on again of a different character; this is very easily done. One should draw attention to the work of da Fonseca (1966) and other workers in the field who have produced a wide variety of nets showing a wide variety of different characteristics.

It is interesting to compare the neural net development with the general automata development, because with the neural nets as one might predict they have been used for trying to predict structural considerations which are relevant to the actual anatomy of the nervous system. It is well understood by all concerned that neural nets are not the same as actual nerve networks, but it is also to be remembered that so-called 'actual' nerve nets are themselves to some extent conceptual since they are a way of depicting what actually happens in the human central nervous system and this we do not know with absolute certainty. This last point is mentioned to emphasize the fact that there is less difference than one might suppose between a neural network representation of an actual human nervous system activity, provided of course that something like a structural similarity is achieved.

Classification systems

We must now describe one important aspect of logical nets; it is that part which is closely concerned with perception, and the sensory systems of organisms, although also relevant to the conceptual processes.

Figure 29 shows a simple *classification* system for positive events, as we shall call it. We believe that this is the *basic* principle on which perception works, even though a very powerful set of economies is certainly employed in living organisms to reduce the necessity for complete classification. Indeed, classification is seldom complete; it is built up in stages involving different sensory modalities. Of course the same sort of argument applies

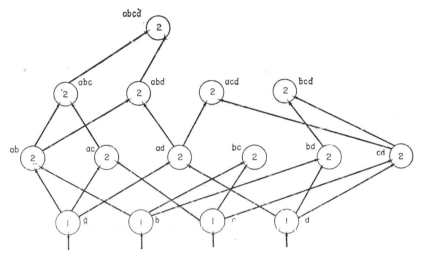

FIG. 29. A CLASSIFYING SYSTEM. This is a simple illustration of a classifying system with respect to four inputs. This is not of course the only manner in which such classifying systems can be constructed.

to our association net or *B*-net. All we have wished to show here is the beginnings of an effective method for the construction of learning systems. We do not think that this is necessarily *the* method employed by the organism, but it is a method in terms of which we can reconstruct theories of cognition, and this we shall do in later chapters.

The order of presentation of the argument will now be to proceed from sensory processes, or input systems, to control and storage systems, and finally to the output systems.

The input system is in some sense a classifying system. This matter has already been dealt with to some extent elsewhere (Uttley, 1954), so here the description will be somewhat limited. Let us conceive, initially, of a large number of 'primitive' inputs. These are equivalent to the simplest distinguishable elements in our world. They record, in the form of the firing of, say, cones and rods, spots of yellow, green, black and white, and so on. They are very simple in that they merely record, or do not record, characteristic elements of the environment according to whether or not the appropriate inputs are stimulated (Price, 1953). From these primitive inputs, by classification processes, we build up the sense-data and the physical objects and concepts with respect to our environment and ourselves. It will later be seen that this picture of perception is probably over-simplified, and it is probable that classification, as here depicted, begins at a later stage in the organization (see Chapters 11 and 12).

Let us name these primitive inputs a, b, ..., n, or, where we have to consider very large numbers of them, a_1, a_2, ..., a_n, b_1, b_2, ..., b_m, c_1, ..., and so on. We may separate the different sensory modalities by saying that the sets

$$\underset{i=1}{\overset{n}{X}} a_i, \ \underset{j=1}{\overset{m}{X}} b_j, \ldots$$

represent the different special senses, viz. seeing, hearing, touching, etc., where X means the set of all for $i = 1$ to $i = n$. Although this represents a theoretical interpretation of the model, it obviously entails no difficulty of any sort at the model level. The set Xa_i may be made up of elements of the visual classification system, Xb_j made up of elements from the auditory system, and so on.

In the above manner we can acquire the mathematical means of defining a classification and control system that may have as many inputs as we please, and cater for every combination of the input. It will be capable of counting as many of the conjunctions and disjunctions of any of the combinations we please by the illustrative methods already described.

We shall need, in order to discuss the actual construction of particular finite automata of biological interest, to have certain simplifying concepts. The use of molar inputs and outputs has already been described. (We shall generally use the same letter for the output as for the input where the output letter is primed. Thus, if a has a directly connected output then it will be a', b will have b', and so on.)

The next simplification will be to call any set of counters that connect any combination of inputs a B-net. The words B-unit have also sometimes been used instead of B-net (George, 1957a, 1957d), the idea being that these B-nets, in keeping with our use of molar and molecular stimuli, can occur on either the molar or the molecular level, and are the organs which, in iterated fashion, make up almost the whole automaton; they are somewhat similar to the packages that are used in the construction of digital computers. In practice, we may wish to add a further long term memory store to the system, but this need depend on no more than what could be 'tapped' from the looped elements, although, by applying 'logical' principles, it will be able to derive information from that 'tapped' input, which will greatly increase its stored information.

A further word of explanation is here appropriate, although still couched in general terms. The storage system will derive its information directly from the input classification and the other parts of the storage system. These bits of information will be in the form of events (or, in an obvious sense, *event names*) of various lengths. The central store will then be able to put these events together to form new events (or event names), as illustrated in a very simple case, for events of length 2, in Fig. 30. This figure, of course, shows only a sample of the possible elements and connections.

The principle is straightforward. An event name of length 2, A/B (where '/' means 'followed by'), can clearly be stored, as can event names

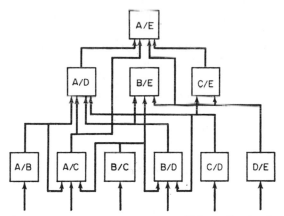

FIG. 30. AN EXTENDED CLASSIFYING SYSTEM. This applies the classifying principle to events that are already at least of length 2. Thus the classifying principle permits of drawing inferences by association. As an illustration, if A/B and B/D have the common element A/D, this may be fired if A/B and B/D have both fired together or even if they have been fired at any time at all. The figure only shows a few sample connections.

A/B, B/D, D/B, etc. Now it seems clear that there is an important relation between A/B and D/B, for example. Both lead to B, and therefore must be associated. Similarly, if we set up the association C/E, then A/C and C/E taken together may define an association A/E.

If we can now associate 'words' with event names, and construct sentences, then we have the possibility of deriving logic and language in our automaton. So far, this task of the reconstruction of a complete language on these lines has not been attempted, although we may expect to find such attempts being made in the future.

The need for economy in storage space will also demand a process of generalization that depends upon recognizing similarities among differences and differences among similarities; this is implicit in a classifying system. This general principle of classifying events, besides enabling recognition to occur, also enables reasoning to occur, although here we are not actually suggesting which of many possible forms the actual associative processes necessary to reasoning may take in the human organism.

We must also have a motivational system (M-system in the model language) which, in keeping with the basic 'needs' of the organism, decrees what is useful to it, and what shall be retained by the conjunction-and disjunction-counters, and what shall not. In this respect the equations (and all that has been said so far) are oversimplified, since there must be added the motivational inputs and outputs which fire into all the inner elements of a B-net. There is therefore some increase in the complication of the necessary and sufficient conditions for an element to fire.

A B-unit will exist to connect any subset of inputs whatsoever, and these units will be elicited in a definite temporal pattern. Let us consider a definite pattern of events, and suppose the occurrence of the following combination of stimuli:

abejdki-fridt-abelopq-

or more briefly

B-D-G-

In fact such patterns will be frequent and in enormous quantities so let us make up a longer slice of behaviour:

B-D-G-B-T-U-B-U-K-L-O-U-B-F-P-U-E-

which might be a short series of discriminable activities, say the mere recognition of some familiar object. This sort of series should immediately remind the reader of a Markov process (Chapter 2), and suggest a whole field of new possible interpretations.

It will be appreciated that many hundreds of counters will, on the theory, be fired even for such a simple action. Many B-units will register a large number of conjunctions, and also a certain number of disjunctions.

It should be noticed that, with the simple use of delay elements, we can, on our c- and d-counters, count events that fire *as remote from each other in time* as we please. 'Together', therefore, does not necessarily mean 'simultaneously'.

But there are many complicated considerations that must be discussed before any progress can be hoped for from the mathematical methods. First, it is essential to try and fix the ideas implicit in the theory.

Before pursuing our interpretation of the cognitive aspects of our automata, we should perhaps give a block diagram (Fig. 31) of the machine we are describing. The cognitive system or control is, it will be noticed, somewhat similar to (or analogous to) the cerebral cortex in so far as it is the highest level in the automaton. We shall discuss the motivational system, the emotional system (part of the rest of the internal environment) and the memory system (also really a part of the cognitive system) later, and in the meantime we shall discuss the cognitive system, or immediate classification and control system.

The automaton conveniently divides up into a control-system (this is referred to as a cognitive-system, or C-system at the level of the model), a motivational-system (M-system), and we may include an emotional-system (E-system) which is closely related to motivation, apart from the permanent memory store referred to above which, as we have already said, is a part of the cognitive-system. The classification of inputs and outputs, involving perception and organized responses to stimulation, will be regarded as being a part of the control system, as will be the high-speed memory store.

We shall start by describing the most important part, which is the C-system. There will be some obvious point in saying that the C-system is the name of that section of the model which will subsequently be interpreted as the control or cognitive system in the automaton.

Clearly, if we restrict ourselves to the memory of the loop elements of our control system (Fig. 27), then we would have to face the fact that the

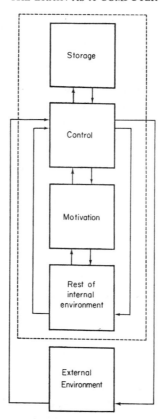

FIG. 31. THE BEHAVIOURAL MODEL. This shows the fairly arbitrary
distinctions that have been made between the store, the control and
the motivational system. All in the brain is really in storage except for
incoming and outgoing messages.

number of loop elements available directly affects the nature of the
probability on which the automaton will operate. Before clarifying this
point, let us make explicit the importance of the conditional probability
on which the automaton will operate.

Let us suppose that a particular 'physical object'—using that term in
the broadest sense that philosophers of perception would use it—is
represented by a combination of primitive inputs *abcdef*, say. We shall
call this set *A*, for short. Let us suppose further that some number of

physical objects B, C, ..., N follow each other in that order. Then there are relations of an important kind that connect these physical objects.

The first important sort of relation that our system has to consider is the perceptual one, and this means, in the main, the problem of recognition. Given some properties a, b, ..., n, what is the probability of their belonging to some particular set A, say? This implies the use, by counting as above, of probabilities which suggest the appropriate set, of which what is sensed at any instant is a subset—possibly, of course, an improper subset.

We think of the operation of *perceiving* as a definite process of analysing and classifying the environment ('sampling' is perhaps the best single word to describe the perceptual operation), and as being spread over a finite time. It is an ordering process in which the probabilities vary as the information about the members of the set increase, wherever that is possible. The tachistoscope on one hand, and the close analysis with ruler and calipers on the other, represent two extremes in this regard. Ideally, however, the process of perceiving—the word 'sensing' will be regarded by some as more appropriate for this series operation—can be represented by a series of probabilities

$$p_1, p_2, \ldots, p_n$$

tending to 1 in the limit, where ultimately each and every property of the finite set is identified. In practice, of course, this hardly ever happens, and we recognize objects (to think now of our interpretation) by small parts of them, or at a glance, in a manner familiar to those acquainted with Gestalt theory. Roughly speaking, the more familiar the object the more quickly we recognize it, and this is simply because a certain subset of properties $abcd$, say, is nearly always a subset of A. This model will be somewhat modified later, when we consider problems of perception in greater detail in Chapters 10 and 11.

Now the basis of this mechanism is clearly supplied by the counting and classification system described—the model of the cognitive system. In practice, however, recognition will also depend on *context*. All that this means is that the probabilities associating different elements with different sets must be the basis of further probabilities associating different sets with each other. This, of course, will cut across the different sensory modalities.

The automaton's behaviour at any instant clearly depends on two factors: (1) the current state of the environment, both internal and external, and (2) the whole past of the organism, *as stored* in the memory store. We must, then, conceive of the counting as leading to responses that are purely classificatory. This storage operation does *not* cause overt response, although naturally overt responses occur as a result of these classificatory responses after classification (perception) is complete.

All that has been said in this chapter so far is aimed at showing a method of describing artificial organisms or automata. These automata are capable of being described precisely in logical terms, and of being constructed in terms of two-state switches. The methods so far discussed are quite general, and designed merely to show the reader that the associations necessary to learning and perceptions are easily obtainable in such a system.

From this point on, most of the rest of the book is concerned with bringing such general methods into line with the empirical facts of behaviour and physiology. This is not to be done by writing specific equations for larger and ever larger nets—this would become too complicated—but by making the principles of more complex operations of behaviour clearer, in terms of these simple associations. Ultimately, no doubt, the more complex nets must be specified, but this may necessitate the use of a computer, probably with the help of an automatic coding procedure.

Theory of perception

The theory for the above model for perception is, strictly speaking, the interpretation placed on the model. In fact, the theory was formulated first and the model provided subsequently. The theory of perception here stated, and now to be briefly described, is molar, and is itself subject to reinterpretation on the molecular level. It will be seen to be generally adequate as an interpretation of the net model, and is believed to be consistent with many of the observable and intuitively known facts of perception. We would remind the reader again that this model and theory are intentionally general, and are not yet being discussed in detail; we are now mainly concerned with illustrating method.

Perception is regarded as being the process of interpreting the messages that arise from the various sensory sources. This implies that we would regard the operations of sensing, perceiving and believing as on a sort of continuum in which the individual is not necessarily able to distinguish various points or intervals.

The act of perceiving is represented as an organic process of selection and interpretation. The selection is partly due to the limits of application of the various senses, and partly due to the 'set' of the individual, which means that the information in the store (representing his previous experience) will operate in conjunction with what is momentarily perceived.

Perceiving is thus interpreted as a process of elaboration of sensory input, where there is a selection from all the potential stimuli in the environment, and where there is a counter system (store) for each of the items perceived. The counting, it should be noted, may well be approximate (Culbertson, 1950), and certainly recoding of the store and other factors mainly concerned with the economy of storing information, will also arise (Oldfield, 1954). The responses for this system are classifactory and are themselves stimuli to the overt response system. We have chosen to describe this in the terminology of *beliefs*. We say that perceptual beliefs are aroused as a result of the categorizing process that perception serves. These are ordinary beliefs, although distinguished from beliefs-in-general in so far as they are directly concerned with what is perceived whereas other beliefs may be derived, by other cognitive or logical operations, from what is already stored.

The word 'belief' is used here as a theoretical term and in the behaviouristic manner, although it is hoped that it will be capable of being interpreted as a formalization of the 'belief' to which we refer in ordinary language. To avoid confusion, let us think of *belief* as a purely theoretical term which is closely related to a *hypothesis* (Krechevsky, 1932a, 1932b, 1933a, 1933b) or an *expectancy* (Tolman, 1932, 1934, 1939, 1952). We shall in fact use the word 'expectancy' for an activated belief. For example, we shall want to say that there are various beliefs stored at various levels of generality, and that at any instant an activating stimulus will arouse some of them, and those aroused are called *expectancies*. The arousal of beliefs, as well as the strengthening of beliefs by confirmation, will depend on the motivational system as well as on the perceptual and storage systems (George and Handlon, 1955, 1957).

Motivation

Before completing our general description of the control system it would be convenient to summarize the role of motivation. The M-system at the model level, as exemplified by the logical network, is fairly simple, and in fact needs no more than the designation of 'values' to certain inputs. This particular point will become clearer after the analysis in the next chapter.

The need for a motivational system in the model is clear if we want the system to be selective, and since our model is to be interpreted ultimately as an organism, it is obviously necessary that it should be selective. In the first place, selection must be on the basis of survival; those activities which are bad for survival are omitted, and those which are good are included. Connected with this basic idea of two sets are many other basic motivators such as food, drink, sex, etc. In the model these are built-in, as they represent activities that are instinctive or innate, and thus passed from generation to generation by genetic means, and they are elicited by stimulation which will occur in the appropriate environment.

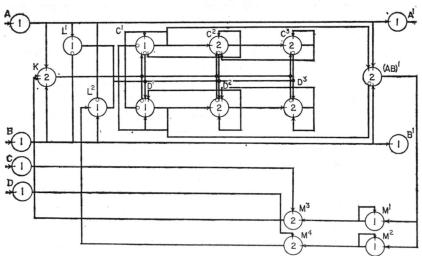

FIG. 32. A MOTIVATION LOGICAL NET. A simple example of the way reinforcement could be introduced into a belief net of the kind drawn in Figs. 26 and 27.

We can think of the model as having two sets of motivation chains made up of loop elements, so that any response which is followed by a reinforcing or non-reinforcing stimulus will, in effect, associate that response with either one or the other of the two sets. This will mean that the C-system will not operate its counting except in conjunction with the motivational effect of the response. Figure 32 shows a sample M-system (with only two loop elements) connected to our original C-system. Activity of the C-system, now modified, is dependent on the outcome of the response. It is again emphasized that these models are illustrative of the method, and that alone. In fact, all that is required is that some stimulus in a conjunction set be *necessary to* the conjunction. That extra (though necessary) stimulus can be designated the 'motivational stimulus'. A simpler example will be given later in this chapter (see Figs. 37 and 38).

At the level of the molar theory, we shall say that stimuli will not be effective in eliciting a response unless they are satisfying a need. Clearly this is not true of the perceptual system, which cannot tell whether a need is likely to be satisfied until recognition is carried through. However, here there is some reason to suppose that the classifying system of perception is influenced by the motivational state, at least in the 'choice' of events classified. This suggests the relevance of 'attention'.

Behaviour may be initiated in some obvious sense by motivational needs, or it may be initiated by external stimuli which have the effect of creating a need, and this implies a complication that our model can easily be shown to cater for. This means that further input elements —presumably from internal sources—should activate the system by firing the inputs initially in a random manner. After learning has occurred, these internal activators will be themselves selectively associated with other particular inputs. The present association system can clearly be extended so that a loop element will fire until such time as a particular input fires and stops the loop element from firing further. Figure 32 shows such a simple system, in which D represents the 'need' stimulus, and C the stimulus that satisfies the need. For learning to take place we must now introduce the same counters between D and A, B and C as exist in our C-system (Fig. 27).

Any system of counters that we have described as a cognitive system would systematically count everything that occurred that it was capable of discriminating, unless there was some system for selectively reinforcing certain events at the expense of others. This is the principle of motivation, and it is necessary for selective or purposive behaviour in an automaton.

Now to consider briefly the linkage between the M-system and the C-system. There are many equivalent ways in which this can be done, and perhaps the simplest now is to dispense with the k- and l-elements, and join the wires from the left-hand selector directly to the conjunction counters, and the wires from the right-hand selector elements directly to the disjunction counters as far as excitation is concerned, and the other way round for inhibition. This is not a vital matter since there are many methods, and these will model many different processes. One alternative method is shown in Fig. 32.

We shall not give the logical net equations for the new system, for it is obvious that these could be derived as has been shown previously.

Emotion

In brief, we can say of the E-system that it is concerned closely with the M-system, being a signal of different degrees of satisfaction which the organism is experiencing. It has the job of facilitating the purely organic aspects of behaviour, but it also has overt manifestations that make it of importance as an index of the feelings, etc., which are part of our awareness. The whole problem of consciousness could perhaps be introduced into the system and regarded as an extra stimulus–response activity (probably connected with the reticular system, see Chapter 10), but we shall not attempt to deal with this here.

Machines in general do not have either motivational or emotional systems, simply because they are not normally *purposive*. However, there are certain purposive and selective systems in being, and for them the M-system is vital, even the E-system is vital, if the systems are to be in any sense autonomous and are to survive.

As far as the human being is concerned there are various theories about the effect of emotion on his activities. It seems certain that they have both a disruptive and a facilitating effect. The main problem is to decide when one and when the other.

Our E-system could easily be constructed in a manner similar to the M-system, so there is no purpose in drawing up a network for it. Its role would be to exhibit a set of specified signals as the appropriate states arise. Clearly, emotion is a factor that will have to be considered in any model (and therefore theory) of the individual; but we shall not attempt to take this argument any further at the level of our logical networks.

Memory

Something must, of course, be said of memory in the theory and in the model. It seems reasonable to suppose that there will need to be *at least* two different stores, roughly comparable to those in a digital computer: (1) a high-speed counting store which will be associated with perception and recognition, and (2) the more permanent store where as much as possible of everything that ever happens to the organism will be recorded. We would like to make it plain here that *we tend to think of the cognitive operations, such as 'thinking', as being the process of transfer to and from the stores, although also involving language.* This will be discussed later.

Our molar theories of behaviour tell us that in recall there are simplifications and distortions of memory that make the remembering process almost one of reconstruction rather than of reproduction. Bartlett (1932) and others have shown these characteristics in operation, and they can be seen to be connected with *set, attention* and *perception.* The storage can be organized in a variety of different ways and, from the point of view of human organization, the correct method can only be arrived at by experimentation, presumably at the neurological level. Our purely molar behavioural account here must be regarded as limited and suggestive; however, more will be said on this matter in the next chapter.

We shall now say a little about the possible range of models. Culbertson (1950) has listed some of the network devices that could be used, and we shall simply say that a system such as that in Fig. 33 would obviously have the capacity to accept information and release that information on stimulation.

It could, of course, also be arranged to circulate the information released so that it returned to the store again, if necessary. Such a net is a simple equivalent of the delay line storage system in computer design. Instead of handling words as impulses in mercury tubes, the words are handled by sets of elements, and the number of elements in the set dictate the length of the word handled. It is an open question as to whether what is remembered is coded as an instruction connecting sets of input elements, or as a number indicating the conjunction or disconjunction of sets of input elements, where the actual inputs referred to are localized by the anatomical location of the store, or both. Matters of this sort can only be settled by further neurological experiment.

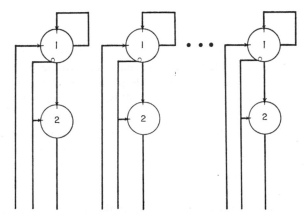

FIG. 33. A STORAGE SYSTEM. The simple principle of storing binary digits by logical nets. All sorts of variations on the same theme are possible.

Obviously we could store information in a logical net in a variety of ways; even without loop elements we could arrange for chains of elements to circulate information indefinitely, and this again would be similar to the delay line form of memory store. We shall next consider one or two examples of hardware automata that are closely associated with logical net theory.

Flebus

Figure 34 shows the logical net of an input and output classification system combined. This was the basis of Stewart's automaton which he has called 'Flebus'. Stewart's aim in building this automaton was partly influenced by the inverse of the well-known Turing game which was concerned with answering the question: 'Can automata behave like humans?'

Flebus has four input channels, each of which may be in one of two

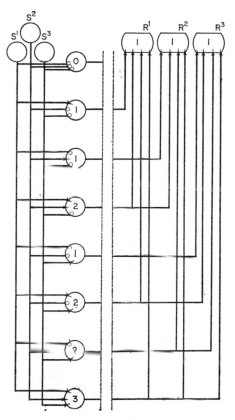

Fig. 34. A STIMULUS–RESPONSE NETWORK. A stimulus classifying and response classifying system. The text should be consulted to understand its significance.

discrete states. Figures 35 and 36 show the hardware of the input and output classification system.

The programming of the automata sets up plugboard connections between the sixteen output sockets of the input net, and the fifteen input sockets of the output net, but of course the automaton can be programmed in a variety of different ways. Stewart then used the automaton for a series of experiments involving the human operator, the automaton being used to simulate a number of different situations, such as the use of

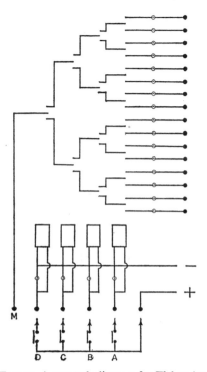

FIG. 35. FLEBUS. A network diagram for Flebus (see text).

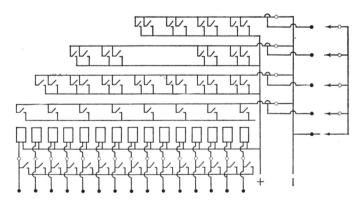

FIG. 36. FLEBUS. A further network diagram for Flebus (see text).

binary controls in a binary display situation, routine checks, fault diagnosis, and so on.

The use of the automaton as a simulator involves further special input and output material, and the realization of simple logical functions and stochastic processes that can be made as complicated as we like.

The automaton has great versatility, and realizes some of the properties we should expect to find in a human organism, although in a very simple form. One of its most interesting features is that it was constructed directly from logical net diagrams.

George's models

These models, like Flebus, were built directly from logical nets. The first model is a direct realization of Fig. 27, and shows a particular classification and conditional probability system. Only two inputs are classified, and the memory is only over six events, but the model can easily be extended, by the use of additional relays, to include any number of inputs and any length of memory. It can also be extended to deal with temporal sequences as in Fig. 28, and logical associations as in Fig. 30.

This brief statement applies to the first model made (George, 1956a). The second model was built in units whose logical net diagram is as in Fig. 27, but whose memory has now been extended to something near eighty events. There were some twelve of these units available, and they could be connected in any way whatever to realize a wide variety of different automata. These automata are capable of realizing all the characteristics already described, and could be shown to demonstrate many of the characteristics of simple learning. Some of the units could be regarded as M-units, and thus the effectiveness of any association may be made to depend on their firing at some time t.

General

The model and theory we have been outlining from the general point of view can be manufactured in a variety of different ways, both digital and analog; but the interesting thing about logical nets is the fact that all the essential features of an organism seem to be capable of being reconstructed in them in terms of simple two state switches. Hence there is a distinct resemblance between the structure of such a switching system and the nervous system. This, we have argued, is the way models should be constructed: with the theory and the intended interpretation in mind. It is this property that places logical nets among the most important of the list of models of behaviour theories that have so far been created.

In this summary we have outlined a model (or method of model construction) of the human organism in a form that is still idealized and contrary-to-fact in many ways, but which can gradually be brought more into line with the empirical facts as these facts are yielded by experiment. We have briefly discussed an interpretation of the logical net model in the form of a molar theory of behaviour, and this was derived independently as a direct result of molar behavioural experiments. In constructing the molar theory, however, we had methodological as well as behavioural problems in mind. We want to advance by slow but careful, and accurate, degrees towards a model that could be interpreted as a human organism, and the rest of the book will be concerned with development towards this end. The model and the theory need the sort of flexibility that allow them room for expansion both in detail and on various levels of description.

A further point about the many-levelled methods employed is that the theory (or theories) itself could, of course, be formalized. We think of theories and models being connected in a definite way, and the process of formalization would be the process of showing the precise logical structure of the theory. There can be no doubt that all theories should be capable of formalization, but theories can be formalized to different extents, and this is where we investigate the coherence, precision, and logical consistency of a scientific theory. *The logical net is a ready formalization in logical terms of a behaviour theory*, although many other formalizations, all logically equivalent, are possible. In a sense, indeed, they may not even be logically equivalent, since the use of theoretical terms in the theory or theory language is vague enough to allow a variety of possible interpretations.

We may now summarize the methods briefly. A theory in science—certainly in the behavioural sciences—may occur at many different linguistic levels which represent different sorts of levels of investigation. Behaviour can be described introspectively, in molar observable terms, or in molecular terms. This means, roughly: in terms of private experience, in terms of the behaviour of the organism-as-a-whole, or in terms of the physiological and biochemical variables. A complete theory will plumb all these levels and thus allow workers dealing with all aspects of human behaviour to draw on all the available information. These theories can all have their logical structure and consistency analysed, and are all subject to confirmation, and with the possible exception of introspective language, this means empirical confirmation by public test.

In discussing these methods of theory construction we have introduced a few empirical statements, usually of a fairly general character, and we have not tried to show very much in the way of the detailed predictions and applications that follow from these empirical statements. Space forbids this, hence we have been able to give no more than a skeleton theory of behaviour which would, for any particular application, need to be greatly expanded in detail, and of course be supplied with the individual constants or boundary conditions that may be applicable.

The idea behind these methods has been that we should have a flexible framework which would serve as a scientific tool for research to encompass the experimental work in progress, and also be precise enough to avoid the pitfalls of ordinary language; and yet again, be capable of being used as approximate models for theories, and to answer questions of varying generality at any time.

Some points from controversy in cognition

Since what has been said so far may seem unduly empty to the experimental psychologist, it should be added that there are various questions that are to be discussed with reference to the model-making methods so far outlined.

The first set of problems comes from learning theory, and surrounds the nature of reinforcement. The manner of our references, so far, to motivation—hinting that this is a need-reducing process of the Hullian kind (see Chapter 7)—is intentionally limited; however, we have also mentioned that 'external' stimuli can themselves produce needs, and for the time being we shall leave open the discussion as to whether stimuli can be associated, or patterns of either stimuli or stimuli-responses can be learned without any reinforcement through need-reduction. This whole

matter must wait, for the benefit of those not familiar with this controversy, until the end of our introduction to learning theory.

There are other problems that arise in learning theory that are obviously not going to be settled by the method of model construction alone,
such as the continuity–non-continuity theory of learning, and the closely
associated matter of discrimination learning and ordinary learning.
These, and our second group of problems which are concerned with
perception, will also be considered later. The perceptual problems are concerned with the various models of the recognition process.

In general terms it might be said that a variety of different models
could be constructed to perform the operations of learning and perceiving,
and the difficulty is to decide between them, although that is by no means
the whole question.

So far we have dealt with classification and conditional probability
as if they were essential to the final model, and in some form this is probably so; but there is no certainty that the problem is as simple, even in
principle, as it has been made to appear up to now, and later we shall
certainly seek to fill in the detail, and modify what has been previously
said. It seems likely, for example, that the Broadbent concept of a filter
will be desirable in some form, and also possibly a more sophisticated
relation between response activities and the central store.

In this last respect Deutsch's learning theory should be mentioned.
Broadbent has argued that Deutsch's model—we can call it a model in
so far as it seems to be capable of realization in logical net form, which
is to say that it is capable of being actually constructed—has links of
elements that allow neatly for a need to be set up with the result that a
certain element or set of elements is kept live until the need-reducer
occurs, whether by being seen, tasted, or whatever it may be, at which
moment the link stops firing, or is switched off. This is something that
lends itself well to logical net treatment. Figure 32 shows, in simple form,
precisely this principle, whereby stimulation by motivational stimuli
would be capable of activating the system, causing it to search for appropriate stimulation. It could, of course, also be done by regarding a particular response as a searching response which gradually fires the set of
relevant inputs.

Figures 37 and 38, which Stewart (1959) calls 'reward type connecting
net' show even more clearly this same type of feedback characteristic in
a response system. At the end of Chapter 10 it will be seen that his argu-

ment links directly with what is said there by Pribram on current neuro-physiology.

In Fig. 37 it is assumed that S is an input element, S^M is the motivating stimulus, and R is the output element. If S and R fire together and the

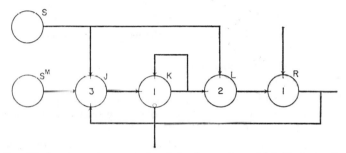

FIG. 37. A REINFORCING NET. A reinforcing system which illustrates the simplest sort of reinforcement.

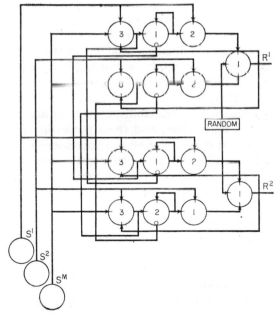

FIG. 38. A STIMULUS–RESPONSE NETWORK WITH RANDOM ELEMENT. A variation of Fig. 34 (see text).

result is to modify the external environment so that S^M fires, then J will be fired, and the feedback loop will be kept active until inhibitory inputs stop it. Figure 38 is a simple generalization of Fig. 37, and also shows the characteristic of simple learning.

Probabilistic considerations within the deterministic network

The design of the counting system already outlined is intended to realize an inductive logical machine or automaton, and it follows, therefore, that the basis of the network is probabilistic. Indeed, the method of connecting the counters for scoring and erasing purposes will be a direct influence on the sort of probability that will be realized by the network. A further influence on probability considerations will be the number of counters available relative to the number of events to be counted.

It will be easy to see that such a machine or network as the one under discussion, even with many more counters, will remember only the recent past if the number of events it has to count is large relative to the number of counters. If the number of such events is relatively small, then a frequency probability of the Laplacian kind will be the outcome.

In the above connection careful attention will have to be paid to various approaches to probability, induction, degree of confirmation and degree of factual support (Carnap, 1952; Hempel and Oppenheim, 1953).

That our automata will be probabilistic, and may also have the properties of 'growth', is fairly clear, and these properties must certainly be considered in the next stages of cybernetic development.

Pask (1958, 1959a, 1959b), Beer (1959) and Chapman (1959) have considered and built systems that are concerned with learning and perception, and which have the properties of growth, and some of these will be referred to again in Chapter 9.

Chapman's model of a classification system, described briefly in the previous chapter, is very similar to the logical nets we have described, but differs in that the degree of connectivity of different elements of the classification system is a function of the experience of the system. These growth nets are probably more nearly a model of what actually occurs in the nervous system, although they sacrifice the logical description and have a mathematical description in its place. Furthermore, it can be shown that anything that Chapman's nets can do can also be done by logical nets. This is an important point in that it suggests that logical nets are an effective method for description, even if what is described is contrary to biological fact. However, Chapman's methods are certainly of the utmost importance to the next development in the subject.

Multiplexing

The method of 'multiplexing', which means the replicating of messages in a system, could be applied to the nets we have described. This would increase the probability of their working, even though the basic components were not always working effectively. Again, we are not intending to give a detailed analysis of a multiplexed net system, but it is clear that we can follow up the principle of the executive and restoring organ (von Neumann, 1952) if we duplicate the network wherever it is possible.

In considering Fig. 27 we can see that a duplication of both the inputs from a and b to k, with an increase of the threshold of the k-element to 3, would permit the failure of any one of the inputs to fire at any instant while still bringing about a correct count. This is an example which can be applied without much difficulty to all the other elements; only the l-elements would be recalcitrant under such changes, although even these, despite some malfunctioning, would still be capable of keeping a proper record.

Another matter that will receive no detailed consideration is the use of random elements. These can be used almost anywhere at any time, and the predictability of the network will largely be destroyed as a result. Their use in explicit design may be somewhat limited, even when the network is explicitly intended as a model of organic behaviour, since the fluctuating interference of the emotional systems on the cognitive system is not a random matter, but a systematic causal one, and random elements would at best be a makeshift device, for which a deterministic substitute should ultimately be found. The indeterminacy of the system would be sufficiently supplied by the interference between one system and another, and the attempt to retain proper communication would be made in terms of multiplexing.

Hierarchical nets

All that we have said in the last chapter makes it clear that the sort of neural net or logical net picture that we have in mind is essentially hierarchical and is also spread out over time. The spreading out over time is fairly obvious; it refers to events which happen sequentially and relationships between those events which can certainly be catered for by a logical net system however far apart in time those events are.

The hierarchical nature of the networks is a reminder that we have to try to simulate activities at different levels of abstraction. The $B(6,2)$ net that we have made the paradigm and basis for generalizing on logical nets is a simple association between two items. This same basic principle applies to all sorts of items even on different levels of abstraction, thus words are associated with 'things', and words with words so that you have a whole hierarchy of levels in which at the ultimate level we are able to reproduce, for example, all that we will discuss in the next chapter on theory of games. Games, whether n-person games or games against nature, or empirical games, all have equivalent nets which are able, provided they are structured in hierarchical form, to mirror the activities that occur. In fact, we want to argue that granted any problem-solving activity which we can formalize and sufficiently well define, that we can always construct a logical net to solve the problem. The word 'always' here is not meant to mean that every problem is necessarily soluble, but that we can always construct a net which will attempt to solve the problem and sometimes will. If the problem is one of a class which has an algorithm, it necessarily must be able to solve the problem, if it is one that demands heuristic treatment, then, of course, it stands the same chance of success as a human being does, unless we can take steps to ensure that the logical net system which is solving the problem is that much more 'intelligent' than the human being.

A point to emphasize is that in talking of logical nets we have talked about a system which can be made as complex as we need for whatever purpose, and this is not true of the evolution of the human brain, and this is a basis for arguing that we can sooner or later manufacture artificially intelligent systems which would have a greater degree of intelligence than human beings.

This whole argument harks back to the earlier chapter where we discussed the philosophical problem of 'whether or not "machines" could be made to think?' The answer clearly as far as we are concerned is 'Yes' and we also have introduced methods by which this could be done. It goes without saying that it is assumed here that we only need to sufficiently well define, and that does not necessarily mean in the most intimate detail, any cognitive activity and we can then draw up the appropriate logical network to simulate that activity.

Summary

This chapter follows up the general approach to finite automata which was started in the previous chapter, and further narrows the interest to logical net systems.

These logical net systems are then brought into line in a general way with the generally known facts of behaviour. This means that it is convenient to consider a general model having an input classification system, a cognitive system, counters and association units (which we have called B-nets), and storage systems, as well as a motivational system which selectively reinforces the associations to which the system is exposed. Finally, some mention is made of the presence of emotion in the system.

The Braithwaite distinction between model and theory is utilized here, and we use such terms as B-net with the 'idea in mind' that it could be interpreted as a *belief*. Although this belief should be regarded as a theoretical term, like *hypothesis* or *expectancy* in Tolman's theory of learning, it is intended that it could perhaps be eventually interpreted in the sense of the word 'belief' as we use it in ordinary language, but the whole matter is complicated by the fact that the way we use words in ordinary language can be too vague to be more than a rough guide to usage in a well-defined system.

The methods of logical nets are used to illustrate various systems or units which might be useful to mirror behaviour, especially, of course, cognitive behaviour, with which we are mainly concerned. Some models in hardware constructed by the author and Stewart are then described.

CHAPTER 6

THEORY OF GAMES

THE theory of games is closely involved with cybernetics and many of the concepts are used as descriptive tools by cyberneticians. This particularly applies to empirical games which are descriptive of either actual or possible goal-directed situations. There is a direct link here with empirical axiomatic systems and applied logic.

The classical theory of games (von Neumann and Morgenstern, 1944) describes the situation where one-off strategies could be played in situations involving coalitions for n-person zero sum or n-person non-zero sum games.

First of all, let us consider the relationship that exists between the classical theory of games, as we now think of it, and logical networks. We should first of all notice that the various strategies are related to probability estimates and guessing behaviour and necessarily applied to a whole range of behaviour at the level of uncertain information. This means that theory of games will be of special interest at the initial stages of learning, but in network terms represents the competitive processing of two or more nets representing two or more (n-person) games. Processing of the environment by a single net implies 'a game against nature'.

The behavioural question is with respect to which strategy will be employed under a variety of different conditions and the answer would appear to be that we may work out a best strategy on well-founded empirical evidence, but we also want to see how the changes might be expected to occur in practice. This underlines the point that theory of games deals with a certain type of rather abstract situation, although such situations have a counterpart in reality. But it does not deal with ill-defined or realistic games of the empirical kind, which we shall as a result be discussing in a separate section.

The occurrence of beliefs of roughly equal value will give rise to states of uncertainty, but where equality of beliefs exists—that is, an equality of strength in terms of some motivational principle of maximum reward–minimum effort (George and Handlon, 1955)—there will still remain the component variables that will generally differ. An individual will evaluate a particular state of affairs in terms of giving one sort of variable priority over another, resulting perhaps in the pessimist's or the optimist's strategy, or in other variations that reflect the varying experience of individuals.

In short, strategy techniques may represent individual differences (differences in experience) between the same logical nets; they are individual constants or boundary conditions in behaviour. They may be brought about in nets, all of which have the same starting conditions, as a result of a different segment of environment being encountered, or they may be due to differences in the stability characteristics of the net, or both. By stability characteristics we mean the extent to which 'rapid counting' takes place when environmental conditions change a reinforced to a weakened connection. The motivational system hastens the slow counting change in the C-system, and makes it possible to change habits quickly. 'Rapid counting' is one way in which response choice could be changed very quickly with changed circumstances. Probably this occurs through the use of *language* in human behaviour. By 'rapid counting' we mean literally the same effect as would occur by stimulation of a counter every single instant over many successive instants.

In psychology the random activity of a Thorndike cat (a cat confined in a box but able to escape when it solves the problem of opening the escape door) is followed by a definite strategy in escape as a measure of success enters the picture. If we change the reward conditions slightly we may change the connections slightly, which will make the difference between the use of one particular technique and the abandoning of that technique and the use of another in its place.

The problem which now has to be described in detail, for any particular net, is: how does the net acquire the strategies it uses relative to a particular environment? This again is further described in terms of computer programming in the next chapter.

Theory of games (see Luce and Raiffa, 1957), which we do not intend to discuss in any great detail, contributes towards higher cognitive activities in that it formalizes a certain range of situations and optimum strategies to be utilized in those situations. That information is still required to describe the situations as a clear-cut one, is clear. Therefore there is a direct relation between game theory and information theory, and the strategies themselves have to be worked out as a reminder that learning has taken place at some level.

In fact, the formal strategies simply imply that the learning has been taken care of by the research workers whereas in the case of empirical games this learning has to take place within the actual situation itself, and is usually, as a result, somewhat less formalized.

Games against nature

While theory of games deals with formal games between people, whether of a zero-sum variety or otherwise, games against nature are concerned with inanimate opponents. This means that one is in the position of guessing as to a state of nature under conditions, for example, of equiprobability for each possible state. There is no question of bluffing taking place in these circumstances, and the problem of the game player is to estimate what the chances are of being right and bet accordingly.

The following matrix:

$$\begin{pmatrix} 2 & 0 & -1 \\ -1 & 0 & 1 \\ -1 & 0 & 1 \end{pmatrix}$$

illustrates the distinction made between three different strategies, the optimist's, the pessimist's and Laplace's strategy.

The problem is to 'guess' which of three equiprobable rows represents a state of nature. In the case of Laplace, the strategy is based on the highest arithmetical mean of a particular column, in the case of the optimist it is based on the maximum pay-off, and in the pessimist's case, it is based on minimizing risk so that you lose the least if you are wrong. There are a whole variety of strategies that have been built up along the same lines (Hurwicz, Wald, Savage *et al.*; see Thrall, Coombs and Davis, 1954) which contribute to our understanding of the probabilities or estimates of chance under conditions of uncertainty.

Again, we are concerned with relating this to learning theory and information theory. It is easy to see that games against nature are complementary to the theory of games and fill up another domain in which decisions have to be made and higher cognitive activities operate.

We should mention (Jeffrey, 1965; Chance, 1969; White, 1969) a whole series of methods which have been developed which refer to matters of choice and decision, where there is a process of weighted deliberation which comes from the conjoining of desirabilities, probabilities, and expectations. Bayes Rule, Inverse Probability and conditional probabilities generally should be mentioned here, but we shall not attempt to reproduce any part of the rapidly growing literature on the subject.

Dynamic programming

Whereas the theory of games deals in one-off situations, there is another field of activity sometimes called dynamic programming which deals with sequential games. Even in the field of sequential games, or sequential processes, no complete theory yet exists which covers all the possibilities. And even in so far as dynamic programming covers a number of sequential activities, degenerating into stochastic processes or Markov nets in particular cases, the theory of dynamic programming represents one attempt to formalize the situation involved in sequential activities and their associated probabilities.

It is important to make the point clear that dynamic programming is not an effective technique to be used as such in describing situations or allowing us to make sensible bets or decisions in situations, rather is it a prior formalization from which ultimately applications may emerge. Dynamic programming (Bellman, 1957; Bellman and Dreyfus, 1962) is a relatively recent development with a considerable potential, but so far the degree of application which it has had to cybernetic problems has been minimal. Far more important in practical terms is the use of Markov nets and other stochastic processes in collecting information, particularly as a basis for inductive inferences and hypothesizing. Nevertheless it is important that the cybernetician should be aware of the existence of the method and see its potential for future development.

Empirical games

We have already mentioned that there is a gulf between the formalized descriptions of limited cases covered by theory of games, or the equivalent model which is interpreted as a linear program, games against nature and dynamic programming. We should now add that by virtue of heuristic methods, which will be discussed in the next chapter, we can provide strategies and decisions in a whole world of ill-defined, under-informed and other non-conventional and non-formalized circumstances.

Any situation whatever involving either one person making bets against nature, or against the state of reality, or any number of people making bets against each other, all with respect to information of some kind or another, can always be modelled in an *ad hoc* manner by heuristic methods.

We shall say little more about this particular matter here since the developments of the next chapter make clear what heuristic methods are and also as a result makes clear how heuristic methods can be used for informal game playing of an empirical kind.

A recent development (Watt, 1970) has been that of imposing the full range of heuristic problem solving and decision making into the context of 'real' games where a degree of formalism is involved. The formalism applies to the description of the game and not to the game itself which may be as haphazard as one wishes, provided only it is not 'completely random' and is goal orientated. Watt considers the capabilities of the players as well as the rules (constraints) and strategies of the game. This is the beginning of a fuller description of a behavioural kind and in effect welds the considerations of the psychologist together with the considerations of the mathematician and statistician and this is a large part of what cybernetics is about.

More precisely we should point out that, for example, when learning has occurred and a specific 'choice' has to be made between a series of alternatives, we 'weigh up' the payoffs and the cost of achieving that payoff ('means-ends' relationships). If we are choosing, for example, between two restaurants we might ascribe weight A to one and weight B to the other, and then say but B has only X units of effort to be achieved, while A has $3X$ units and we assert

$$XB > 3XA$$

where $>$ means 'is more worth while than'. Now we only need to push these simple beginnings into a more formal mode and we have our first empirical games, and then as abstractions from such games, the more idealized situations of theory of games and games against nature.

Like most other chapters in this book, this chapter could become a book, or several books, in itself, so with a re-emphasis on the references for further reading we shall leave this topic and its very brief description and go on to consider cognitive models on the computer in the next chapter.

CHAPTER 7

PROGRAMMING COMPUTERS TO SOLVE PROBLEMS

IN THIS chapter we consider the problems of learning, planning, decision-taking and problem solving, from the point of view of computer programming. This means in terms of the programming of a general-purpose digital computer.

Oettinger (1952) showed that the EDSAC computer could be programmed to learn certain quite simple operations. It is important that in doing so it acts on information that has not yet been obtained when the original program has been stored in it, and thus the behaviour of the computer is conditional on certain events not initially known. Let us give a simple example of the Oettinger type of program.

The easiest way to regard the computer as an analog of the outside world is to think of the input tape as being the computer's environment. But since tape-reading on the EDSAC is its slowest operation, Oettinger has divided the machine into two parts, letting one part play the role of learning machine and the other the environment.

The description of the learning activities can be interpreted in terms of a series of shopping expeditions, where the shops are described by an $m \times n$ matrix. The elements $a_{ij} = 1$ if shop i has article j, otherwise $a_{ij} = 0$. Any row of the matrix is a row vector defining the contents of a particular shop (shop vector), and any column represents the article and all places where it may be found (article vector).

Now the learning machine selects a shop number i_k, say, at random, and forms the address $m + i_k$ of the corresponding shop vector, and from this and EDSAC order C_{m+i_k} (C_m means contents of storage location m) which collates the shop vector with the given order vector. If C order is obeyed, then $a_{inj} = 1$ if the article is in stock; if $a_{inj} = 0$, it implies that i_k has not got the article j in stock.

165

An 8×7 'stock' matrix

$$\begin{bmatrix} 1 & 0 & 0 & 1 & 0 & 0 & 0 \\ 1 & 0 & 1 & 0 & 0 & 0 & 0 \\ 0 & 1 & 1 & 0 & 0 & 0 & 0 \\ 0 & 0 & 0 & 0 & 1 & 0 & 0 \\ 0 & 1 & 1 & 1 & 0 & 0 & 0 \\ 0 & 0 & 0 & 1 & 0 & 0 & 0 \\ 0 & 1 & 1 & 1 & 1 & 0 & 0 \\ 0 & 0 & 0 & 0 & 0 & 1 & 0 \end{bmatrix}$$

describes 8 shops selling 7 articles. The mth shop vector is stored in location $m+i$ in EDSAC, where m is the reference address.

This process goes on until a shop is found with the desired article. Now the computer stores the information, and also a little extra information about other articles in the shop besides the one searched for, and this in turn means that a future search will often be unnecessary, even if the article has not been searched for before. This is an example of what cognitive psychologists call 'latent learning'.

This simple sort of learning has obvious limitations that were recognized by Oettinger, and he sets out some methods by which the relative inelasticity of the program might be overcome. It is sufficient for our purpose that we can point to the fact that programs of a contingent character have actually been constructed.

Somewhat similar programming has been undertaken by Turing (see Bowden, 1953, and Shannon, 1950), where this sort of learning was involved in the playing of chess.

Shannon programmed a computer to learn chess, but neither he nor Oettinger paid any attention to the parallel problems of learning as dealt with by experimental psychologists working on both animals and men. Since those early days of learning programs, a large number of learning programs have been written, and the whole notion of heuristic programming has grown up.

In this chapter it is intended to *outline* a series of programs for a general-purpose digital computer, showing the problems that occur in getting the computer to learn for itself. In discussing computer programs there is some difficulty that surrounds the actual terminology in which a computer program has to be stated. This varies with each machine, and we shall therefore represent our programs in the form of flow diagrams from which it would be easy to write the detailed program for any computer whatever.

The difficulties that have been experienced in programming computers to learn are mainly due to the fact that, in programming them to play a game like chess, you can assume no background information whatever; it is the equivalent of a newly born child. Everything it knows has been told it expressly for the purpose of playing the game.

Shannon says that the computer lacks 'insight', and in such cases this is inevitable, since insight can hardly be able to operate over a single problem considered in isolation. But Shannon went beyond this; he said that computers were at a disadvantage because they lacked 'flexibility, imagination, inductive and learning capacity'.

Now it is certainly true that the form of most general-purpose digital computers is inconvenient for many purposes; nevertheless, with a sufficiently large store a great deal of flexibility can in fact be achieved. Imagination we can leave for the moment, but induction and learning capacities can most certainly be attributed to them, indeed, given them by virtue of the program.

A computer does what it is programmed to do, and it can be programmed to perform inductive operations, and to learn. It is this that is the main purpose of our investigation.

Programming the computer to play a simple game

In Chapter 2 we outlined the basic idea of programming a computer, and now we must consider the problem of programming it to learn. This will be dealt with in roughly the same historical order as it has occurred, starting with simple, special cases.

We have already implied that what has been called 'insight' seems at least to depend upon taking over information from one situation and using this information in another situation. Or it may be thought of—and this is in essence the same thing—as building up general principles which can be seen to apply to more than a single isolated case.

The result of this consideration is to make it seem artificial to program the computer to play one particular game, such as chess, or noughts-and-

12*

crosses. However that may be, it will serve as an example to illustrate the method to be used.

The computer starts with empty registers, which means with no knowledge at all, so for its first game it must be explicitly told what it has to do. The comparison even with a new-born child is perhaps somewhat misleading, for that which is innate in the human is, by analogy, already built into the computer.

We shall first consider noughts-and-crosses, since it is a simple and well-known game. The first thing is to number the squares of what we may call the noughts-and-crosses board, using the numbers one to nine inclusive, but of course in binary form. This numbering seems to raise a problem, and the actual choice of the numbers directly affects the *statement* of a winning position, or rather, a won game. There are many ways of carrying out the numbering, but this turns out to be a matter *of no importance* since the computer, provided it is told which game is won and which lost, will still be able to learn to play the game, regardless of the numbering system used.

This point about numbering the board state is important in that we want eventually to program the computer to learn anything, and not simply restrict the performance to one particular game. This means that every game must be capable of being stated in terms of an array, and that the notion of a 'game' must be extended to what is usually regarded as learning, the game being simply to learn what the environment is.

A further point to notice is that, even for noughts-and-crosses, the computer must be able to discover the results of the games it has been playing; it must know whether the final position is a winning or a losing one, for this represents the necessity for confirmation or disconfirmation in terms of what motivates the organism.

The computer program must also provide means for avoiding moves that lead to a loss, and encouraging moves that lead to a win. This is the very problem of motivation, and it goes back to the law of effect. More generally, where games are not necessarily won or lost, we can substitute some principles of optimization.

To return to the board state, it will be clear that, for the game of noughts-and-crosses, this is simply the whole of the sensory field of the computer, and if we seek generality we must avoid giving the computer special means of looking at certain situations (e.g. particular games) which are of no use for other situations. We have, then, a set of quite general elements, as we shall call them, which we refer to by numbers, any nine of which represent a noughts-and-crosses board.

The computer must now learn the tactics that allow it to win, assuming that it is given direct instructions as to how to select the elements. It will learn that certain ways of carrying out this process of selection are called 'winning ways', and others 'losing ways'. This, however, implies the existence of concepts in the computer, and it would be better to say, more simply, that when the number 10, for example, is punched at the end of a game, the moves of that game are avoided in future; and when the number 11 appears, the moves are repeated. Number 12 is a draw, and will leave the 'tactical values' unchanged. In one sense the whole process is quite automatic.

The method of storage must be considered next. Clearly, the registers of the computer must be used in such a way that the order in which the moves are made is recorded. Associated with each order there must be a number, which we shall call the 'value number' (the 'tactical values' referred to above), which increases or decreases according to the success or otherwise of the particular play. We can, say, add 1 for a win, subtract 1 for a loss, and leave unchanged for a draw. We shall not, in fact, need to take the whole nine moves of a game together and give an evaluation to that; rather, we shall want to break down the total sequence into subsequences, say, just three, or five, successive moves, starting with the opponent's move, followed by the computer's own move, followed in turn by the opponent's.

Among a number of further points that arise is the necessity to keep a record of the complete set of moves making up a game, in order that it will be possible to decide whether the moves are good or bad. This merely represents the fact that we cannot tell whether a hypothesis is good or bad (true or false) until we have tested it and seen the outcome. This process of confirmation is simple in the game situation, but will be more complicated in general. It is true that we shall want to regard the business of living in an environment as being much like playing a game; and thinking, under these circumstances, is much like the computer playing a game with itself, playing both for itself and for its opponent. In this case we may wish to associate two numbers in the interval (0, 1) with each sequence of moves, if one number is the probability of one event following another, and the other number is the 'value' to the organism of this particular sequence.

The object of the experiment with simple games is to see if the machine learns the tactics after being told the rules. There is, however, rather an arbitrary division between rules and tactics, and it should be said that rules can, of course, themselves be learned, provided that the computer is able to watch the game being played, or that a sample of games is fed into it for analysis into component values. This implies the use of the computer as a sequential analyser of a stochastic kind (Bush and Mosteller, 1955), and since this is so, it is convenient to regard a tactic as a rule for the purpose of our example.

The rule we will now illustrate is well known in noughts-and-crosses, but to make it, and our subsequent discussion, clearer we will select a numbering scheme for our board and play some games.

The board will be numbered in the following rather special way for purposes of illustration:

$$8 \quad 3 \quad 4$$
$$1 \quad 5 \quad 9$$
$$6 \quad 7 \quad 2$$

This has the added convenience—against which there is certainly a loss of generality—whereby a game won is a game in which three numbers adding up to 15 are selected by one player before the other. Indeed, from the computer's point of view, noughts-and-crosses can be redescribed as a game of playing in turn, the winner being the first player to select three numbers that add up to 15.

In terms of the above numbering our rule, then, is to check the board state to see whether two numbers have already been selected such that there exists a third number, not yet selected, which will collectively add up to 15. If so, then this number should be selected, either to win the game or to stop the opponent winning.

A further problem arises in the course of the game. Since we wish the computer to learn about its environment, or learn to play a simple game (which, we have asserted, is the same thing), its speed will be greatly affected by the slowness of its input and output as compared with its computation speed, to say nothing of the comparatively enormous delay created by its human opponent's thought. In practice, therefore, it has been found convenient to divide the computer into two parts, which we will call α and β (Oettinger, 1952), programming α with all the rules *and* the tactics, and β with only the rules, and letting β learn the tactics by playing the games. Figure 39 shows the flow chart for the complete operation.

We next see a series of games played, taking for granted the fact that the original randomly chosen set of values was attached to the registers. These can be stated as follows, where the symbol / means 'is followed by', and the value tables from which we start have the last number in each case representing the initial random value.

5/1/1	5/8/4/1/1
5/2/0	5/8/4/2/5
5/3/-4	5/8/4/3/0
5/4/2	5/8/4/6/4
5/6/4	5/8/4/7/-3
5/7/1	5/8/4/9/6
5/8/12	
5/9/-2	

If we assume, for the sake of illustration, a fairly regular pattern of play in α, then, letting L stand for lost and D for drawn, the following games may result. Note the convention assumed for taking the first of two tied value numbers.

5/8/4/9/6/L
5/8/4/2/6/L
5/8/4/9/6/L
5/8/4/2/6/L
5/8/4/6/1/9/3/7/D

After this point the game remains constant for α playing consistently. Exactly the same process occurs for α varying, although it takes much longer to reach a stable state.

It remains to add that the computer can easily perform the operations described, and it very quickly learns the important tactical steps, after which it *never* loses. One more point of interest should be noted: the computer β *never* has exactly the same statement of the tactics as α, since α plays on a purely deductive basis following a rule which is verbal, whereas β carries through the steps of checking the maximum values from the tables in store. In practice, of course, this will lead to exactly the same result. What is missing to β is the language in which he can provide a statement of the game's algorithm.

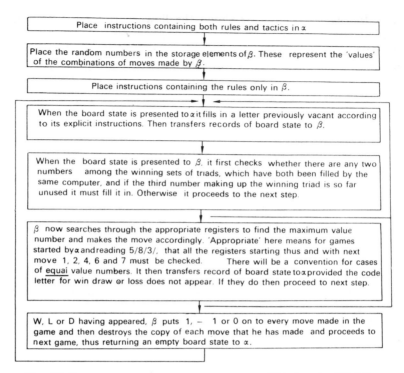

FIG. 39. FLOW CHART FOR NOUGHTS-AND-CROSSES. This is a simplified flow chart for the game played between two computers, both of which know the rules of the game, while only one knows the tactics.

This point is connected with the statement that we should not yet want to claim the full meaning of 'insight' on the part of either α or β, since there is no possibility of taking over a result and using it in another situation. To grant the circumstances for this to be a possibility, the computer must be taught at least one other sufficiently similar game, with the record of the noughts-and-crosses experience still available to it. For these results to be utilizable we should need the computer to generalize its results.

It can be shown that such generalizations are possible. One example is offered by teaching the computer to play noughts-and-crosses and to follow this up by teaching it—or getting it to learn—three-dimensional noughts-and-crosses. The learning of the latter game can be shown to be facilitated by having learned the former. An extension of this same principle will suggest itself for all learned material.

A simple explanation of how such a generalization may come from noughts-and-crosses alone is afforded by considering an alternative numbering scheme for the board, say,

$$1 \ 2 \ 3$$
$$8 \ x \ 4$$
$$7 \ 6 \ 5$$

and then examining the following games:

$$x/1/2/3/L$$
$$x/1/2/4/L$$
$$x/1/2/5/L$$
$$x/1/2/7/L$$

It is clear from this short sample that all sequences of moves which follow the starting move of x will have the general form

$$xm \ n(n+4) \tag{1}$$

if they are not to be losing.

The principle which can now be directly extended to all the moves of the game is completely general, and eventually states in the form of (1) a decision procedure sequence. It should be noticed that the statement of (1) implies the cyclic nature of the number. Thus, 11 is the number 3.

The ability of the computer to make the above generalization depends upon the ability to recognize numerical differences and to state general mathematical forms; this is something which it must separately learn, unless it is already programmed in.

We should say that the above example of a very simple type of learning situation now goes back several years and many techniques have been added to the programs outlined above.

The question of representation of problems or games to the computer is one of considerable importance. In the above example it was seen that the method of generalization depended on the way the information was represented. Amarel (1960, 1965, 1967, 1968) has shown that by mapping one representation of the game onto another or by changing the manner in which the game is represented, the nature of the problem is also changed. Obviously, therefore, one of the most important single features of problem solving will be to try and represent the problem in a manner which either trivializes it or makes it very much simpler to solve. This suggests that one of the main factors in computer programming of the problem-solving kind is to change the representation around a bit to see if one can find a simpler representation and thus find a simpler way of solving a problem. Perhaps it is best to say that however it is represented one will try to solve it and if one finds difficulty one will change the representation as well as change the attempted hypotheses which have been used to try and solve the problem.

Generalizations on game playing

We should say a few words now about the generalizing of the simple noughts-and-crosses example. The next program which was written for three-dimensional noughts-and-crosses and some subset of the correct solutions or sequences for three-dimensional included the solutions to two-dimensional noughts-and-crosses, therefore there is a positive transfer between the two and having learned two-dimensional noughts-and-crosses it is that much easier to learn three-dimensional. The notion of 'transfer of training' plays a very important part in problem solving and learning, since information is bound to be cumulative, we learn much of our information through language which is essentially cumulative and we learn even from our direct experience things which we can use in other situations and this is how we build up a reserve of hypotheses. Where positive transfer exists between two situations, then of course previous learning plays a very important part in the solution. However, the other side of the coin is that where negative transfer exists, then when hypotheses are drawn from one situation to one to which it is negatively associated, then of course a great deal of interference occurs. This principle is a simple logical principle which simply says that if one thing is sufficiently like another, that what will solve one will solve the other and if it looks like it but is in fact basically different, it will interfere.

Other games were also played besides three-dimensional and two-dimensional noughts-and-crosses and these included halma, ludo, draughts and chess. We shall be saying a little more later about draughts (Samuel, 1963, 1967) or chequers as it is sometimes called, although the principles utilized apply in exactly the same way to all these games as they do to noughts-and-crosses. All games seem to have a somewhat similar structure and there nearly always seems to be a positive transfer between them, therefore it might be supposed, and we have some evidence to support such a supposition, that all domestic games of the kind we have discussed have some sort of positive transfer.

It is quite clear that there are also differences between these games, a random element being introduced in the form of a deal of cards in one game, a throw of the die in another game, and so on, where some games like chess and draughts are completely deterministic and have no random components. Nevertheless, all the games also have something in common; they all involve pieces (in some sense) and all involve spaces (in some sense) and there is a sort of structural relationship that is a link between them all.

It should be noted that although we have talked about playing noughts-and-crosses by playing one computer against another, this is clearly unnecessary; one computer could play the role of both players and could collect evidence in store for both players and thus greatly speed up the learning operation. This is the equivalent presumably of contemplation on the part of the computer and reminds us of the fact that when we, as humans, learn to play games we do tend to combine reading the instructions and contemplating them and therefore presumably making deductive and inductive inferences about the games and, on the other hand, playing from time to time and mixing the two seems to be a typical human way of solving the problem of playing the game efficiently.

A question soon arose over this game-playing type of operation. It was concerned with what made it more restrictive than the way humans learn to solve everyday games or everyday problems. Admittedly one can have the cumulative effect of playing a whole range of games which will give you a store of information on which one could draw one's hypotheses or heuristics for everyday occurrences, but even so it did not seem enough. The answer to this must lie in language, the thing that is missing can be pictured this way from the point of view of noughts-and-crosses. One player continues to play from his 'Markov tables', while the other player plays from the statement given in the form of an algorithm. So it is necessary to translate the Markov tables into the algorithmic statement. This is just a particular case of a more general procedure which is characteristic of all human cognitive activity to translate into communicable language (ordinary English) that which is being structured in the nervous system in a language like symbolic logic, say. So the development of language plays a critical part in computers' learning and computers' problem solving.

We have already mentioned the fact that Banerji and others have developed languages for concept formation and distinguished them from the language which people communicate with each other. We want to make the same distinction here. Some sort of symbolic language seems appropriate for collecting the information about games and transfering it from one game to another to provide the internal representations of this game in terms of basic concepts. And it is the translation of this language into ordinary English, say, this is involved if one has to communicate with other people. Bearing in mind all the time that much of what we learn about any game, whether real life or domestic game, is learned by other people telling us either in the form of written instructions, from books or by ordinary conversation. We shall be returning to this central and crucial issue of language again in Chapter 13 where we are talking primarily of languages for external communication as opposed to languages for internal representation.

It is hoped the reader will see that in considering learning and problem solving on the computer, even in terms of domestic games, we have something which is a paradigm of the ordinary human learning and problem-solving situation. It should be noted in passing that learning is only distinguishable from problem solving in the sense that it is more specifically goal directed, that is the problem solving is more specifically goal directed. One can obviously learn things which are incidental to the goal at any particular time (latent learning) as we saw from Oettinger's program, but once we come to the internal representation of events and making deductive and inductive inferences about the internal representation, we are in the field of thinking (George, 1970) and although this may be accompanied by what we call images and therefore some feedback between the images and the representation, this does not alter the basic fact that in talking of learning we are talking of the essence of the whole of cognition which is built up as an edifice upon the basic notion of learning or adaptation.

General inductive programming

Let us use the following notation: A, B, ..., N will represent stimuli or input letters, and Q, R, ..., Z represent overt responses or output letters. These letters may be suffixed if necessary, giving a potentially infinite stock of input and output letters. The mode of generation may be quite general, so that at any instant whatever, although the number of input and output letters is finite, the number of letters can always be increased.

We can now state the problem as being one of setting up a dictionary which relates input to output letters, according values and probabilities to such relations by virtue of differential reinforcement.

Now for every input letter M there will be an output letter Y, and for every choice of M and Y there will be a probability of some further input letter N, and an assessment of the value of N is made by the computer. The 'assessment' is not itself an easy matter to decide in the full scale learning of human beings, but it at least involves the reinforcement of associations which are in temporal contiguity with 'pleasurable' outcomes, by designation.

This temporal interval of reinforcement could be graduated and extended over any number of time intervals. It could also, in the more complex programs, be associated with the occurrence of anticipated outcomes, even where these are remote in time from the reinforced associations.

It has to be the case that the motives, or some motives, are built in. For human beings, the main motive is undoubtedly survival of the organism. For the computer we will normally designate some input or output letters as positive or negative, motivationally.

The question of whether or not the computer can construct new goals for itself must be left for the moment, but it will be returned to after a further discussion of the general inductive programming procedure.

In practice, inductive programming is best illustrated on the computer by dividing it into two parts and letting one part play the role of the environment and the other the organism; *in thinking of the matter*, however, it is easier to think of it as a tape that is punched with the details of the environment and passed into the computer, and it is with this analogy in mind that we shall consider the matter. (Figure 40 shows a generalized flow chart.)

We shall have a tape made up of input symbols and representing the environment, and the problem of the computer will be to categorize the relationship between the letters on the input tape, and modify them in terms of its previous experience. For example, if A is followed by B if and only if the computer prints R after A, then we say that the occurrence of B is contingent on the occurrence of R on the output tape. This means, of course, that the input tape must be a function of the output tape. This is what logicians call a contingent relation, and it represents the fact that what people do may change the nature of the environment in which they live.

Computer α is stocked with instructions for generating outputs (i.e.,βs input letters) and responding to βs output letters. The original instructions for these operations are random.

↓

Computer α records its input letter and responds according to the principles outlined in Figs. 39 and 41 of this chapter.

↓

α has to go through the ordered set in storage appropriate to the input letter (see Fig. 41) and if there is no such event letter it makes either a random response, or if there is another event letter similar to the missing one, it will respond as if that one occurred. This last principle of stimulus generalization depends upon the inputs being themselves complex patterns of letters.
Whichever takes place the result is recorded in a separate storage register.

↓

If α now receives another input letter before a response has been made to the last letter, it checks blocks I and II of the store (see Fig. 41) and if the input letter does not occur there then the input letter is put into a temporary storage and the computer returns to the scanning prior to making the response still not made to the letter. If the last letter was involved in block I or II, then the second input letter would be put directly into temporary storage without a preliminary check of I and II.

↓

α now associates a new value number with the input-output relation last processed according to the satisfaction or otherwise subsequently derived. This also means that a certain range of effect may occur so that the input before that and perhaps also the one after has its value number changed. With language in the computer it will also change its description of its environment as a result of these value number changes.

↓

The computer α is now in a position to process the next input event, and may if there is a delay before the next input arrives derive the logical consequences of the information already in its storage system.

FIG. 40. A GENERAL FLOW CHART FOR COMPUTER LEARNING. This is a generalization on Fig. 39 and shows in simplified form a game in which one computer plays the environment and the other the organism.

It may also be the case that the machine's response to a particular input letter will have no effect whatever on the next input letter, and in such a case the logician will say that the two letters on the input tape— say, C and D—are necessarily related.

Quite obviously these are two limiting cases, and in between we have relations of varying degrees of complexity. Thus, E may follow F if and only if some combination of R, S and T is printed on the output tape. This could be regarded as the analog of the machine solving a problem; indeed, a scientific problem could be regarded in just this light as a particular set of relations existing between input and output letters. The idea of controlling the environment emerges when the computer is in the position of being able to anticipate every input letter by virtue of the previous input letter, and change the next input letter whenever that is desirable; this depends directly on the selective reinforcement of the system.

This is the way in which a computer can learn. It stores information made up of the occurrence of successive combinations of symbols or events and, by ascribing probabilities to these combinations, ensures that a control is maintained, assuming always that the ability to control the succession of events is in fact possible.

The storage registers themselves are not fixed in their length, and this caused some difficulty. Obviously we shall want to store events of what are sometimes called length three (cf. Tolman's *expectancy*, discussed in the next chapter), which means an input followed by an output followed by an input letter, e.g. $A/R/B$. But this may not be enough, since the probabilities associated with an event of length five, say, are not the same as the product of the probabilities associated with events of shorter length that make up the event of length five. That is to say,

$$p(A/R/B/S/C) \neq q(A/R/B).s(B/S/C)$$

where p, q and s are probabilities. In a special case, of course, they may be equal.

Problem-solving behaviour calls for an extension of the length of events used when the problem is not soluble with events of too short a length. This implies that there must be means for generating events of greater length as they are needed.

Statistically speaking, this matter of storage represents the well-known methods of a stochastic type. It is a matter of associating probabilities with successive elements of a sequence, where these probabilities are changing regularly as a result of each successive input. In fact it is probably undesirable that all the probabilities should change quickly, and there will be some method available whereby, once a particular relationship is well established with probabilities approaching 0 or 1, these 'certain beliefs' may be moved to a separate store, or at least to a set of well defined registers. At the same time we must use some method of 'rapid counting' to undo quickly an obviously inappropriate response due to changed environmental conditions. This might be achieved by heavily weighted reinforcement, or through language.

All this links up with work that has already been done on 'heuristics' (Minsky, 1959), which demands the use of fairly well-defined generalizations as partial or intermediate solutions. 'Heuristics' here really means analogies (i.e. generalizations) taken over from one situation and used in another in order to solve the problem presented by the new situation.

A tactic in noughts-and-crosses can be learned by the differential reinforcement of moves in a game in which all the moves in a game lost were scored -1, and all moves in a game won were scored $+1$, even though some of the same moves may occur in either game. This does not matter in noughts-and-crosses, where the range of possible moves is small, and discrepancies in move-evaluation are soon worked out; but in a long game like chess it would take time of astronomical proportions to evaluate every move in a game, and a similarly excessive period to learn a decision procedure by such a method. We must therefore look for intermediate or simplifying principles.

Obviously, just these sorts of heuristics, or simplifying principles, enter into chess as played by ordinary humans. They have rules of thumb that guide the strategy or tactics of the game, and these tactical generalizations could be formulated in an inductive programme in the same way as in the generalizations which we have already discussed; but we shall try to show that language leads to an alternative formulation. Let us now discuss heuristics in more detail.

Heuristic programming

Heuristics are best thought of in contrast with algorithms, since they represent *ad hoc* methods, approximations or rules of thumb, which will not normally give you a completely precise solution to a problem. In playing chess, one plays from the rules of thumb, where the better set of heuristics used characterizes the better player. No doubt, given the 'complete' set in some sense, the algorithm would be available but an incomplete algorithm is a sort of heuristic.

There is no point here in trying to be precise about the definitions of 'heuristic' and 'algorithm', since they probably differ in matter of degree as much as such terms as 'analytic' and 'synthetic'. We are thinking of heuristics as rough guides such as 'Keep the ball in the centre of the field whenever you are a goal up', 'Try and control the centre of a chess board', 'If you get overfilled with production, always delay some period of time and keep a customer late before you build up a new production line', and various other good (or bad) guides to rather ill-defined and ill-structured behaviour which human beings manifestly deal in and for which they use decisions.

We know we can program computers to perform heuristic operations, and we do so by providing models, and from these models providing interpretations which are themselves algorithmic. The relationship between limited forms of deduction and induction illustrate the method. A probability, for example, refers to an event with some degree of uncertainty; the chances of some event $Ap_A(H1)$ is calculated to be $\frac{23}{41}$ at any particular moment in time, but although the uncertainty applies to the event, the compilation of the probability itself was done by straightforward counting which is algorithmic, so we have the model which is heuristic being one level above the machine code program in the computer context. It remains to show how it is possible to construct what turns out to be axiomatic systems of this empirical kind which allow for adaptive heuristic programming and the possibility of generating new heuristics.

Heuristic generation

In this section we will first outline the general principles on which we are going to operate. We have to set up an axiomatic system, which therefore will have axioms, rules of inferences and be capable of generating theorems. However, the axioms refer to specific features of an environment and we are not pretending at this stage that the environment is a system which has the properties of completeness, consistency, etc. We do, however, assume some modest form of consistency since if we are able to generate theorems which are inconsistent we shall have to decide which one is correct and in an empirical context we can do this by actually investigating the statement, or the alleged theorem, and seeing whether it correctly depicts the facts. This is the kind of test which is not, of course, open in the case of formal axiomatic systems.

The system can be constructed in terms of operators, $A, B, \ldots, N$ which can take as many suffixes as necessary and have a number of reversed words. These reversed words are such letters as are given specific semantic rule; so if $A1$ equals ADD, $S1$ equals SUBTRACT, say, then these have become reversed words.

The rules of inference will be the entailments which the operators carry, thus if we had R referring to a relationship, then if this is interpreted as '... a brother of—' then we know that the entailment here is such that given that the two gaps are filled by x and y and given another statement with y and z filling the two gaps, then one can draw the conclusion x and z. In other words, it is the entailment of the operators which includes all verbs and connectives which decides what are the logical possibilities within the system. This is so, of course, apart from constraints which are further imposed by the proper words representing things, object words, usually nouns or possibly adjectives, which are used to fill the blanks which go with the operators. In general we shall expect these to be variables and constants and they can refer to classes or individuals. We shall not expect here to refer to propositions because we are referring to a more 'atomic' structure.

We now have to build up a statement of a purpose or goal to the system, since without some sort of forcing function which determines the end point of behaviour we have no way of effectively learning or measuring the degree of learning with respect to which the system means to operate; this is always possible, though.

This whole question of how human beings solve problems is not our first consideration, since, it will be remembered, we were taking a cybernetic view, and therefore we would say that if we oscillate between particular cases and the development of a general deductive argument, the first really is inductive and the second is deductive, then it is only because it is empirically more convenient to do it this way rather than try to push through a detailed deductive argument which, with this sort of loose empirical axiomatic system, might prove to be exceptionally difficult. In fact, it is probably necessary to do it by deduction alone, in general, to have anticipated the full strength of the argument before one applies it.

Language for the computer

We now wish to add words X_1, X_2, ..., X_n to our system, and we wish the computer to have a potentially infinite number of words at its disposal. This implies that it has the means of constructing an indefinite number of words. The method, which is learned by example in humans, may also be so learned by the computer.

The principle of association, by which words come to be associated with physical objects (or events), is exactly the same as the manner in which events have already been shown to become associated with each other. Indeed, it will be apparent that our input tape may contain words as well as event symbols, and furthermore, there is really no need to distinguish these outside the machine, since the word will associate with an output, say, and precipitate an action in the same way as an event.

This raises many interesting problems for the programmer. It can be shown that computers can learn simple languages in this way, and of course the natural languages for them to use are those languages which we call 'logical'. They are the logics of empirical classes and empirical relations (Chapter 3), since they are descriptive and probabilistic. It is from this that ordinary language can then be derived.

We can see here a clear link between this sort of programming and auto-coding, although at present virtually all auto-coding is essentially 'deductive'. This is a matter we shall discuss briefly later, in connection with an inductively programmed computer changing its own goal.

The argument about inductive or learning programming seems to suggest that no distinction, except one for purely linguistic convenience, need be drawn between words and concepts. The word 'concept' might be used to apply to the development of a state, represented by a Markov Chain table in the register in the computer, up to the stage at which it reaches verbal reformulation as a result of the computer now having a language with which to describe everything and anything that occurs to it. This includes relations between output events, between input events, and between output and input events. These inputs and outputs must also themselves include words, for it is now well understood that we shall want to distinguish between words about events and words about words.

It should be noticed that generalizations may occur in linguistic form representing events that may never have occurred in the computer's

13*

experience. This is closely linked to what is called 'imagination', and reminds us that this imaginative process, closely allied, one suspects, with what is called 'creative thinking', can most conveniently be handled in language, although, if the tables of the computer generated new strings of symbols, it would seem to be largely an academic matter to inquire whether these were verbal or not.

A computer that has gone this far can, in principle, surely deal with the problem of transferring findings from one situation to another, and thus satisfy a condition which seems to be much the same as is needed by human 'insight'. We can now bridge the gulf between the two computers α and β, where they could be shown to perform the same responses on different bases. These different bases refer to the fact that although one computer learns to do the same thing as the other, it still does it on the basis of tables rather than verbal instructions.

Earlier in this book we represented the material on which a computer works as a set of numbers. This means that all the operations of a general purpose computer are mathematical operations. From this point of view, games like noughts-and-crosses are problems of set theory. The same argument exactly applies to other games like draughts, chess, and even card games, although there may be additional conditions to be satisfied.

The significance of all this is that we want the most complete basis for all possible arithmetical operations, and this we find under the name of primitive recursive functions (Davis, 1958).

Primitive recursive functions are the general class of functions that include everything that normally occurs in classical mathematics; the operations of addition, subtraction, and all other mathematical operations can, of course, be exemplified in this way. This means that if the computer has the power—by virtue of being programmed—to carry out any primitive recursive operation, it would seem that it could do as much as anyone could hope to do by way of learning.

Changing goals

There has been some argument among cyberneticians as to whether a computer can or cannot change its own goals. Semantics are certainly involved here, but in particular terms which will be explained, it can most certainly be said that a computer can change its goals. This is, of course, necessary if the model is to be useful to psychologists interested in learning.

If the computer is differentially reinforced it will perform, with respect to a certain subset of variables, optimalization operations. This is like putting survival above all else in a human being; but these are by no means the only goals, since in the inductive associative process we can evaluate every association with respect to its contribution to the optimalization of the basic variables. A simple example of this is to say that when an event is associated directly with something obviously good for survival, it becomes thought of as itself good for survival. We may call these other goals secondary goals, and these of course will change according to the changing circumstances upon which the computer is making its inductive inferences. Similarly, there is no reason why we should not ascribe specified values to the basic goals, and allow these to change if and when a secondary goal exceeds the basic goal in value; such things seem to happen with humans when they are prepared to sacrifice their lives for some cause.

Cybernetics and learning

Much of what has already been said in this book may be taken as summarizing some of the results of cybernetic research, and forging a link between learning and cybernetics. Something more explicit must now be said on this subject.

In the first place we must consider the relation between the learning theories, such as those of Hull and Tolman, and cybernetic research. It will be remembered that Hull's theory dealt with stimulus–response units (see next chapter) which are strung together into a stochastic process of the same kind as the one analysed by the computer. In fact the resemblance goes deeper than that, because the concept of differential reinforcement that we have used is very similar to that of Hull's concept of primary and secondary reinforcement.

In the computer program we have assumed some such concept as a primary drive, and further, that initially neutral stimuli take on this drive, or motivational characteristic, by virtue of their association with primary drives.

Tolman's theory is essentially the same in its interpretation of needs and cathexes (this means 'values', roughly speaking; see the next chapter), where the secondary cathexis that becomes associated with an originally neutral stimulus is simply an alternative rendering of what the computer may be said to be doing. This confirms in part the belief that Hull and Tolman represent two different interpretations of the same model.

Tolman's basic association unit is stimulus–response–stimulus, rather than stimulus–response and, as with motivation, we might say that the emphasis has gone away from the habit type of learning and towards the more sophisticated type where the emphasis is on the *next* state, rather than a mere response to a stimulus.

In our computer learning, the same stochastic methods are used, but we shall not lay heavy emphasis on stimulus–response, nor on stimulus–response–stimulus, as a 'basic unit', since learning can be clearly seen to depend upon very complex associations, of which stimulus–response and stimulus–response–stimulus seem rather simple special cases; and this is true regardless of the interpretation we place on the words 'stimulus' and 'response'.

Our computer experiments point to the fact that our methods of describing learning must be *effective*. We must consider what our assumptions (Woodger has called them zero-level statements) are, and make them explicit and give them an operational definition. The use of the computer lends further emphasis to this point.

To return to the essentially Markovian (Markov chain) nature of learning, it seems clear that the length over which our conditional probabilities must spread is a function of the complexity of the problem to be solved (or the operation to be learned), and the extent to which the organism is motivated to learn it, and the organization of the memory store.

The principles of the input and the output depend, no doubt, upon a classification principle (Uttley, 1954; George, 1956a, 1957d), whereas the central problem is that of organizing the information for storage.

The details of the storage organization have by no means been worked out in detail, but Fig. 41 shows a suggested scheme of organization. Programs have already been designed which order information such that the most valuable comes out in the first registers to be scanned, and the ones with high probabilities come next; this simply means that urgent matters are dealt with first and habits next. If the input does not demand an urgent response, but merely elicits a habit response, then it enters into the bulk of storage where matters are still 'more obviously' *being learned*, with the exception that the first set of this large set has been generalized into 'beliefs', so that some arbitrariness may have been enacted on the facts. This will not matter if the degree of arbitrariness is not too great. In other words, it will not matter if we treat Mr Smith exactly as we treat Mr Brown, provided the difference between them is sufficiently small, so small that we shall get similar sorts of results from the same response to either.

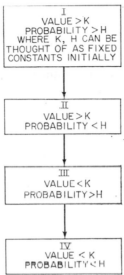

FIG. 41. THE STORAGE SYSTEM. The storage systems may be regarded as being responsible for ordering stored information. This figure shows the simplest priorities and there will also be a variation in degree of generality of information.

Finally we come to those matters where learning is still occurring, which will naturally lead to the longest delay in responding. Those of high value and probability are the most important, but these variables also partially cloak the other factors of *recency* and *frequency*, except in that value is a direct function of frequency, and that, among equal values, the most recent will appear as the top item in the subset. Motivation is represented by built-in stimuli, and the development of secondary motivation is brought about by association.

The pattern of learning is clearly beginning to emerge from studies of this sort, and it is perhaps not too much to claim that we now understand how learning occurs (or could occur), although we do not understand either the biological or the social details sufficiently well to allow us to make predictions for individuals beyond a very limited range.

Looking again at what we have said in the light of modern learning theory, it might be guessed that both stimulus–response and stimulus–response–stimulus elements occur. The first represents the 'habits', or events of high probability, where no emphasis on the next response is needed (since the stimulus–response connection has a high probability). In the stimulus–response–stimulus element, the automatic nature of the response does not occur, but the 'urgency' (very high value numbers) may or may not be high. What is important is that much longer sequences may occur, indeed need to occur, for reasonably accurate learning and problem solving.

It is also interesting that the presence of neither primary nor secondary motivation is necessary to associate with any novel input to bring about a response, since the value numbers associated with all input sequences are relative to the others of the same set, and thus a response will still be made, although of a random kind. This brings out the point of trial-and-error learning.

This trial-and-error is subsequently reinforced, and thus prepares the way for the sort of 'insight' in another sense which recognizes the appropriateness of a response as a result of selective reinforcement.

As a result of this we may say that objects subsequently have a 'cathexis' and an 'induced cathexis' (a value imposed by association on an otherwise neutral event. See next chapter). But this, as in Tolman's theory, will be relative to the context in which they may occur. For the computer, the context is given by events of greater length that have already a high probability associated with them. To take a case: for event A, the probability and value numbers may be such as to predict not just $A/R/F$, but $A/R/F/S/C/T/D$, or some such longer event.

Generalization will occur if we say that each input is really a combination of subunits—which it surely is in organismic learning—and this means that two sets may be identified if they have common numbers and are such that no distinction is forthcoming with respect to one input as opposed to the other. A special case of this—more convenient in the nomenclature of this book—is the simple identification of two different input variables. It will be noticed that this argument of generalization can clearly apply to inputs, outputs, or input–output relations, of any length whatever.

Other aspects of learning can easily be explained in terms of this computer organization, so that 'transfer of training' occurs simply as a result of generalization over events of length greater than two.

Memory is such that frequency and recency are necessarily factors, since this is the way we have ordered the events to be remembered, subject, of course, to the other conditions of value and probability.

'Set', by the same sort of argument, depends simply on the context of events of length greater than two—often, indeed, much greater—where the response is made to a stimulus with the expectation of another stimulus, simply because of its high probability.

'Learning sets' will be accounted for by saying that a particular relation that is well learned does not interfere with the same input letter being associated with a new output, since the first is now of high enough probability. This means that it would be immediately responded to were it not for the explicit instruction *not* to respond to it. To remember *not* to respond is thus something that is a function of the degree of learning; or in other words, the discrimination (as opposed to generalization) can be carried through better where the probabilities are wholly separated.

This last point is brought out more clearly where the system works on an approximate basis, and comparison of probabilities is approximate, and thus glosses over discriminations dependent upon only a small amount of learning.

In this chapter we have not attempted to bring out the full significance of computer programming for learning theory, for it is intended that this significance shall be noticed more fully in later chapters. It is hoped that, without really taking up in detail the point of language in the computer, enough has been said to indicate the possibilities inherent in this approach. It should be remembered that many more programs have been run on the computer than could possibly be shown here, and much more has been learned about learning than can now be stated.

Summary

This chapter is really complementary to the last one, and deals with the whole matter of learning from the point of view of programming a digital computer.

Contrary to many opinions, the general-purpose digital computer can be shown to learn, or behave inductively, if suitably programmed. The type of stochastic organization needed is essentially the same as the type of organization used in the logical net models of the previous chapter.

Although in a short chapter it has not been possible to illustrate the full range of experiments that have been carried out in computer programming, enough has been said to illustrate the method and its great potentiality. Programs have been undertaken over other games besides those mentioned, and the methods used are the same. The most interesting points that arise in learning programs are connected with the power of the computer to generalize and to use heuristics and to use language. These matters have been discussed all too briefly, but the possibility of both aspects of computer programming being greatly extended is fairly obvious.

The second half of the chapter is also concerned with forging a link between the established theories of behaviour, such as the learning theories of Hull and Tolman. It is in fact possible to see that both the Hull and the Tolman theories could be restated in a manner making them suitable for a computer program, and such effectiveness is exactly what Cybernetics needs.

One point comes quite clearly out of the programming of computers to learn, and that is the fact that there may be a considerable difficulty in dealing with the build-up of input information. Learning is a selective process, but so is perception, and we may expect input information to be put in short term storage while other information is being handled.

CHAPTER 8

PSYCHOLOGICAL THEORY OF LEARNING

OUR main aim in this book is to show the part that cybernetics can play in helping to solve the traditional behavioural or psychological problems within the field of cognition, and the first cognitive problem with which we shall deal explicitly is that of *learning*. Before we can try effectively to employ logical networks, inductive computer programs, or any other cybernetic model, to the solution of a problem, we must consider what has already been done in the field, and where solutions are already forthcoming, and where they are not; otherwise we cannot make the necessary comparison with what is actually known of human behaviour. We shall, in passing, be referring to those aspects of learning that have already been met in previous chapters.

We shall necessarily have to rely on a *brief summary* of the major work done in learning, since this is not a text on learning theory as such. The reader who seeks to develop cybernetic methods in learning in more detail must do so with a more specialized analysis of learning. This, of course, applies to the whole of cognition, indeed, to the whole of behaviour, and on physiological levels as well as psychological. We shall start with a discussion of the meaning of the word 'learning'.

'Learning', as Humphrey has pointed out (Humphrey, 1933), is a recently introduced term. It is not mentioned in the indices of either Kulpe (1893), Stout (1896), or Ward (1918), nor is it mentioned explicitly in Baldwin's *Dictionary of Philosophy*, or William James's treatise on psychology (1890). Wundt regarded learning as approximately the same as memorization of words. William McDougall, in his *Outline of Psychology* (1923), only once mentions the word 'learning', where it occurs under the title 'primitive learning'. In fact, of course, the processes were studied under different names, such as 'memory', 'habit', 'framing', and 'apperception'. These terms, in so far as they are still used, are regarded as referring to special cases of learning, developed in the formative years of the subject; they have now largely disappeared.

Various attitudes towards 'learning' will now be noted. McDougall himself describes a primitive learning process, among animals low in the scale of intelligence, as a modification of present actions through past experience, and he quotes, as an example, his experiment with crayfish. If some food is placed at one end of a long trough of water, and the crayfish is put in at the other end, he will swim towards the food. Now if the trough is divided into two parts A and B, so that by A he can reach the food and by B he cannot, then after some number of trials, he will always take the path A. This is a particular case of *learning*.

Humphrey insists on using 'learning' to apply to behaviour modification that is *useful* to the organism (part of the survival need). A seagull whose behaviour is modified to the extent of following ships to get food is said to have 'learned'. If, on seeing a ship, the seagull always flew in the opposite direction, it would have had its behaviour modified, but would *not* be said to have 'learned'. In this connection it is worth quoting Humphrey's own words (Humphrey, 1933):

> A gull, let us say, has learned to fly after the ships as they leave the harbour. Clearly the learning rests on the fact that the bird is able to obtain bigger and better meals, and easier ones. That is to say, its energy intake is more economically effected. If, after finding food behind a number of ships, it had so modified its reactions that it flew in the opposite direction whenever a ship appeared, we should hardly say that learning had taken place.

The special sense in which the word 'learning' is being used here should be carefully noted. Humphrey goes on to differentiate between different types of learning, and places them on a continuum with simple negative adaptation (habituation, or accommodation, and tropisms, which are orientating responses and are known to be mediated by fairly simple physico-chemical means) at one end, and maze-learning, puzzle-box learning (Thorndike, 1898, 1911, 1932; Adams, 1929; Guthrie and Horton, 1946), and ape-learning (Köhler, 1925; Yerkes, 1916), in stages of increasing complexity, leading to human learning at the other end. The conditioned response (Pavlov, 1927) falls somewhere towards the middle of the continuum.

By a 'conditioned response' we mean here, as before, the simple associative principle involved in 'classical conditioning'. The unconditioned response might be salivation at the sight of food (which is the unconditioned stimulus), and then, when the food is presented and a bell rings at the same time, the bell may be called the 'conditioned stimulus'. Conditioning occurs when the response of salivation is elicited by the bell alone (now called the 'conditioned response'), without the presence of food.

From this starting-point Humphrey goes on to analyse the whole subject in great detail. So far as our present knowledge of cybernetics goes, it suggests that the main distinctions are, in fact, likely to be between 'learning' and 'having learned', where the learning may vary from trial-and-error to insight, and the 'having learned' overlaps that which is built in and also that which is acquired by maturation, or in the course of growth and development.

Into the depths of the verbal problems are soon drawn other terms which are used to refer to modified organic activity. These terms include 'instinct', 'purpose', 'insight', and 'maturation', and the whole matter becomes much more complicated. Some attempt to clarify it can be started by saying that maturation and instinctive behaviour are usually distinguished from learning.

At a certain level, the distinction may be made between behaviour depending on special organic development (of which Coghill's (1929) salamanders are a very good example) and learned behaviour. The working out of inherited, relatively fixed, probably electro-chemically mediated, behaviour patterns (instincts), and behaviour which is in some way modified by external or internal changes towards the survival of the organism, or towards a state of homeostasis (Cannon, 1929), demand the closest attention (Tinbergen, 1951). The verbal distinction between 'involuntary' and 'voluntary' behaviour is in some ways an analogy, although very limited, to the above distinction.

Now it can be seen that there are large possibilities for confusion in our basic understanding of 'learning', and more careful definition is necessary. If one turns to some modern definitions of 'learning' it may be seen that greater clarity has been only partially effected. Hull states (Hull, 1943, p. 68):

> The essential nature of the learning process may be stated quite simply. Just as the inherited equipment of reaction-tendencies consists of receptor-effector connections, so the process of learning consists in the strengthening of certain of these connections as contrasted with others, or in the setting up of quite new connections.

Hull's work may be taken as one cornerstone of modern learning theory, and it will need careful analysis. For Hull, 'learning' can be defined in terms of conditioning, and the problem of learning is reduced in essence to the problem of *reinforcement*. However, before looking more closely at any one view, it is necessary to continue our survey of definitions a little further.

Hilgard and Marquis (1940) define 'learning' thus:

Change in the strength of an act through *training procedures* (whether in the laboratory or in the natural environments) as distinguished from changes in the strength of the act by factors not attributable to training.

This can be regarded only as a working definition as, of course, the real difficulty is shelved, since 'training procedures' are not defined, nor is the method of observation for distinguishing between behaviour modified as a result of training or non-training. The Hilgard and Marquis (1940) definition of Thorndike trial-and-error learning may also be quoted:

The mode of *learning* in which the learner tries various movements in its repertory, apparently in a somewhat random manner, and without explicit recognition of the connection between the movement and the resolution of the problem situation. Tentative movements which succeed are more frequently repeated in subsequent trials, and those which fail gradually disappear.

This form of definition leads to the famous law of effect and to a discussion of reinforcement, and it is fundamental to our inductive programming.

Three further definitions of 'learning' may be quoted; they are due to Guthrie, Hilgard and Thorpe respectively. Guthrie's (1935) reads:

The ability to learn, that is, to respond differently to a situation because of past responses to the situation, is what distinguishes those living creatures which common sense endows with *minds*. This is the practical description of the term 'minds'.

Neglecting the totally unnecessary introduction of the word 'mind', we see that the definition is exactly the same as the implicit definition of McDougall.

Hilgard's (1948) avowedly working definition reads:

Learning is the process by which an activity originates or is changed through training procedures (whether in the laboratory or in the natural environment) as distinguished from changes by factors not attributable to training.

This, of course, is only a slightly modified form of the Hilgard–Marquis definition.

Thorpe's (1950) definition is:

> The process which produces adaptive change in individual behaviour as the result of experience. It is regarded as distinct from fatigue, sensory adaptation, maturation and the results of surgical or other injury.

Separate definitions of 'trial-and-error learning', 'reinforcement', 'latent learning', 'insight learning', 'instinct', etc., are also worth noting (Thorpe, 1950).

The problem of learning is, plainly, thought to be a central one for experimental psychology. The difficulty has been to earmark what is essential to learning and what is not, and this may merely represent the fact that learning is really a more or less complex process of association units working together, as we suggested in the previous chapter, and if this is so, this is vital to the cybernetic approach, which is especially well equipped to deal with such complexity.

Within the compass of learning there are certain essential distinctions between different sorts of learning; for example, some organisms can learn without immediately manifesting their learning in a changed performance. This is called 'latent learning', and is very typical of human beings. The fact that some learning may occur when obviously initiated by purely random behaviour (trial-and-error learning) does not blind us to the fact that other learning may show 'insight'. This word does not necessarily mean something mysterious; it is used here to indicate that what is learned in one situation, or previously learned in general, perhaps through language, may be applied in a new or particular situation. Such refinements and distinctions do not, it seems, invalidate the essential unity of the concept of learning itself. But it does look as if learning is dependent on a 'forcing function' or selective operation such as reinforcement.

Reinforcement has generally been explained in terms of one of the following three principles: (1) Substitution, (2) Effect, and (3) Expectancy, and for most theorists it remains the essential factor upon which learning depends. Although these three principles may appear to be different aspects of some more general principle, they have not, as yet, been integrated. The principle of substitution springs from classical conditioning (Pavlov, 1927, 1928; Bekhterev, 1932; *et al.*), and a first working definition might be:

The principle of a substitution states that a conditioned stimulus, present at the time that an original stimulus evokes a response, will tend, on subsequent presentations, to evoke a response.

The first important question is that of the generality of the principle. Pavlov and Guthrie are its principal supporters, but they differ as to its generality. Pavlov (1927) says that substitution occurs only under certain circumstances, while for Guthrie substitution always occurs, and occurs completely. For Pavlov, the factors determining the degree of substitution are: (1) The time interval between the conditioned stimulus and the unconditioned response, (2) The intensity of the conditioned stimulus and of the unconditioned stimulus, and (3) The number of repetitions of the stimuli; but these factors are not necessarily regarded as being exhaustive.

To consider Guthrie first (Guthrie, 1935, 1942; Hilgard, 1948): it is a general criticism of Guthrie's behaviour theory that it oversimplifies the facts. The basis of his theory is contained in his two basic laws:

(1) A combination of stimuli which has accompanied a movement will, on its recurrence, tend to be followed by that movement.
(2) A stimulus pattern gains its full associative strength on the occasion of its first pairing with a response.

Since these do not allow the necessary predictions, because of lack of detailed analysis, the laws must be considered inadequate to explain learning on a sufficiently general basis. We might guess that it is not that the model is incorrect, but that it is inadequate by reason of its lack of detail. To put the matter another way, Guthrie's theory, as stated by him, lacks generalizability. There is a further objection: it is a principle that does not allow of verification nor does it readily suggest further experiment. On these grounds Guthrie's formulation will be put aside, and provisional acceptance given to the Pavlov formulation. However, this does not appear to be a vital issue; indeed, in a sense it is a sub-issue of the more general problem of selective learning, which still needs definition.

Although we appear to be dismissing Guthrie in a somewhat cavalier fashion, we are very ready to admit that, apart from other important features, his theory has laid emphasis on the principle of contiguity as primary and motivation as secondary, and this has served to draw attention to an aspect of learning that might otherwise have been obscured.

The influence he has had on this score alone is quite considerable, and can be detected in Estes' model of learning (1950) as well as in more recent theories of learning such as those of Sheffield (Sheffield and Roby, 1950; Sheffield, Wulff and Backer, 1951; Sheffield, Roby and Campbell, 1954) and Seward (1950, 1951, 1952, 1953).

From the point of view of logical nets this question is one of special interest. We have said that the motivational system may initiate response activity *and* stimulus–response associations may occur to change the internal (motivational) state of the organism, but only—according to the view stated—in the presence of a secondary or primary reinforcer. If we drop this condition we are in difficulties in explaining why learning is selective. Even if we granted the presence of a selective filter, and that some part of that selection was based on conditions of attention, which was based, in turn, on the relevance of some stimuli for existing needs, this would in no way change the basic need for differential reinforcement, although, as we might expect, it would mean that we must take a broader view of motivation than is implicit in Hull's theory of need-reduction. The same argument applies, of course, to stimulus–stimulus associations.

We shall leave this knotty point for the moment, and return to our summary of the principal features of learning theory.

The distinction between Pavlov's and Guthrie's substitution must now be regarded from the point of view of logical nets. Consider Fig. 27 of Chapter 5, which represents our logical net model of the conditioned response in its simplest form.

We can see quite easily, in comparing Guthrie's and Pavlov's notions, that the first question is as to whether we should regard the association as being set up at once, or by degrees. The answer is not unambiguous, since our logical net could be interpreted from either point of view. If we consider the matter from Pavlov's point of view and ask ourselves whether the time interval between the conditioned stimulus A and the previously unconditioned response (the bell and salivation in classical conditioning) makes a difference to the effectiveness of the associations being made, the answer is a complex one. We can certainly arrange for events to be associated directly, however far from each other in time, but we may expect that pairs of contiguous events are normally associated during learning. It would therefore seem to be difficult for the organism to *learn* the relation between events widely dispersed in time. This does not mean that, having learned an association, there may not be considerable delays in the subsequent associations, although these delays would, according to Pavlov, weaken the association.

What emerges from this picture is that we have not as yet made clear the full workings of our automaton, particularly with respect to its timing, so we shall look further at this aspect of the development. In the first place, the designs of Figs. 26, 27, and 28 in Chapter 5 are not intended necessarily to accept only single stimuli but, rather, volleys of stimuli (this matter of volleys could of course be restricted to peripheral mechanisms in which sensory classification occurs, although they may take the form of specialized analysers, or be of a very particular form such as that suggested by Osgood and Heyer (see Chapter 10)), and we may expect that a particular volley represents, by its size, the intensity of stimulation. If an event, A say, so represented, occurs, then the subsequent state B will normally follow quickly, dependent or not on some response A'. This leads to the *belief* $A \to B$, say, where ' $\to$ ' simply represents the association of an event name A with an event name B such that we say A *implies* B, but—and this is now vital—there may be many interesting stimuli and responses in the repertoire of the automaton that occur concomitantly on $A \to B$, and these are what Guthrie would call 'maintaining stimuli'. These maintaining stimuli are mostly automatic in themselves but may need to be given some organization, particularly at the motor classification level, to permit $A \to B$ to occur at all.

This argument is important in bearing out Guthrie's points about an association being immediate and occurring at full strength, where practice has the effect of organizing the *maintaining stimuli*. At the same time, the sketchy explanation given is also consistent with Pavlov's idea that delays in temporal contiguity affect the efficiency of the association. In other words, *beliefs* occur as *expectancies* in a very complex way, many occurring more or less together, and where the A part of $A \to B$ may be quite remote from the B part. Thus, if A occurs, the proper response may be of the form

$$A \to C \to D \to E \to F \ldots N \to B \qquad (1)$$

where the successful association is only established after many, even necessary, intervening responses have been made. In other terminology we could write (1) as

$$A \, | \, | \, C \, | \, | \, D \ldots | \, | \, B$$

or $$A \, | \ldots | \, B$$

here '/' means 'is followed by', and we shall sometimes use '//' to mean 'is followed immediately by'.

From our assumption (above) of volleys we may see that Pavlov is certainly justified in saying that the strength of the conditioned stimulus will be important since, very simply, the more intense each stimulus is, the stronger will be the association, provided they become associated at all.

We might next try to compare Guthrie and Pavlov with respect to motivation. Here we are in agreement with Pavlov in believing that a motivational system must selectively reinforce the conditioning (associative) process. Guthrie maintains that motivation is not of primary, but of secondary importance. Unfortunately Guthrie's position over reinforcement is very vague, and something like Skinner's in its adherence to operational (sometimes called positivistic) tendencies (Mueller and Schoenfeld, 1954). In experimental psychology this usually means that the attempt has been made merely to restate observed results, with little or no interpretation, and therefore with little use for theoretical terms. It is this consideration that hinders a detailed analysis of the situation, but it does look as if Guthrie and Pavlov could both be talking of the same logical net, with a difference in interpretation (their difference is in their theory language), at least as far as we have gone.

According to Mueller and Schoenfeld (1954, pp 368–9), Guthrie disputed with Pavlov about the importance of pairings in conditioning, Guthrie insisting upon the importance of the temporal relation between the conditioned stimulus and response. The above writers show the doubtful nature of these conclusions, and though from our logical net point of view the association is important, it seems perhaps to be less fundamental than that between the conditioned stimulus and the unconditioned stimulus. If $A \rightarrow A'$ and $B \rightarrow B'$ are two unconditioned reflexes, and A is to be the conditioned stimulus with respect to B, then $A \rightarrow B$ and $A \rightarrow B'$. But clearly $A \rightarrow B$ is false in that, although the association is between A and B, A will yield the response to B, which is B', and therefore what occurs is actually $A \rightarrow B'$. This is perhaps the source of a misunderstanding since, in a sense, $A \rightarrow B$ and $A \rightarrow B'$ are both vital connections that will necessarily go together.

Consider for a moment the case of language in humans: A is a word whose reference is B, and the response to the name A or to the referent B (these are not necessarily identical, hence our use of $(AB)'$ in our B-

circuits) is similar. It seems reasonable, though, to argue that the 'fundamental' connection, in some sense is between A and B and not A and B'.

We cannot take this comparison any further now, but we may return to their explanations later, in the discussion of anticipatory responses. Up to now we might say that the differences between Pavlov and Guthrie are largely due to lack of detailed analysis, but there is one more point: in order to explain certain aspects of learning it seems important to make a firm distinction between items *already learned* and those *being learned*, and this, at any rate, Guthrie does not seem to do.

From the operational point of view, the principles of Guthrie and Pavlov are virtually indistinguishable, but Pavlov might be preferred for the reasons stated, i.e. it would appear that the principles of Pavlov involve the necessary generalizability. On the other hand there will be the suggestion that this includes only a limiting case of behaviour.

Before any more can be said about the principle of substitution, a brief review must be made of the law of effect. This is invoked as a principle of reinforcement, in the context of instrumental conditioning, where emphasis is placed upon the consequences of certain activities. One should perhaps start by giving Thorndike's original definition of this law (Thorndike, 1911):

> Of several responses made to the same situation those which are accompanied or closely followed by 'satisfaction' to the animal will, other things being equal, be more firmly connected with the situation so that, when it recurs, they will be more likely to recur; those which are accompanied or closely followed by 'discomfort' to the animal, other things being equal, will have their connections with that situation weakened, so that, when it recurs, they will be less likely to occur. The greater the satisfaction or discomfort, the greater the strengthening or weakening of the bond.

This principle is clearly bound up with 'rewards' and 'punishments', again involving us in the dangers of circularity (Postman, 1947; Meehl, 1950).

We must just remind the reader at this point that the law of effect is explicitly incorporated in the design of the automaton in the form of an M-system which is to be interpreted as a motivational system that selectively reinforces associations in terms of the law of effect. This fact does not, however, exclude *substitution* and *expectancy* as appropriate principles to explain behaviour, as we shall see.

The law of effect has sometimes been criticized as being 'circular'. Meehl has argued that the law of effect *need* not necessarily involve us in any circularity in either of two senses he gives to the word 'circular'. It is a legitimate form of definition, analogous to Newton's definition of Force, or Hooke's law in physics. Two versions of the law of effect are quoted by Meehl; one he calls the weak law and the other the strong law.

The weak law states:

(1) All reinforcers are transituational (a transituational reinforcement law states, 'The stimulus S on schedule M always increases the strength of any learning response'). A definition of 'learning' is needed here.

The strong law states:

(2) Every learned increment in response strength requires the operation of a transituational reinforcer.

In his discussion, Meehl says that the law of effect is not circular in either of two ways that 'circular' can be interpreted, (1) the term defined in terms which are themselves defined in terms of the original term, and (2) proofs which make use of the probandum. He further states that the Skinner–Spence type of definition of effect is clearly immune from these pitfalls. The Skinner version is as follows:

> A reinforcing stimulus is defined as such by its power to produce the resulting change. There is no circularity about this; some stimuli are found to produce the change, others not, and they are classified as reinforcing and non-reinforcing accordingly.

Now we can begin to see the full force of our concession in avoiding circularity. We are to equate learning with performance in a positivistic manner, or certainly to regard 'reinforcement' as applying strictly to performance in a simple stimulus–response (S–R) system; and now one is pushed into the difficulty of explaining the data which come under the heading of 'latent learning' and 'place learning'. Skinner introduces theoretical terms for such purposes: 'reflex reserve', 'secondary reinforcement', and a distinction between *operant* and *respondent* behaviour. This last distinction attempts to distinguish between behaviour that is *emitted* and behaviour that is *elicited*.

With these aids, of course, it should be possible to give some model,

TABLE 1

Type of experiment	Abstracted process	Substitution	Effect	Expectancy
Classical conditioning	Homogeneous reinforcement	Substitution principle is directly applicable	Conditioning depends upon drive and heterogeneous reinforcement	Learning occurs only if response is part of a behaviour-route to a goal
Instrumental reward and escape	Heterogeneous reinforcement	Reward (or escape) terminates conditioned stimulus and the last response made remains conditioned	Effect principle as directly applicable	Reward (or escape) confirms expectancy; appears to be a spread of effect as a gradient of uncertainty regarding the probability that expected consequences will materialize
Instrumental avoidance and secondary reward	Derived reinforcement	Conditioned stimulus evokes anticipatory responses learned by substitution. These are the surrogates of expectancy	Heterogeneous reinforcement is necessary to produce and support derived reinforcement	Expectancy principle is directly applicable

although generally Skinner attempts no more than a restatement of experimental results. He makes two further points: that primary reinforcement and *habit strength* are not the same, rather it is the patterning of reinforcement that matters, and also the derived secondary reinforcement. All this leads to difficulties in assessing the relative value of reinforcers, and although it would not appear to be circular, it is necessarily arbitrary, and allows of little or nothing in the way of prediction. The law of effect itself is a basic issue in all learning theory, and in some form it seems inescapable.

The third principle of reinforcement is the principle of *expectancy*, and this is used in the context of instrumental conditioning to explain the varieties of conditioning known as 'avoidance' and 'secondary reward'. According to the principle of expectancy, reinforcement must be such as to confirm an expectancy (or expectation), and the expectancy itself is said to depend on previous learning. We can say that an *expectancy* is a theoretical term which implies the combination stimulus–response–stimulus, where the emphasis is 'forward looking' and illustrative of 'purposive' action.

We must now consider a little further this central problem of reinforcement. Broadbent (1958) doubts the validity of primary and secondary reinforcement as a principle of selection in learning. Many writers have suggested that novel or strong stimuli are themselves effective motivators (Berlyne, 1950; Miller and Kessen, 1952) and there is some neurophysiological support for this idea (Sharpless and Jasper, 1956).

We would re-emphasize here what we have already said about these matters, and in particular that in our logical net models we have assumed that motivation may initiate searching behaviour as readily as it may itself be built upon selective reinforcement. We would also want to include here curiosity as a drive, and certainly we must accept the fact that needs may be set up by conceptual means. On the associative principle, then, we may expect needs to occur because of an association with something else that leads to the organism producing searching activity. This is like saying that thinking about food will make you hungry, or rather, that it may do so under certain circumstances, the additional circumstances being that some need of an organic kind must also exist, although on its own it would not have led to drive reducing behaviour until later. It is the association that 'makes the person think about food' that leads to the production of searching activity.

It may seem that this extension of reinforcement spoils the Hullian theory, but in fact we would argue that it merely calls for an expansion.

To take up one particular point made against reinforcement theory by Broadbent (1958, pp. 245 *et seq.*), when he asks why the rat does not learn to go down 'blinds' in maze-running when the trial as a whole is rewarded, this is, clearly, not to be taken too seriously, since there are various ways out of the dilemma so presented. Perhaps the most obvious one is to remember that, while we may regard the total running of a maze as a trial that may be reinforced, the rat may well regard each bit of maze as something that is separately reinforced, and these blinds are of course non-reinforcing because they stop the rat, however hungry or curious or both he may be, from moving forward.

In fact no great problem really exists here since the selective nature of learning can only be explained in terms of selective reinforcement, wherever and however that principle is to be applied. The problem is, to make the details of its application clear, and to explain why a degree of stability occurs in behaviour in spite of the vast range of possible stimulus–response connections. It is perhaps over this last point that we must add the amplifying effect of selection by attention to the mere application of secondary reinforcement.

Table 1 (page 202) illustrates well that the distinction between the various models of learning proposed is a matter of the theoretical terms used, and of their interpretation, and we are interested to know whether this implies a difference in the underlying model. We add two definitions to those already given; they are by Hilgard and Marquis.

(1) *Heterogeneous reinforcement.* The strengthening of a conditioned response through reinforcement which depends on a response which does not resemble the conditioned response. This is a characteristic of reward and escape learning, but not limited to it. A simple example would be the rewarding of a head movement by the presentation of a carrot.

(2) *Homogeneous reinforcement.* The strengthening of a conditioned response by reinforcement with an unconditioned stimulus which evokes activity similar to the conditioned response, required according to the substitutional principle. Here, a simple example would be the salivation of a dog leading to food. It is *homogeneous* in that the salivating is something normally connected with food, whereas in heterogeneous reinforcement, as we have seen, it may be completely unconnected.

Obviously, crucial experimental tests are necessary to distinguish the above systems if they are to be taken over in all-embracing fashion. Brogden (1939) has carried out an experiment that claims to discriminate between the principles of *effect* and *substitution*.

In this experiment dogs were trained in conditioned response technique, in pairing a bell and shock stimulus to get conditioned leg-withdrawal response, and rewarded with food when the correct response was made. Omission of the unconditioned stimulus (shock) on 1000 trials led to no extinction on conditioned withdrawal. This may be taken to favour the principle of effect as opposed to substitution in this situation, but whether on the strength of it one can be any nearer saying that the effect is more general than substitution is open to manifest doubts. In fact, one can remind oneself again that the attempt is to distinguish between different theoretical terms, and that only. The above table does not disagree over performance, but only on the constructed theory designed to explain it.

It will be well to note what is involved here. Different sorts of experimental situations promote different sorts of behaviour, and these can be categorized as in Table 1. The scientists's problem is to find the common elements, and integrate such a set of elements into a theory which covers each type as a special case of a general theory; and while as yet this may or may not be possible, it is certainly necessary at some stage if there is to be a scientific theory of behaviour. In much experiments it is always being assumed that *individual difference* as a variable is cloaked by *general similarity*, i.e. that individual variation is markedly less than the factors in common, in the particular aspect of behaviour being considered. If this were not so, it would be almost impossible to have a science of behaviour; or at any rate a deterministic science in the sense of classical physics or chemistry.

Is it then possible to glimpse, at this stage, some integrative aspects in learning? Are the explanations of *substitution, effect* and *expectancy* really mutually exclusive? Do they refer to the same levels of behaviour? In this respect it is important to consider the comparative factor; have all the experiments been on the same sorts of organisms? This last point may be important when it is recalled that, in the early Gestalt–Watson differences over insight, and trial-and-error learning, Köhler's work was largely on apes, and Watson's on rats. It seems possible that the character of behaviour is more complex as we ascend the evolutionary scale, and this is another barrier to generalization.

No adequate statements can really be made until more of molar behaviour theory has been investigated, but it is instructive to consider the
Hilgard and Marquis table of comparisons further. According to this
table, classical conditioning can be *explained* by substitution; what, then,
is substitution? The definition given by Hilgard and Marquis (p. 76) is:

> A conditioned stimulus, present at the time that an original stimulus evokes a
> response, will tend on subsequent presentation to evoke that response.

In tentatively accepting Pavlov's rather than Guthrie's principle, it is
accepted that substitution occurs as a matter of degree, and stimulus is
defined independently of the conditions.

But Hilgard and Marquis try a further, and more adequate, definition
of substitution:

> An activity initiated by a stimulus, occurring at the same time as another activity
> which results in a response will tend on subsequent occurrences, to evoke that
> response.

The penultimate word 'that' in this definition may result in this being
dubbed a special case. Instead, *similar* (with conditions to be specified)
might be a step towards generality.

This point is brought out, we shall remember, in our logical net (see
Fig. 32, Chapter 5), where a distinction was made between either the
B'-element or the A'-element and $(AB)'$-element. Obviously this network
is constructed in terms of the distinction made independently and proves
nothing, except perhaps the simplicity and the naturalness with which the
response to $A.B$ should be somewhat different from that to A or B alone.

A comparison of the *effect* principle and the *substitution* principle of
conditioning might be taken to imply that homogeneous reinforcement is
a special case of heterogeneous reinforcement.

There is a brief reference to the expectancy theorist in the phrase,
'learning occurs only if response is part of a behaviour-route to a goal'.
What one knows is that a pattern of performance takes place, and from
this the theoretical term 'learning' is introduced, and the organism is
modified. The expectancy theorist's description in this case is identical
with the other two if only it is said that, in these very limited conditions,
the part of a behaviour-route is a limiting case, and happens here to be
the *whole* of the behaviour-route to the goal.

It may be tentatively suggested that the three explanations of classical conditioning are by no means as different as they may appear at first sight, encouraging further the notion that it is at the level of the theory language, rather than at the level of the model that differences occur. It seems perfectly possible that a *rapprochement* can be brought about between expectancy and effect, with substitution as a special case of either. The real point here is that when the vague verbal propositions of the various protagonists are tested by the construction of models, it becomes clear that their differences are differences of interpretation, or of philosophical directives that are being brought to bear on the subject. This belief is further encouraged by the fact that the molar type of explanation is based on overworked theoretical terms. They are, in fact, propositions that invite vagueness, and the maximum interference from the methodological or philosophical prejudices of the particular theorists and experimentalists.

Hull's theory of learning

In considering Hull's position in reinforcement theory, we shall draw on his restated postulational position (Hull, 1950). There is, of course, more detail given by Hull than it is proposed to discuss here, but the basic postulates III–IX which refer to the problem of reinforcement will be quoted immediately. Hull (1952) further modified his theory but only to a minor extent and these further modifications will not be considered here.

Postulate III

Primary reinforcement. Whenever an affector activity (R) is closely associated with a stimulus afferent impulse or trace (s') and the conjunction is closely associated with the diminution in the receptor discharge characteristic of a need, there will result an increment to a tendency for that stimulus to evoke that response.

Collorary (i). *Secondary motivation.* When neutral stimuli are repeatedly and consistently associated with the evocation of a primary or secondary drive and this drive undergoes an abrupt diminution, the hitherto neutral stimuli acquire the capacity to bring about the drive stimuli (S_D) which thereby become the condition (C_D) of a secondary drive or motivation.

Corollary (ii). *Secondary reinforcement.* A neutral receptor impulse which occurs repeatedly and consistently in close conjunction with a reinforcing state of affairs, whether primary or secondary, will itself acquire the power of acting as a reinforcing agent.

POSTULATE IV

The law of habit formation $(_sH_R)$. If reinforcements (N) follow each other at evenly distributed intervals, everything else constant, the resultant will increase in strength as a positive growth function of the number of trials according to the equation

$$_sH_R = 1 - 10^{-aN}$$

where a is a constant, as it will be in other formulae.

POSTULATE V

Primary motivation or drive (D). (A) A primary motivation (D), at least that resulting from food privation, consists of two multiplicative components, (1) the drive proper (D'), which is an increasing monotonic sigmoid function of h, and (2) a negation or inanition component (E) which is a positively accelerated monotonic function h decreasing from $1 \cdot 0$ to zero, i.e.

$$D = D' \times E.$$

(B) The functional relationship of drive (D) to one drive condition (food privation) is: from $h = 0$ to about 3 hr; drive rises in an approximately linear manner until the function abruptly shifts to a near horizontal, then to a concave-upwards course, gradually changing to a convex-upwards curve reaching a maximum of $12 \cdot 30$ at about $h = 59$, after which it gradually falls to the reaction threshold $(_sL_R)$ at around $h = 100$.

(C) Each drive condition (C_D) generates a characteristic drive stimulus (S_D) which is a monotonic increasing function of the state.

(D) At least some drive conditions tend partially to motivate into action habits which have been set up on the basis of different drive conditions.

Postulate VI

Stimulus-intensity dynamism (V). Other things constant, the magnitude of the stimulus intensity component (V) of reaction potential $(_sE_R)$ is a monotonic increasing logarithmic function of S, i.e.

$$V = 1 - 10^{-a \log s}.$$

Postulate VII

Incentive motivation (K). The incentive function (K) is a negatively accelerated increasing monotonic function of the weight (w) of food given as reinforcement, i.e.

$$K = 1 - 10^{-aw}.$$

Postulate VIII

Delay in reinforcement (J). The greater the delay in reinforcement, the weaker will be the resulting reaction potential, the quantitative law being

$$J = 10^{-jt}.$$

Postulate IX

The constitution of reaction potential $(_sE_R)$. The reaction potential $(_sE_R)$ of a bit of learned behaviour at any given stage of learning is determined (1) by the drive (D) operating during the learning process multiplied (2) by the dynamism of the signalling stimulus at response evocation (V_2), (3) by the incentive reinforcement (K), (4) by the gradient of delay in reinforcement (J), and (5) by the habit strength $(_sH_R)$, i.e.

$$_sE_R = D \times V \times K \times J \times {_sH_R},$$

where

$$_sH_R = {_sH_R} \times V_1$$

and V_1 is the stimulus intensity during the learning process.

Postulates I, II, IX (corollaries), XI, XII, XIII, XV, XVI, XVII and XVIII are not needed for our examination of Hull's theory of reinforcement; if needed by the reader, reference should be made to the original paper (Hull, 1950).

The three well-known questions of Postman (1947) still serve as a useful 'prop' for a discussion of reinforcement. They are:

(1) What is the agent responsible for reinforcement?
(2) What is it that is reinforced?
(3) What is the basic mechanism of reinforcement?

Wolpe (1950) aimed his solution directly at (3), and was criticized by Seward (1950) for having oversimplified the problem; he found, indeed, that Wolpe's theory was lacking in cogency. Seward returned to an examination of (1) and (2), which appeared to him to be of first importance. He recognized the many-meaninged nature of the term 'reinforcement', and he built on Meehl's (1950) definition to give the following definition:

> When a stimulus change X, following a response R to a situation S, increases the probability of R to S, X is called a *reinforcer*, and its presentation is called a *reinforcement*.

It will be noticed that this is much more general than Hull's definition (postulate III), and admirably defines the activity of the M-system in our logical net (Chapter 5).

Let us now proceed to Hull's new system. The most striking change is the clear-cut separation between learning and performance. A comparison between Hull's old and new definitions of both $_sH_R$ and $_sE_R$ illustrate the matter.

OLD DEFINITIONS

$$_sH_R = (1 - e^{-iN})(1 - e^{-kw})e^{-jt}e^{ut}$$
$$_sE_R = f(_sH_R) \times f(D).$$

NEW DEFINITIONS

$$_sH_R = 1 - 10^{-aN},$$

$$_sE_R = D \times V \times K \times J \times {}_sH_R,$$

and substituting for K, J, and $_sH_R$ we get:

$$_sE_R = DV(1 - 10^{-kw})10^{-jt}(1 - 10^{-iN}).$$

The resemblance between the old definition of $_sH_R$ and the new definition of $_sE_R$ is obvious. Omitting e^{-ut}, and replacing e by 10, and lastly, put w for W, and the equations are identical. It is clear that K and J no longer enter the equation for $_sH_R$, but they do directly enter $_sE_R$, thus allowing for sudden changes in performances. Seward has neatly demonstrated this point (Seward, 1950).

Now these brief statements must suffice to show that Hull's revision has had the effect of making $_sE_R$, rather than $_sH_R$, the principal variable affected by reinforcement. This was an attempt to meet the criticisms of the neo-Pavlovian S-R theories—made by the expectancy theorists—to the effect that the law of effect applies to performance rather than to learning. The result, then, has been to bring the Hull theory much nearer to the Tolman theory; but we shall be able to see this much more clearly after our review of Tolman.

For Hull, the basis of learning is still the strengthening of S-R bonds, although the actual relationships between the theoretical terms which cover the internal variation have now been changed. It is possible that the problems of *latent learning* are now more susceptible to treatment, and the theory has probably gained in generality and flexibility. However, there is still the question of testing the theory, and that will have to be done before any detailed judgment can be made. One might guess *a priori* that no adequate definition of a theoretical term such as $_sH_R$ can be given as a function of N alone. It suggests an unlikely simplification, of the type associated with Guthrie's theory.

Furthermore, Seward has pointed out that it is at least unlikely that the present place of J and K in the definition of $_sE_R$ is adequate. Indeed, one can go further and question whether such a linearly related system of theoretical terms can adequately mirror the complexities of even relatively simple organisms' performances, under all circumstances, with anything approaching the necessary degree of approximation. The attempt seems thoroughly worth while but, with all its clarity and conciseness, the theory is still open to objections on the grounds of vagueness. The particular interpretation that one gives to 'response', for example, seems vital to the acceptance of the basis of the theory, and in particular, the definition of $_sH_R$ depends crucially on precisely what constitutes a trial, and so on.

Seward (1950) sees the difference between the Hull and Tolman theories as primarily a difference between the habit-builder (rS_G) and a 'mobilizer of demand' (Tolman, 1932), 'cathexis' (Tolman, 1934), or 'progression readiness' (Tolman, 1941). On the other hand, Meehl and MacCorquodale (1951) describe the ultimate non-verbal difference between Tolman and Hull as dependent on the notion of 'response'. In fact, to put it another way, the difference could be stated simply as: Tolman's theoretical terms are more *central* than Hull's. We shall maintain that the *only* difference is in the theory language, and not in the model at all.

Before we discuss Tolman's expectancy theory, we must remark that a formalization of Hull's earlier theory of behaviour has been undertaken by Fitch and Barry (1950) and—although we cannot discuss this formalization here—it takes Hull's theory one stage nearer to the sort of precision we need, for it is a model of the process implied by the learning theory and, although applied to the older Hull theory, it makes it easier to see what sort of blueprint is explicitly entailed by Hull's theory language.

Tolman's theory

Tolman's system will be briefly described. His work has not been systematically stated nor, as yet, put into postulational form, although MacCorquodale and Meehl (1951) have proposed a provisional set of postulates for it.

Let us first outline Tolman's theory in simple terms. The core of his theory, and the equivalent proposition to reinforcement, is the setting up of an expectancy; this is a central theoretical term. Tolman himself talks in terms of *strip maps*, and it is clear that some sort of internal mapping is, in fact, envisaged although as Spence (1950) has pointed out, this map-control-room vs. telephone switchboard way of comparing Tolman and Hull is merely a matter of colourful metaphor, and not relevant to a genuine comparison.

The important points have been impinged on by MacCorquodale and Meehl (1954). They point out that there are certain important aspects of behaviour which are not *necessary* to an expectancy theory, including 'Gestalt-configural stress', 'perceptual field stress', discontinuity in discrimination learning', and perhaps more surprisingly, the distinction between 'learning and performance'.

The essential difference claimed for Tolman's theory is in the fact that it is an *S–S*, rather than an *S–R*, theory. Tolman's system anticipates increments in learning other than by an *S*-then-*R* sequence actually run off in performance. The basic definition of *expectancy* has postulates, as suggested by Meehl and MacCorquodale, for the introduction of an expectancy postulate. These are essentially tentative. The logical net model can, of course, be equally effective in dealing with *S–S* as with *S–R* relations.

p. 1. *Mnemonization:* The occurrence of the sequence $S_1 \to R_1 \to S_2$ (the adjacent members being in close temporal contiguity) results in an increment in the strength of an expectancy $(S_1R_1S_2)$. The strength increases as a decelerated function of the number of occurrences of the sequence. The growth rate is an increasing function of the absolute value of the valence of S_2. If the termination by S_2 of the sequence $(S_1 \to R_1)$ is random with respect to non-defining properties of S_1, the asymptote of strength is $\leqslant$ relative frequency of P of S_2 following $S_1 \to R_1$ (i.e. a pure number). How far this asymptote is below P is a decelerated function of the delay between the inception of R_1 and the occurrence of S_2.

p. 2. *Extinction:* The occurrence of a sequence $S_1 \to R_1$, if not terminated by S_2, produces a decrement in the expectancy if the objective S_2-probability has been 1·00 and the magnitude of this decrement is an increasing function of the valence of S_2 and the current strength of $(S_1R_1S_2)$. Such a failure of S_2 when P has been $= 1$ is a *disconfirmation* provided $(S_1R_1S_2)$ was non-zero. For cases where the S_2-probability has been $< 1·00$, if this objective probability P shifts to a lower P', and remains stable there, the expectancy strength will approach some value $\leqslant P'$ asymptotically.

p. 3. *Primary stimulus generalization:* When an expectancy $(S_1R_1S_2)$ is raised to some strength, expectancies sharing the R_1 and S_2 terms and resembling it on the elicitor side will receive some strength, this generalization strength being a function of the similarity of their elicitors to S_1. The same is true of extinction of $(S_1R_1S_2)$.

p. 4. *Inference:* The occurrence of a temporal contiguity S_2S^* when $(S_1R_1S_2)$ has non-zero strength, produces an increment in the strength of a new expectancy $(S_1R_1S^*)$. The induced strength increases as a decelerated function of the number of such contiguities. The asymptote is the strength of $(S_1R_1S_2)$ and the growth rate is an increasing decelerated function of the absolute valence of S^*. The presentation of S_2 without S^* weakens such an induced expectancy $S_1R_1S^*$. The decrement is greater if the failure of S^* occurs as the termination of the sequence $S_1 \rightarrow R_1 \rightarrow S$ than if it occurs as a result of presentation of S_2 without S^* but not following an occurrence of the sequence.

p. 5. *Generalized inference:* The occurrence of a temporal contiguity S_2S^* produces an increment in the strength of an expectancy $S_1R_1S^*$ provided that an expectancy $S_1R_1S_2'$ was at some strength and the expectandum S_2' is similar to S_2. The induced strength increases as a decelerated function of the number of such contiguities. The asymptote is a function of the strength of $S_1R_1S_2'$ and the difference between S_2 and S_2'. The growth rate to this asymptote is an increasing decelerated function of the absolute valence of S^*.

p. 6. *Secondary cathexis:* The contiguity of S_2 and S^* when S^* has a valence $|V|$ produces an increment in the cathexis of S_2. The derived cathexis is an increasing decelerated function of the number of contiguities and the asymptote is an increasing decelerated function of $|V|$ during the contiguities, and has the same sign as the V of S^*. The presentation of S_2 without S^*, or with S^* having had its absolute valence decreased, will produce a decrement in the induced cathexis of S_2.

p. 7. *Induced elicitor-cathexis:* The acquisition of valence by an expectandum S_2 belonging to an existing expectancy $(S_1R_1S_2)$ induces a cathexis in the elicitor S_1, the strength of the induced cathexis being a decelerated increasing function of the strength of the expectancy and the absolute valence of S_2.

p. 8. *Confirmed elicitor-cathexis:* The confirmation of an expectancy $(S_1R_1S_2)$, i.e. the occurrence of the sequence $(S_1 \rightarrow R_1 \rightarrow S_2)$ when $(S_1R_1S_2)$ is of non-zero strength, when S_2 has a positive valence, produces an increment in the cathexis of the elicitor S_1.

This increment in the elicitor-cathexis by *confirmation* is greater than the increment which would be *induced* by producing a valence in S_2 when the expectancy is at the same strength as that reached by the present confirmation.

p. 9. *Valence:* The valence of a stimulus S^* is a multiplicative function of the correlated *need D* and the *cathexis C^** attached to S^* (applies only to cases of positive cathexis).

p. 10. *Need strength:* The need (D) for a cathected situation is an increasing function of the time-interval since satiation for it.

Upon present evidence, even basic questions of monotony and acceleration are unsettled for the alimentary drives of a rat, let alone other drives and other species. There is no very cogent evidence that all or even most 'needs' rise as a function of time since satiation, although this seems frequently assumed. Even the notion of satiation itself, in connection with 'simple' alimentary drives, presents great difficulties.

p. 11. *Cathexis:* The cathexis of a stimulus situation S^* is an increasing decelerated function of the number of contiguities between it and the occurrences of the consummatory response.

The asymptote is an increasing function of the need strength present during these contiguities. (There may, however, be some innately determined cathexis.)

p. 12. *Activation:* The reaction potential $_sE_R$ of a response R_1 in the presence of S_1 is a multiplicative function of the strength of the expectancy $(S_1 R_1 S_2)$ and the valence (retaining sign) of the expectandum. There are momentary oscillations of reaction-potential about this value $_sE_R$, the frequency distribution being at least unimodal in form. The oscillation of two different $_sE_R$'s are treated as independent, and the response, which is momentarily 'ahead' is assumed to be emitted.

Add to this the fact that Tolman regards 'Maintenance Schedule' (M), 'appropriate goal object' (G), 'mode of stimuli' (S), 'type of motor response' (R), 'cumulative numbers of trials' $\Sigma(OBO)$, 'pattern of preceding maze units' (P), as the set of independent variables. The equivalent intervening variables are, 'demand', 'appetite', 'differentiation', 'motor skill', 'hypotheses' (which he later called 'expectancies'), and 'biases'. The relation of the independent and intervening variables is a function of 'heredity', 'age', 'previous training', and 'endocrine, etc., states'. Finally, there is 'performance', which is a complicated function (generally non-linear) of these three sets of variables.

Tolman regards his intervening variables as in need of defining experiments. The trouble here is that it does not appear possible to apply the usual form of linear experimental situation to define variables that will generally be non-linear. It is probable, rather, that the so-called intervening variables should actually be regarded as full *logical constructs*, as Tolman himself later seemed to suggest (Tolman, 1952).

Now a comparison of Hull's theory with Tolman's shows that there is, in fact, precious little difference between them. Indeed, it is possible that the theories are interchangeable, provided a suitable interpretation is given to the word 'response' by the S–R school. If, however, they insist on interpreting this as an effector event, then it does seem to constitute a definite non-verbal difference (Meehl and MacCorquodale, 1951; MacCorquodale and Meehl, 1954). From the cybernetic point of view our suspicion is again that the differences are at the level of the theory language; it is the same sequence of events, S_1–R_1–S_2–R_2–... that is being dealt with, only the one takes S–R, and the other S–R–S, as the basic unit.

Tolman's system, generally, is a molar behaviourism, as is Hull's, but it tends to emphasize *purpose* in the theory construction in a way that Hull's theory does not. In Tolman there is no direct use of reinforcement, and in place of it we find the notion of expectancy based on sign-learning (cf. *expectancy* and *effect* earlier in this chapter). The strength of Tolman's theory can be seen most favourably in three situations: (1) Reward-expectancy, (2) Place learning, and (3) Latent learning.

Tinklepaugh's (1928) experiments with monkeys are a classical illustration of (1). A monkey saw a banana placed under one of two containers, and was then taken away. On returning later he showed accuracy of choice. When a lettuce was substituted for the banana in the monkey's absence, he exhibited searching activity on his return.

The place-learning experiments, of which MacFarlane's work (MacFarlane, 1930) may be regarded as typical, tend to show that the actual process of running a maze is not a chain of S–R acts, but involves a knowledge of the maze-as-a-whole—a sort of *insight*. Place-learning is exemplified by an organism learning to go to a particular spatial location X, say, regardless of the route taken.

Latent learning supplies perhaps the strongest experimental evidence in support of Tolman's position as opposed to the older Hull theory (Blodgett, 1929; Tolman and Honzik, 1930), and this will be reviewed separately.

A further experiment carried out by Krechevsky (1932a, 1932b) must suffice as an example of the type of *hypothesis* theory that is characteristic of the expectancy or *S–S* theorist, as opposed to the *S–R* theorist.

This particular example of Krechevsky's work is an analysis of individual rat performance. The experimental situation involved the training of rats to discriminate between a path containing a hurdle and an equally lighted path containing no hurdle. A multiple discrimination box was used, and the performance was documented in terms of number of errors, number of right turns, number of left turns, and number of terms in keeping with an alternating scheme. On statistical analysis, it seems that any response occurring above 73 per cent would almost certainly be a non-chance factor. The graph (Fig. 42) shows the cases of greater than 73 per cent response rate very clearly, and is therefore thought to constitute evidence for 'hypotheses'.

Krechevsky (1933a, 1933b) also avers that 'bright' rats use spatial hypotheses predominantly, whereas 'dull' rats are more prone to use non-spatial hypotheses (e.g. visual, in the particular experiment). Control rats appeared to be neutral in this situation. Krechevsky (1935) further reports that the number of 'hypotheses' used by rats is decreased in discrimination learning. In the argument regarding bright and dull rats there exist the seeds of possible circularity in an objectionable sense.

The main fact about Krechevsky's work that will be of importance is the relation between learning and performance. Inevitably, the process is to observe performance, and make inferences about learning, and here the notion of hypotheses does, in fact, appear to fit very well.

Some attempts have been made to decide between *S–R* and *S–S* theory at the experimental level. Two examples will probably be sufficient illustration (Humphreys, 1939a, 1939b).

Humphreys carried out an experiment on eyelid conditioning in humans. Conditioned discrimination was thought to be more rapid when subjects knew which stimulus of a pair was to be positive, which negative, etc., rather than when experience was a necessary prelude to prediction. Humphreys showed that a random alternation of reinforcement and non-reinforcement led to a high level of conditioning, and a greater resistance to extinction than if reinforcement was 100 per cent.

He assumed that changing hypotheses accounted for this and, using humans in a study of verbal expectations, he appeared to get corroborative results. The actual study involved showing two lights, one at a

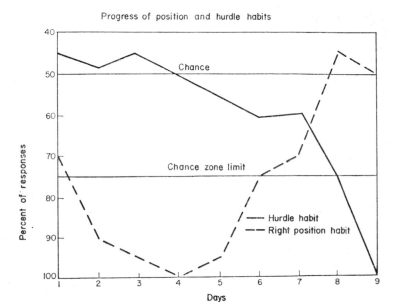

FIG. 42. EVIDENCE FOR HYPOTHESES IN A RAT. The rat was trained to
discriminate between two paths only one of which contained a hurdle to be
surmounted. The solid line represents the percentage of errors made on
successive days, while the broken line represents the right-turning response
of the subject. It should be observed that the right position habit occurs
with a frequency of from 70 to 100 per cent during the first 6 days of training. It then approaches a frequency that could be attributed to chance.
This suggests that the rat was guided by the hypothesis that a right turn
would solve the problem. This 'spatial hypothesis' was finally given up
in favour of the correct 'non-spatial hypothesis', which in fact means
that the correct path is the one with the hurdle. (After Krechevsky.)

time, and when one light was switched on, asking the subject whether
the other light would follow or not. Two groups were set up, and the
first group was always shown light 1 followed by light 2, while the second
group had a random distribution of light 2 or not light 2 after light 1.
The second group guessed at chance level which, so far, was to be expected. The next part was the extinction of these responses, and this was seen
to be much quicker in the first group. These experiments seem to favour
an expectancy theory; in fact, the resemblance to Krechevsky's 'hypotheses' will not be overlooked.

To return to the comparison of Tolman and Hull, one or two tentative statements may be made. Tolman tends to place emphasis on the organism dominating its environment, while for Hull, emphasis is placed on the environment's domination of the organism. It is only a matter of different emphasis, but this difference can be traced back to the differences in philosophical directives accepted by their two viewpoints. They are modern variations on the well-known mechanistic vs. teleological controversy in biology, and their positions have been modified to such an extent they have arrived at situations which differ by only a very little, if at all.

Partial reinforcement, latent learning and some other variables

Before it is possible to complete an assessment of molar theories from a cybernetic point of view, it is essential to consider some of the other principal variables and theoretical terms in the molar psychological field. It is intended to start with 'partial reinforcement', and to make considerable use of the summary made by Jenkins and Stanley (1950) in the discussion. For reference purposes it might be convenient to give a working definition of 'partial reinforcement'.

Partial reinforcement − *df*. Reinforcement which is given on only a certain percentage of trials (or following responses). Thus the limiting cases are: total 'reinforcement'−100 per cent, and no 'reinforcement'− 0 per cent.

In partial reinforcement, interest will be centred on a brief summary of the experimental evidence, and a more detailed study of the suggested theories. Platonov is one of the first experimenters credited with partial reinforcement experiments. In one series of his experiments a conditioned response was *maintained* by application of the unconditioned stimulus on the first trial only of each day. Pavlov, Wolpe and Egon Brunswick carried out early experiments in this field, and Egon Brunswick was led to his interesting probability theory of discrimination (Brunswick, 1939, 1943, with Tolman, 1935).

The most important experiments would appear to be those carried out by Skinner, and—since in this sort of work it is not humanly possible to investigate each and every case separately for slight variations in design—it will be assumed that a certain degree of generalizability is possible, and Skinner's work will be regarded as, largely, typical. At this point it is important to notice that, to him, the *operations* are the principal concern, and not such theoretical terms as 'reflex reserve', which are invoked to explain them.

Skinner's experimental work is on rats. The first experiments (1933) compared lever-pressing performance following a single reinforcement, and following 250 reinforcements. He found that the relationship was, at least, not a linear one.

The actual performance demanded of the rats was that of lever-pressing, and the reinforcement was the pellet of food received from the apparatus.

Using essentially the same lever-pressing apparatus, Skinner has shown two different sorts of partial reinforcement. The first, which he calls periodic reinforcement, involves the use of reinforcers at standard intervals of time (Skinner, 1938). This implies a constant amount of reinforcement per unit of time, and leads to a constant response performance. Over a considerable range, Skinner found a roughly constant response rate of 18 to 20 responses. From this is derived the notion of 'extinction ratio'. (*Extinction ratio = df.* the uniform number of responses per reinforcement.) This is supposed to be a measure of learning under varying conditions of drive. Parenthetically, it may be noticed that the greater maintenance of response-rate observed in partial reinforcement is accounted for by Skinner simply by employing a theoretical term, 'reflex reserve'.

In Skinner's second type of partial reinforcement, which he called 'reinforcement-at-a-fixed-ratio', the pellet is delivered after a standard number of responses, instead of after a standard interval of time, and the result is a very high response-ratio, the extinction ratio changing from 20 : 1 in Skinner's first type I situation, to 200 : 1 in this. Two sets of graphs will illustrate these well-known results.

This work does require some explanation, but before this is discussed we must devote some attention to more general considerations in the design of partial reinforcement experiments. 'Frequency' and 'pattern' may be seen to be at least two of the most important variables, i.e. continuity of reward and regularity of reward are the variables that appear to be most important, and this has been illustrated by Skinner. However, there are two kinds of experimental situation which need to be distinguished: (1) those where the responding is independent of the experimenter and of the environment, circumstances which cover both types

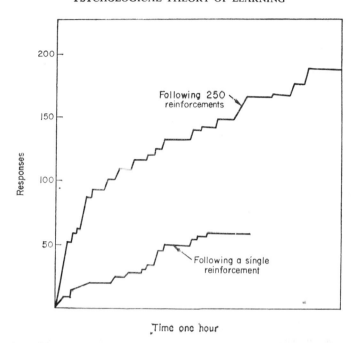

Time one hour

FIG. 43. EXTINCTION OF LEVER PRESSING BY RATS. The graph illustrates simply the different amount of responding after one and after 250 reinforcements.

of Skinner's conditioning, and called, after Jenkins and Stanley, 'free responding', and (2) experiments where trials are involved, and there is control of opportunity to respond, e.g. mazes, multiple-response situations, etc. (this is referred to as 'trial responding'). (1) and (2) differ with respect to a time schedule. Table 2 (Jenkins and Stanley, 1950) is useful in distinguishing the various cases.

It will be noted in these experiments that initial training has always been on reinforcement, and only subsequently has partial reinforcement been introduced. Keller (1940) carried out an experiment in this field. A group of rats were continously reinforced for one period, and then were split into two groups, one of them being subjected first to continuous and then to periodic reinforcement, and the other group being given the same reinforcements, but in the opposite order. Using resistance to extinction

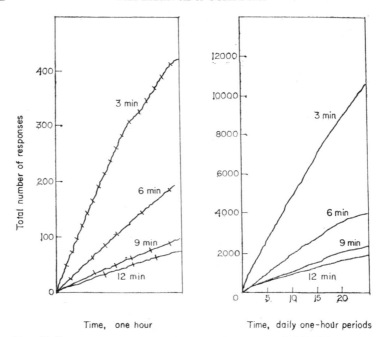

FIG. 44. RESPONSES WITHIN ONE AND WITHIN REPEATED SESSIONS OF PERIODIC
REINFORCEMENT. In the left-hand figure, the situation was one in which a
pellet of food was delivered every 3, 6, 9 and 12 min. respectively. The
more frequent the reinforcement the more rapid the rate of responding. In
the right-hand figure is shown the *cumulative* record over several of the
rats depicted in the left-hand figure.

as a measure, the second group was far superior for the first five minutes
only.

Apart from these difficulties, and suggestions of further complexity,
there are other problems too detailed to enumerate, such as *inter-trial
interval, massed* and *spaced* training, and the complex relationship
between number of trials and number of reinforcements. For example,
a group that has been partially reinforced can be compared with a continuously reinforced group, with respect to number of trials or number of
reinforcements, but not both. Further, there is the variability of response-
strength at the end of learning to be considered, in comparing resistance
to extinction in continuous and in partially reinforced groups. These, of
course, are only the major aspects of the problem.

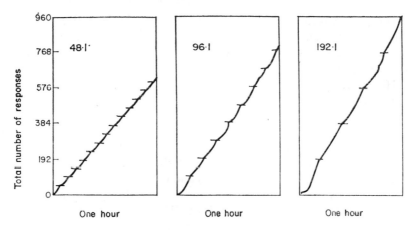

FIG. 45. RESPONSES WITH REINFORCEMENT AT A FIXED RATIO. Responses from individual rats reinforced every 48, 96 and 192 responses. The point of reinforcement is indicated by the short horizontal lines.

TABLE 2

Variations of reinforcement	Situation			
	Free-responding	Trials		
		Simple response	Alternative response	Multiple responses
Time Regular Irregular	Periodic reinforcement Aperiodic reinforcement	Time variation not ordinarily used		
No. of responses Regular Irregular	Fixed ratio reinforcement Random ratio reinforcement	Fixed ratio reinforcement Random ratio reinforcement		

One point worth noting especially is that made by Jenkins and Stanley, that there is a marked skewness in various response sets, especially with respect to extinction, which implies that the use of many standard statistical methods is invalid.

However, to put it concisely, it may be said that the problems of partial reinforcement may be placed under five headings: (1) Acquisition, (2) Performance, (3) Maintenance, (4) Retention and (5) Extinction. As far as acquisition is concerned, the general findings are that there is little apparent difference between the continuous and the partial groups, although the former appear to have a slight advantage. The same state of affairs appears to pertain in (2), (3) and (4), and it is only in extinction that a serious reversal is apparent. Here the partial group were significantly ahead of the continuous group. These results, briefly stated as they are, require explanation. How are they explained by molar psychologists?

In the first place there are certain, as it were, sub-difficulties. Skinner's work on reinforcement at a fixed ratio (see Figs. 5, 6 and 7) shows oddities in graphing that appear to call for explanation on three scores: (1) the very high rate of responding, (2) the delay after reinforcement, and (3) the acceleration between reinforcements. Skinner explains these by saying that each lever-pressing in the early part of a run acts as a secondary reinforcement (this is a very important principle that requires further analysis). (2) is explained by the 'negative factor' associated with reinforcements, and the weakening of what Skinner calls the *reflex reserve*, and (3) is a function of (1) and (2). This sort of explanation by appeal to theoretical terms and functional relationships between them is typical of molar theory, and is often difficult to test. It is these interrelated theoretical terms that we are hoping to model more adequately by the use of logical nets. It should be mentioned in passing that Trotter (1957) demonstrated a major weakness in Skinner's experiments by showing that 'responses' are arbitrarily defined, and that semi-responses made by the rats were simply not counted.

It is not clear that a straight application of *S–R* theory could account for partial reinforcement. The fact that a *reward* strengthens a response, and omission of *reward* weakens it, would be insufficient to account for partial reinforcement, since it would fail to account for the greater resistance to extinction following partial training. Skinner, Sears, and Hull have formulated explanations in terms of secondary reinforcement, although Sears pointed out that the definition of response could be widened to meet the difficulty, and that our treatment of units of behaviour may be at fault. This may be true, but it does not lead to an adequate explanation of the behaviour. Miller and Dollard (1941) have suggested that greater resistance to extinction may be expected to occur when unrewarded behaviour is ultimately followed by a reward, and their argument is essentially based on a gradient of generalization.

Mowrer and Jones (1943) accept the fact that a response removed in time more than 30 sec from a reward is not reinforced, and yet they accept an explanation in terms of Perin's 'temporal gradient of reward', even though intervals far above 30 sec have been found efficacious.

Jenkins and Stanley (1950) make this comment on the above:

> It would seem that some mechanism of the response-unit variety is operating, otherwise, behaviour could not be maintained when reinforcements occur only once in nine minutes, or every 192 responses. A temporal gradient restricted to strengthening only behaviour occurring not more than 30 seconds before reward is, at best, an incomplete account. A temporal gradient may well be one of the factors interacting with several others, but clearly it cannot explain many of the findings that Mowrer and Jones fail to mention.

Sheffield and Tenmer (1950) have compared the acquisition, and extinction, of a running response under the escape and avoidance procedures, and point out that extinction practically always involves a change in the cue patterns, present in training, while escape training does not permit the conditioning of the consequences of failure to respond. Thus, correctly, their theory predicts greater response strength for escape procedure in training, but greater resistance to extinction following avoidance conditioning.

The modern Hull interpretation of partial reinforcement would appear to depend wholly on secondary reinforcement, and, in this context, it will be of special relevance to refer once more to the work of K. W. Spence. Spence (1947, 1950, 1951, 1952) has made the assumption that the gradient of reinforcement is a special case of the stimulus generalization gradient. He goes on to place emphasis on the vital nature of secondary reinforcement. Now secondary motivation (III (i) in Hull's newer postulate system) is said to arise when neutral stimuli are repeatedly and consistently associated with the evocation of a drive, and this drive undergoes an abrupt diminution. Secondary reinforcement (III (ii)) occurs when a neutral receptor impulse occurs repeatedly, and consistently, in close conjunction with a reinforcing state. The *secondary rein-forcing* is the fractional antedating goal response r_{SG}, and this is apparently conditioned, in the Hull view, to the after effects of non-reinforcement in the stimulus compound, during training.

Sheffield (1949) goes on to argue that in extinction following partial reinforcement the stimulus situation, by virtue of generalization, is more like conditioning than after 100 per cent reinforcement. In extinction, as opposed to conditioning, the cue pattern is changed greatly for the 100 per cent group, but is reinstated for the partial reinforcement group.

It is, perhaps, enough at this stage to have isolated partial reinforcement, and noted that explanations can be offered by the representatives of both Hull and Tolman, and also by Skinner, that the differences are not very marked, albeit perhaps it may be thought that Hull's is the most cogent form of explanation.

In terms of logical nets the problem of partial reinforcement can be highlighted in an interesting way. We may ask the direct question: will the automaton which we have so far outlined (Chapter 5) exhibit the properties manifested under partial reinforcement? The answer appears to be 'yes', subject to a condition to be stated.

We shall assume that we are dealing with single stimuli inputs, and that reinforcement is occurring only on 1 trial in n; then the belief which is confirmed is that reinforcement will occur in every nth trial, hence the process of disconfirmation will take longer to occur and the response rate will vary with respect to the belief acquired and the *value* attributed to the stimulus.

Clearly, a stimulus may be made more valuable by its relative rarity; the conjunction-count will therefore be greater for a rare (though valuable) stimulus than it will be for a regular stimulus; but to achieve this end we must assume that the degree of need-reduction is greater when the stimulus is more infrequent. It is easy to see that this can be arranged in a logical net system in many different ways.

Latent learning

In the subject of latent learning, now to be briefly considered, there is a difficulty that does not wholly apply to partial reinforcement. There is, indeed, a doubt as to whether latent learning actually takes place or not—

that is, within the definitions framed by some workers, and both Maltzman (1952) and Kendler (1952), in criticism of Donald Thistlethwaite's summary of latent learning (1951), were suspicious of the evidence. Maltzman suspects the statistical evidence in the Blodgett design, and regards the criterion for 'latent learning' as inadequate, and he proposes an alternative interpretation. The Haney design is also criticized.

It would be as well to enumerate the designs for these types of experiment before following up the Maltzman–Kendler comments. Thistlethwaite classifies latent learning into four groups:

(1) Type I. The Blodgett variety, in which the rats are given a series of unrewarded, or mildly rewarded, trials in a maze, and then a relevant goal object is introduced before further trials take place (Blodgett, 1929).
(2) Type II. The organisms are allowed to explore the maze prior to a trial in which a relevant goal object is used (Haney type, 1931).
(3) Type III. Organisms (rats), which are satiated for food and water, are given trials in a maze, the pathways of which contain the goal objects for which the animals are satiated (Spence–Lippett type, 1940).
(4) Type IV. Organisms (rats), either hungry or thirsty, are placed in a maze with relevant and/or irrelevant goal objects. Rats are then satiated for formerly desired goal objects, and deprived of the previously undesired goal object (Kendler type, 1947).

Further, the term 'latent learning' has the twofold historical usage:

(1) Learning not manifest in performance scores.
(2) Learning that occurs under conditions of irrelevant incentive.

Returning to the question of existence, Maltzman has claimed that type I and type II (Blodgett and Haney types) do not reveal latent learning, and can be explained in terms of the Hull and Spence theory of reinforcement. It will be noticed immediately that there are two quite separate points here. Maltzman's argument appears to be that since there is improvement in performance in the unrewarded period, then any distinction is invalid, and he questions the statistical significance of the results. Later, however, it appeared to him that there was some confusion over the definition of latent learning, resulting apparently from the lumping together of the two separate propositions that: (1) latent learning is not revealed, and (2) the phenomenon revealed can be explained in terms of the Hull–Spence theory of reinforcement. No one, it should be noted, is averring that latent learning is not explicable in Hullian terms.

The Haney design is the one in which a group of hungry rats were permitted to explore a 14-unit T-maze for 4 days (18 hr per day), while a control group spent the same amount of time in a rectangular maze. In this first part of the experiment neither group was rewarded with food in the maze. Then both groups were run, hungry, in the T-maze for 18 days, and rewarded one trial per day. The experimental group having been allowed to explore the T-maze, had of course been able to acquire knowledge which had been denied to the control group, but since there was no statistical difference in performance, the result actually shows that learning can take place without a reward. There is, however, a point here, in that performance is taken to imply learning, and it is therefore presumed that it is possible to identify this in a negative sense. Without bringing out the points of Kendler's criticisms of Thistlethwaite in full, it may be said that there exists the usual doubt that the existence of latent learning is supported by his experiments, for he claims that these include all the stated conditions of latent learning, and yet do not show that it takes place.

Kendler does make a point of logic which is of interest to us. He says of both the Blodgett and the Tolman–Honzik experiments that they led to the conclusion that maze performance did not necessarily mirror maze learning, and he makes the point already mentioned, i.e. that in comparing the food and no-food groups, performance is taken as a measure of learning, whereas the same level of performance does not necessarily imply the same level of learning. This is a serious point, but it is possible that performance can be taken to be the same as learning if, and only if, the motivation and reward-value of the incentive are equivalent. This is precisely the reply that Thistlethwaite makes, and it is also implied in Tolman's writing. The important point is whether or not motivation can be sufficiently controlled, and the burden of proof for this lies with the experimenters. Thistlethwaite's replies to the criticism of Kendler and Maltzman are of interest (Thistlethwaite, 1952). He comments initially that reference to experimental evidence should end controversy. This is obviously over-optimistic in practice, since the results of experiments are rarely so precise as to allow of only one interpretation. His comment on the exclusion of untestable hypotheses is laudable, but not clear cut. He, moreover, appears to consider that the burden of proof, in the matter of Kendler's criticism of his so-called logical point, lies with Kendler, and with this it is, of course, impossible to agree.

The next step is a brief re-consideration of the theoretical interpretations of latent learning. The first point is that reinforcement may be introduced (i.e. defined) in such a way that it is always necessary to every performance, or that it may be independently defined, and thus may or may not be relevant to the behaviour under discussion. The particular convention adopted commits us to one of two very different interpretations of reinforcement; the first being Hullian in type, and the second Tolmanian. The position seems to be that if the hypothesis that reinforcement is necessary to *all* learning is granted, then it is necessary by definition, and the next step must be to show, by operational methods if possible, that such a definition is consistent with the observable facts. This would indeed appear to be an embarrassment to the old Hull S–R theory, but it is important to note that Hull's modified theory (Hull, 1950) might be said to make an explanation easier. There always remains, of course, the possibility that suitable sources of reinforcement may be found; for instance, in the Blodgett type experiment, curiosity and escape are, at the least, such possible sources. There is no need here to summarize this work in detail, as this has already been admirably done by Thistlethwaite (1951); it will therefore be sufficient for our purpose if a general statement is made.

Tolman's theory would appear to have no special difficulty in giving an account of latent learning, since it does not demand an S-then-R type behaviour; and although latent learning is an embarrassment to Hull's older theory, his modified theory (the modifications, one presumes, were brought about to cater for this very effect) can be made adequate by freeing both J and K from 'habit', i.e. by differentiating more sharply between learning and performance, the gap can then be bridged.

Other problems of learning

We shall now move away from the established theories of learning and, in considering some problems of learning theory with which these theories were not primarily concerned, see if our finite automaton can deal with them.

As far as latent learning is concerned, our automaton will, like Oettinger's programme (see Chapter 7), show just this characteristic, as indeed can any system with storage. The interesting question is as to whether we should regard latent learning as Russell (1957) does, and interpret it for the machine as 'unrewarded experience put to use later on'. As far as logical nets are concerned, this involves a decision as to whether or not every bit of information is recorded if and only if, say, it satisfies a need. Is it a matter of secondary reinforcement or not? This is perhaps less important than it once seemed, but we shall continue to suppose that information is not retained unless associated in some way with reinforcing activities; the question is really as to how remote the association can be.

Matrix representation of logical nets

We have already mentioned the use of matrices to represent logical nets. Unfortunately there do not seem to be important matrix properties which would allow us to restate the theory in terms of groups and other abstract algebraic forms; however, for the purposes of clarity of exposition, it is convenient to state the obvious fact that a matrix A made up of the numbers, 0, 1 and -1 can completely define the structure of any logical net; for example, Fig. 26 (Chapter 5) has a 'structure matrix', as it may be called, as follows:

$$
\begin{bmatrix}
0 & 0 & 1 & 1 & 0 & 1 & 0 & 1 \\
0 & 0 & 1 & -1 & 0 & 0 & 1 & 1 \\
0 & 0 & 0 & 0 & 1 & 0 & 0 & 0 \\
0 & 0 & 0 & 0 & -1 & 0 & 0 & 0 \\
0 & 0 & 0 & 0 & 1 & 0 & 0 & 1 \\
0 & 0 & 0 & 0 & 0 & 0 & 0 & 0 \\
0 & 0 & 0 & 0 & 0 & 0 & 0 & 0 \\
0 & 0 & 0 & 0 & 0 & 0 & 0 & 0
\end{bmatrix}
\tag{1}
$$

The form of such structure matrices is always

$$
\begin{bmatrix}
O & A & B \\
\hline
O & C & D \\
\hline
O & O & O
\end{bmatrix}
\tag{2}
$$

where the blocks are of input, inner and outer interconnections. The rows and columns are of course made up of elements $A, B, \ldots, N$.

It is also clear that for each moment of time these connections may be live or dead, which means that a matrix composed of 0's and 1's accompanying a structure matrix (sometimes called a 'status matrix') completely defines a logical net and its history. Such status matrices in one form have already been discussed in Chapter 4. Now we wish to add a further matrix, which we shall call a B-matrix, to add to our collection. This is mainly so that we can quickly refer to the associations or *beliefs* that occur in any logical net and let this matrix show the cumulative state of the associations, so that a positive number in any position a_{ij} designates a belief that will be effective if any of its components fires, while a negative number in that position designates a belief that will not fire unless all the components are present.

This particular B-matrix is consistent with the B-nets we have previously defined, but it should be emphasized that this particular arrangement depends solely on the connections, and the manner in which they are chosen. This point will be seen to be of the utmost importance when we consider the problem of extinction. This is perhaps also an appropriate moment to make the point that we are not committed to one particular form of connection; the problem is simply to make the connections—define the B-matrix—so that they are consistent with all observed behavioural phenomena.

In what follows it will also be seen that if A and B have occurred together more often than A and C, then when A is presented B is assumed, by which we mean that the automaton will respond with AB' and not AC'. In the same way ABC' is elicited when ABC occur together more often than all proper subsets of ABC.

Retroactive inhibition

Consider the following three lists of stimulus–response connections.

List 1	List 2	List 3
A-B	A-D	M-N
C-D	C-L	O-P
E-F	E-B	Q-R
G-H	G-J	S-T
I-J	I-H	U-V
K-L	K-F	W-X

and now consider the change in the B-matrix when List 1 is successfully learnt. Let us suppose, for simplicity, that the only B's affected are in the first row of the matrix, and if there is an increment of 1 for each occurrence, then after n trials (let us suppose that n is fairly large) the matrix will read:

$$\begin{bmatrix} n\ n\ \ldots\ n \\ o\ o\ \ldots\ o \\ -\ -\ -\ -\ - \\ o\ o\ \ldots\ o \end{bmatrix} \tag{3}$$

Now it is clear that there will be a great difference in the nature of the subsequent matrices according to whether list 2 or list 3 is next used. Let us suppose they are represented by the second and third rows respectively of the B-matrix, then they will appear exactly the same in that, after r trials, they will have the form of the matrix above, with either the second or third row filled with r's; but whereas in the case of list 2 the presence of the r's will be completely ineffective in producing response until $r > n$, in the other case it will be effective as soon as $r > 0$.

The reasons for the above are quite simple. The probability of a particular stimulus is given wholly by the previous experience of the system as reflected in the counting devices attached to the classification system. Thus, for associations like A-B, given A there will be a response B and therefore not D, whereas M will be responded to immediately by N since it has no other association.

The above argument, which simply says that a conditional probability system *of the type we have defined* will lead to *retroactive inhibition*, can be given two different interpretations in practice, according to whether or not it refers to the use of conditional probability in recognition (or perception) itself. In the perceptual case, the tied nature of associations giving the probabilities could be said merely to cause confusion as to the identity of the object perceived since, to put it simply, there would be many different physical objects with many of the same properties. Alternatively—and if one has to choose, this seems the more likely—it is the relation of consecutive perceived events (already composed of many subproperties) that become confused simply because they are similar in that some part of an association is already tied to another event.

The present discussion has been straightforward, but we must now turn to a more complex and more interesting question. Granted the above argument is correct—and this merely assumes that a conditional probability operates in a particular inductive manner—what are the means by which we can predict closely related phenomena? Let us first consider 'transfer of training'.

Transfer of training

Transfer of training is merely a way of describing the empirical fact that similar tasks have a degree of 'carry over'. It is a complementary fact to retroactive inhibition, and has been neatly summarized by Osgood (1949) in a simple geometrical model.

From the point of view of our machine model it is easy to see how transfer would occur. The interesting fact is that it could be as a result of either of the two well-known principles: (1) by virtue of some large task involving whole sequences of events, where two sequences had many common pairs, or (2) by virtue of stimulus generalization, which means that two sequences of events are treated as the same, or as being two subcases of some more general relation; this depends on the fact that our conditional probability machine will be capable of deriving consequences, by inductive and deductive processes, from the relations that are observed through its perceptual processes.

The first explanation is self-evident, but the second needs some elaboration. We should note, though, that here we have a case in which what have appeared as two rival explanations could both be appropriate to a learning machine; furthermore, they smack of the sort of distinction that might be made at the 'habit level' in the first case, and the more 'cognitive level' in the second.

Stimulus generalization

A further discussion of our second method in which transfer of training takes place means that we must look again at stimulus generalization. This, and the fact that certain events are classified together as if they were identical, must be a characteristic of any system, and it means that differences are either intentionally neglected or not observed. The only situation in which such generalization could be revealed or discard-

ed would be one in which the outcome of the generalization was unex-
pected or undesirable, and this would be revealed in its effect on the motivational system. Need-reduction would fail to take place, and the
necessary condition for registering a conjunction count (a positive association 'to be encouraged') in the machine would not occur.

Now it is obvious that what has been said does not tell us what any
particular automaton will generalize with respect to, at any time. In so
far as it is general, it will depend on *set* and *value* for the organism. Set
merely represents the fact that the probabilities associated with perception will interact with knowledge of context, which is simply saying that
the probability with respect to the perceptual process is never independent of its place in the temporal sequence of events; it is the conditional
probability over the larger interval that will lead the organism to expect
some particular outcome to its responses (this will particularly depend
on the machine's use of language). Value will arise in so far as different
stimulus–response activities will be associated with different degrees of
need-reduction (change in state of motivational system, or rather, rate of
change). This matter is obviously complicated, and no further discussion
of it will occur here.

We must also bear in mind that the automaton will have the capacity
to draw logical inferences, and again we can illustrate the principle only
by saying that within the machine two pairs of events may be seen, or
perceived, to be independent. Consider the following scheme of events
involving A, B, C and D, where the same letters primed imply organismic
responses to the molar stimulus of the same name:

$$A/B \qquad (4)$$

and

$$C/D \qquad (5)$$

and let us suppose again that '---/---' means 'is followed by'.

Now suppose B is *always* followed by C. This means that the relation
B/C is a *necessary* relation, necessary, that is, for the organism; it still
remains a problem to confirm that A/B or C/D are necessary relations.
$A/B/C/D$, as we should now write it, is a slice of behaviour that involves
one necessary relation with or without the other two relations being
necessary, and this means that the conditional probability for B/C must
be 1. This necessity, and indeed the probability for the other purely contingent relations, may be said to be dependent upon, or independent of,

some response on the part of the organism. We can substitute '---/---'
for '---//---', thus including the word 'immediately' if we wish, then we
can write the necessary and contingent relations

$$A / / X' / / B / / Y' / / C / / Z' / / D \tag{6}$$

and

$$(AN') A / / N' / / B / / N' / / C / / N' / / D \tag{7}$$

respectively, where $(A\text{-})$ is the universal operator taken from the lower
functional calculus, and N' may range over all possible responses in the
organism.

The above interpretation is simply that of a typical Markov process,
where the sequential conditional probabilities are stored with stimulus
and response letters.

The process of generalization arises whenever two subsets have common letters. Thus *abcdefg* and *abcdefh* are 'common members' of the
set *abcdef*, and if we write A for this set, it is easy to see that if g and h are
properties that, while possibly recognized, are independent of the outcome of the response, they may lead to generalization. Indeed, such set-
theoretic inferences can be drawn on any of the relations existing in the
store.

We can now state once more that it seems plausible to add a permanent store to the simple counting device with its temporary storage
system. A logical net can be drawn in pencil and paper, or built in hardware as in a general purpose computer, wherein information in temporary storage will at some time, and according to certain conditions, be
transferred to the permanent storage. What are these conditions? One
might guess that there are two sorts, and that they interact with each
other: (1) Where the degree of confirmation is high, and in particular (2)
Where the association is at the habit level. This last phrase, 'habit level',
can be the source of much discussion, but what is intended here is that
there are certain relations that involve no interference, and association
is actually known. The problem here is to know the correct response for
some desired outcome; the system apparently does not know it inexo-
rably until some number of trials have taken place, and this may reflect the
presence of random elements in our connections. We are, indeed, merely
drawing attention to the fact that the *learning* process—which is perhaps
dependent on the temporary store—is different from the *learned* process,

which is dependent on the permanent store. This is exactly the same problem that arose when we were considering the programming of computers to learn.

The distinction is usually drawn between temporary and permanent storage registers in digital computer design, and although it is not obviously necessary in uneconomical automata, it is precisely through economy of space and elements that this distinction comes about. Here it is suggested that all the counters are in multi-stage storage, and some small subset of all the counters is used for all actual counting. When associations have passed a certain level of count (all of which are in agreement), then no further counting will occur, and the production of the stimulus elicits the response. The recurrence of a doubt about an association would then renew the counting process. Such a counting and transfer arrangement is very simple to reproduce in our network terms or in a computer. Confirmation of this distinction is considerable, and one special case must be quoted, that of 'learning sets'.

Learning sets

Various experiments have been carried out on learning sets, and results of an apparently inconsistent type have sometimes been discovered. It appears, however, if we may generalize, that with overlearning, interference from retroactive inhibitions is wholly overcome. This implies that our matrix (1) applies only to the learning period, and that the first row of n's is replaced by zeros after some finite time t.

What is now the basis of this transfer? It seems plausible to say that transfer will take place when all the counters, or counting capacity, of the machine will be used up, it being assumed that there is only the possibility of a finite count taking place. We might guess that value has a bearing on this, and it would doubtless have the effect of merely filling up the counting elements more quickly where greater value-for-the-organism occurs. At any rate the finite automaton will have just this property of a finite set of counters and can be given the property of precisely discharging its probability into a permanent store after the counters are filled up.

Let us now look a little deeper into this matter. Suppose A/B (or $A/X'/B$) is a well-learned association, we must be careful to remember this means that some response, X' say, is appropriate to A to produce satisfaction B, where A represents the letter A in list 1, and X' the utterance of the letter B from the same list. Now learn list 2, and we have the association $A/Y'/B$ where Y' represents the utterance of D. Now when A occurs during list 2 one might expect that X' would be the response, and this would indeed be so were it not for the fact that some rule intervenes. This rule is the experimenter's instruction which occurs and is stored, and this—*granted* that the first list has been learnt sufficiently to ensure it being taken off the temporary store—replaces the belief derived from the previous direct learning.

The above explanation depends upon one very important fact, which is that the effect of a verbal instruction can completely undo a 'certainty' relation, and is far more effective than a count that arises through direct acquaintance with the environment. This argument depends upon the distinction between *description* and *acquaintance*, and yet we shall certainly wish to argue that language is learned by the same associative process (by counting) as any other learning activity. The implications of this very important point go deep, and demand an analysis of language in the automaton, and this cannot be undertaken here. Let it suffice that there is every reason to suppose that, while language signs are associated with their referents in the same way as all other signs, when a coherent set of signs is learnt and a language therefore known, the effect of utterances in that language can be different from a direct experience of an event, in that it will bring about a large and quick change in the count. It is as if another person's large experience (count) were transferred to the listener's storage where, subject to certain other considerations of confidence, it will have the effect of concentrated experience.

The rule can only operate on the permanent store where it itself is stored, and this reflects the fact that any attempt to pursue this course before the transfer has taken place will cause precisely the interference of retroactive inhibition.

It should be emphasized that what we are trying to do here is to build up a precise machine—a blueprint from well-understood principles—for constructing switching devices, keeping within the fairly well-validated evidence from experimental psychology. Clearly, it is the hope that such automata that fit some of the facts of experimental psychology can also be shown to fit others for which they were not explicitly designed, and other tests should be suggested from which psychological experiments could be designed. This attempt is no more than a beginning to the process, which is necessarily very complicated.

In the matter of learning sets, James' (1957) results suggested that the order of presentation, as well as the nature of the stimulus, will materially alter results. This one might expect to be the case in a finite automaton, given only that they had already built up a fair number of beliefs (associations and generalizations); it follows that no simple automaton could exhibit this behaviour, which is an extension of stimulus generalization, wherein sets of associations and relations—what we commonly call theories, hypotheses, or general beliefs—are already effective.

It will generally be the case that, after a longish period of time, the automaton will acquire many different scores in its B-matrix. The only problem that now arises for a matrix such as

$$\begin{bmatrix} n\ n\ \ldots\ n \\ r\ r\ \ldots\ r \\ s\ s\ \ldots\ s \\ -\ -\ - \\ w\ w\ \ldots w \end{bmatrix}$$

where $n, r, s, \ldots, w > 0$, is involved if the components of the B's in the later rows have common components with the B's of the top row. For the input matrix this will cause confusion in the recognition process; but for the B-matrix this will not cause confusion, even though there are components in common, unless events that are incompatible occur together, and this, presumably, would make nonsense of all processes.

We should notice that, to explain learning sets, we assume that after n trials the information (now learned) is transferred to a permanent memory store, and that the reason that a new response to a stimulus already in store does not occur is because there must also be the rule (experimenter's instruction) in store, and this is effective in suspending the original count.

Two questions have to be considered here. The first is the nature of the memory store used by humans, and its reproduction in the machine, and the way the selective process of perception works with the memory store in the first place.

We shall say that the facts observed and the rules under which these facts are observed (the experimenter's instructions) are coded economically from the initial stage of the experiment. The events being coded for store are effectively infinite, and we may therefore expect that gross abbreviations occur. These will occur, according to our empiricist viewpoint, in terms of the effectiveness (value) of the coding in previous cases. Having said so much, it is easy to see how this—as well as many other oddities—comes about as a sort of artefact, in that the coding was too abbreviated to allow a success, due to the need for more information than such a situation normally demands.

Thus, to take a simpler case as an example, if you show a subject a simple diagram such as a black square on a sheet of paper, he will probably remember the words 'black square', and in a future recognition test he will easily pick out the figure from a group of such figures if it is the only black square of about the correct size. If, however, you ask him to choose from *a set of* black squares he will probably fail. This is partly because he may find it difficult to code the actual size if he is not allowed actually to measure the square, and partly because he will not have stored anything more than a rough visual estimate which is inadequate in the subsequent fine test. Essentially the same thing would certainly occur with a machine that coded its perception as 'arrow pointing to the right', and then applied that rule directly in the new situation when facing the opposite way. The conceptual contamination situation of Piercy's (1937) is more complex than this, and depends on the inability to carry through what is a fairly complex transformation. The possibility arises in this case, therefore, that the capacity to reason logically has also failed. Certainly we can easily show that people are not able to draw simple, logical conclusions in easy mathematical or logical puzzles. Here, it is more in the nature of a geometrical puzzle, and failure to see what is required is the cause of coding into storage the wrong information.

This whole question raises difficulties for our machine design because, if our explanations are correct, then the fault is a very high level and complicated one, very closely related to the nature of the machine's experience. But if we put the machine in an environment where somewhat similar operations are ordinarily performed (the natural process of turning around in a room), then the economy of coding would soon necessitate a coding habit that would be adequate in the difficult Piercy conditions. Random elements would be introduced into a realistic machine so that there would be a certain percentage of blockages to ordinary reasoning, and this would account for both sorts of error, the ambiguity over axes (stimulus generalization) remaining, as Piercy suggests, the cause of more errors in the one direction than the other.

Two consequences of interest follow from the above. It seems a clear prediction that if Piercy had instructed his subjects in a simple routine method for retaining the information necessary to the successful performance of his task, then he would have eliminated errors. The error is clearly one of performance, which could be remedied by learning. Secondly, the relation of perception to memory is thrown into relief, and the question of the selective memorizing of perceptual processes is clearly connected with experience. This last point becomes more obvious when it is realized that a machine without the earlier similar (but also different) experience would not have made the Piercy errors, because the making of the error, on our hypothesis, depends on having learned to do something different in the past from what is now demanded. This point relates it to the other matters of stimulus generalization and retroactive inhibition already discussed.

We also see from what has been said that it does not in the least matter what memory storage system we use for this machine; any one would yield the same results, since it is not in the storage method but in the selective coding that the error occurs.

These few samples must be sufficient to show the methods of application of finite automata theory to learning theory, as compared with its use in giving an effective model for existing learning theories.

We must remind the reader that molar psychological theory—and this is what we have so far discussed with respect to learning—is a particular example of what is called 'black-box theory', the essential principles are to give a predictive account of the behaviour of the black box under a range of different conditions, *without* opening the box to see the internal mechanism. However, the use of theoretical terms makes it clear that we shall need, for the purpose of constructing effective theories, at least to guess at the internal mechanisms, and this will later be supplemented by an actual study of the mechanisms under the name 'physiology'.

We have only been able, in spite of the lengthiness of our present chapter, to outline some of the principal examples of learning theories, controversies over theories, experiments and controversies over experiments; and there are other theories—especially the mathematical ones—

and many other experiments, that should be carefully considered by the reader in this context (Estes, 1950; Bush and Mosteller, 1955; *et al.*).

Extinction

We will now consider the problem of extinction from the cybernetic point of view. Here it will be easier to follow the argument if we illustrate a succession of stimuli by a status matrix wherein rows represent a succession of times, $t_0, t_1, \ldots, t_n,$ and the columns represent the set of elements and whether they fire at any particular instant or not. Unfortunately we cannot conveniently represent in one matrix the current firing state *and* the cumulative past history of the automaton; to simplify the discussion we shall therefore leave the cumulative matrix out of the discussion and, unless otherwise stated, it may be assumed that the cumulative state is positive if the particular combination making up the element's firing has more often fired together than not. To illustrate the point, let us say that if x and y have occurred together more often than not, then the firing of x receives a response as if both x and y fired.

Broadbent, writing on this subject and describing Uttley's (1955) explanation of extinction, concludes that it is inadequate, and that therefore the problem of extinction requires more than the storing of conditional probabilities. This argument is not necessarily true and should be restated in the form that *if* extinction is inadequately catered for by Uttley's explanation, then this is only inadequate for *his particular version* of a conditional probability system.

We consider it extremely important to make it clear, even at the risk of boring repetition, that whether or not Uttley's particular model is correct, conditional probabilities *are* not necessarily incorrect on that account. There are a number of different ways of computing conditional probabilities, not just one, and the possible inadequacy of Uttley's explanation does not necessarily imply the inadequacy of conditional probabilities.

Broadbent's description of Uttley's explanation is based on a series of tables, and we shall briefly consider some of them.

The first one takes the following status matrix form for inputs X, Y and Z, which are represented by the first three columns, and $X.Y, X.Z$ and

$Y.Z$, which are represented by the last three columns:

$$\begin{bmatrix} 1 & 1 & 0 & 1 & 0 & 0 \\ 1 & 1 & 0 & 1 & 0 & 0 \\ 1 & 1 & 0 & 1 & 0 & 0 \\ 1 & 0 & 0 & 1 & 0 & 0 \\ 1 & 0 & 1 & 1 & 1 & 0 \\ 1 & 0 & 1 & 0 & 1 & 0 \\ 1 & 1 & 1 & 1 & 1 & 1 \end{bmatrix}$$

In this matrix it is assumed that a short finite number of associations for all the desired pairings is enough to illustrate the method basic to the argument.

Now the first thing we should notice about this matrix is that it represents a particular set of logical nets in the same way as we have described them in Chapter 5.

The second thing is to realize that we could have changed many of the items in the present matrix and still have preserved our logical net representation, and indeed, our conditional probability principle. This point can be quickly illustrated. If X had been regularly paired with Y it must have taken on a positive count for $X.Y$. If this is so, then the counter for $X.Z$ could be either 0 or $-m$ after m associations of X and Y. Either is possible, and either will depend—or may be made to depend—upon whether or not the associations are 'reinforced'. The next point in the example given, taken from Broadbent, is that it appears to be assumed that X and $X.Z$ are different stimuli, and that if X/Y fails through lack of reinforcement, or through the failure of Y to occur (these might be the same thing), then it is assumed that $X.Z/Y$ is unaffected. But again this simply depends on whether or not the firing of the elements $X.Z$ and X have the independence which they could easily be given, and which could equally easily be granted.

The following matrix illustrates an alternative conception of the conditional probability* net:

---

* A conditional probability machine can be defined in terms of connections where each connexion is defined by a fraction m/n where n is the total number of occurrences and m the number of favourable outcomes, but this system can be constrained or differentially weighted in any way we choose.

$$\begin{bmatrix} 1 & 1 & 0 & 1 & 0 & 0 \\ 1 & 1 & 0 & 1 & 0 & 0 \\ 1 & 1 & 0 & 1 & 0 & 0 \\ 1 & 0 & 0 & 1 & 0 & 0 \\ 1 & 0 & 0 & 1 & 0 & 0 \\ 1 & 0 & 0 & 1 & 0 & 0 \\ 1 & 0 & 0 & 0 & 0 & 0 \end{bmatrix}$$

Here the failure of X to elicit Y is really independent of the presence of X, and depends merely on the decaying association of X and Y, which itself could account for extinction; and indeed we could always account for it by firing a stimulus of any kind and at any time with an inhibitory association.

This last point brings out another matter that we should bear in mind. The lack of need for an inhibitory activity to account for spontaneous recovery, disinhibition and, in general, extinction, does not in any way mean that the concept of inhibition is unnecessary. Here, in the light of empirical evidence, especially from neurophysiology, Occam's razor is inappropriate; it is simply failing to pay attention to the probabilities implicit in the empirical evidence.

Leaving this aside, and returning to logical nets or finite automata and the conditional probability explanations of extinction, brings out again the failure of Uttley's model to fit the plausible empirical evidence suggested by Pavlov. But again, of course, there is no problem in general; we can easily arrange for our system to fit the facts. Extraneous stimuli can be made quite ineffective, as in the second matrix (above), and in many other possible matrices representing a whole set of finite automata.

What we are saying here does not deny that Broadbent may be right in believing that Uttley's theory of learning may need supplementing by further principles; indeed this is likely to be so. One further principle is that suggested by Broadbent himself: the principle of the selective filter; but what is important to notice is that the effects described *can* be quite easily accounted for without going beyond conditional probabilities.

The foregoing is an excellent example of the value of a methodological analysis and of the reduction of a problem, in part, to a mathematical form. From what has already been said about logical nets it is obvious that one could be constructed with the desired properties, and that the problem of learning, indeed of all cognition from this point of view, is the mathematical problem of whether or not there exists a set of matrices that satisfy each and every piece of empirical evidence and are at the same time consistent with each other. Such a net is precisely the conceptual description for which we are searching.

Our last task in this chapter will be to give a brief interpretation, in terms of finite automata, of those terms in cognition which have not already been sufficiently discussed. Various terms such as 'taxis', 'kinesis', etc., do not obviously need interpretation; and 'instinct' can be taken to refer to those *beliefs*, or associative connections (*B*-nets), that are *built into* the system. A 'displacement activity' would seem to be an example of an activity that involves the blocking of a particular response in such a way as to return the pulse into some other response channel, rather than merely stopping and destroying it. A 'releaser' is a stimulus for a built-in belief or association; 'imprinting' (see Russell, 1957) is the acquisition of *detailed basic* behaviour from experience; and so on.

There are many other terms in common use in learning theory (see, for example, the glossary of terms in Hilgard and Marquis, 1940), and it should be possible to reinterpret each and every one in terms of our own finite automaton, and to carry through this program rigorously. It is confidently hoped that the reader will now understand what the process entails, for it is not the intention in this book to carry through the program in detail.

Recent advances

The bulk of the work that has gone on in recent years in the field of cognition has been addressed at the detail of learning and memory and the higher cognitive functions of the central nervous system, and the old disputes as between Hull and Tolman have been largely forgotten. The reason for this is itself of interest and rests on the fact that the broad framework of learning and the higher cognitive functions is broadly agreed, and it is the detail that needs to be worked out now because it is only by working out the detail that we are likely to make any sort of final decisions, if that is an appropriate way of looking at it, between such theories as Tolman's and such theories as Hull's.

In practice, it should be re-emphasized that the differences between Hull and Tolman's theories of learning are far more imaginary than real. The most important difference is the unit which we take to be the basis of the explanation and almost everyone would agree today that there is no need to take such a simple unit as Hull took; it was in fact much more sensible to take a central and cognitive type of unit of the Tolman kind. Yet it is also true to say that most of Hull's theories still more or less apply to cognition. The disadvantage of both theories, and indeed of most other theories of learning, is that they are too limited in their approach since it is the higher cognitive faculties that need to be explained, especially in human beings, and these can be tackled directly. In a sense learning is a special case of higher learning activities rather than the other way round.

One concept which has come to the fore in recent years has been that of secondary motivational systems. The concept of secondary motivational systems has come to permeate current accounts of both human and animal behaviour. On a stimulus response view, these interpretations relate to the acquired capabilities of particular conditions or events to energize, punish or reinforce, various classes of behaviour. The present review is an attempt to evaluate the applicability of this concept to the explication of behavioural phenomena, mainly in animals in simple situations customarily subsumed under the headings of conditioned needs, fear, incentive motivation, frustration, conflict and sensory reinforcement. The energizing or activating effects of motivation in which avoidance behaviour to extinction is powerfully resisted is confounded with such factors as the reinforcement produced by fear reduction and the after effects of shock escape training.

If the motivation association is a result of classical conditioning, for example, the outcomes of the criteria test should vary systematically with presumed increase in the conditioned response during acquisition, with such other phenomena of classical conditioning as extinction, spontaneous recovery and dis-inhibition.

Secondary motivation is still the primary concept and one we have already completely grasped and understood. One thing we have to bear in mind is to what extent the emotional system (the E-system) and the M-system are themselves interacting in the conditioned picture, in the form of providing ordinary stimuli.

As far as memory is concerned, and we see this of course in terms of storage elements in the B-net, both looped elements and internal loops involving a number of elements, then the concept of 'chunking' (Miller and Dilara, 1967) is one by which the subject recodes X strings of ordered units into shorter strings. This suggestion has also previously been made by Oldfield (1954). This information theoretic approach to memory is fairly typical of the way things have been going and again is wholly consistent with our own cybernetic approach. In fact, it *is* a cybernetic approach for all practical purposes, and it was also an extremely straightforward problem to draw the necessary logical nets to perform the chunking operation. We shall now try to make some sort of integrated statement as to the interaction of the various fields of cybernetic approach to cognition.

In the first place, it is quite clear that we need our nets to be hierarchical in fashion and we certainly need them to be partial partitioned classifications systems. The fact that they are adaptive is obvious and the only question is whether we need actual growth of neural tissue to make the necessary connections after maturation is complete or whether all that is needed is a functional change. This is a matter that can only be decided in the course of time by more experimental evidence. The main point to appreciate is that in building up the models in logical net terms, we have the ordinary statement of an automaton which could just as easily have been put in scanner and paper terms. If we abstract from this structural system, and consider only the functional relationships between inputs and outputs, then we have something that can be defined in terms of either information theory or in stochastic processes. The ordinary verbal learning theories, theories of learning stated usually in ordinary verbal terms or semi-formalized terms, represent an attempt to put the flesh of verisimilitude on to the bones of the statistical facts.

If one at this stage questions the effectiveness of cybernetics on the grounds that there are no predictions they have made that could not have been made without it, the answer is that this may well be true but this is not the object of cybernetics, we must not get caught up in the old misunderstanding of trying to challenge some discipline on the grounds that it did not achieve something that it never set out to achieve. What cybernetics wants to achieve is a systematic description of artificially intelligent systems and there is in fact every reason to suppose that you can build a cybernetic system, either in functional terms such as a stochastic model, or in structural terms, either by using logical nets or suitably programming a computer, which again is the equivalent operation, or even programming a computer in terms of logical nets probably in a matrix form.

All of these things can be done to provide the model of any cognitive activity one cares to mention and as a result can in fact predict a number of activities which are far from obvious in terms of experimental evidence alone, and certainly quite independently can predict things that have already been known to happen in behavioural terms.

To this extent the use of hierarchical B-nets tells us something about the organization of information processing which is extremely suggestive for future experimentation. The first and most obvious example is the nature of the memory filter; this clearly depends, among other things, on recency, frequency and the evaluation of the information.

The notion of chunking that we have just referred to is a method of recoding information rather as one abstracts information with respect to books and journals to ensure not too much memory space is taken up with irrelevant detail. We cannot be absolutely sure that this happens in the central nervous system, but there are some reasons in terms of dimensional analysis for thinking something like this happens. This immediately suggests a form of experimentation or a form of interpretation which helps to clarify one's understanding of behavioural problems. The notion of latent learning comes directly from Oettinger's computer model of learning and something that makes it obvious straightaway that latent learning is not something which should surprise us, when found by experimental evidence, but something that is inevitable by the nature of the design of the central nervous system. We could multiply examples indefinitely but there should be no need; it is obvious now that we have got to the point of sophistication in model construction that makes much of the earlier disputations between molar theorists of learning seem fairly irrelevant.

As a result of this, most of the recent work on cognition has been at the higher levels where language plays a vitally important part, and this is a field which was much neglected by earlier psychologists. It was treated most naïvely and now we have come to the point where verbal learning plays an important part and we are beginning to understand verbal learning in terms which cohere much more closely with that of the logician and philosopher.

Perhaps nothing would be more appropriate at this point than to quote E. B. Hunt (1962) who has worked in the same field of cybernetics and cognition and makes the following observation, with which we would wholly agree.

17*

Concept learning has been presented as a topic for logical analysis, a behaviour to be explained by psychology, and as a desired capability of intelligent automata. When stated together in a single sentence, it seems obvious that many common problems face researchers in each area. They should be able to support each other. However, in the view of research that has already been done, we found that they cannot. More often than not, the empirical work on logic, psychology and artificial intelligence aspects of concept learning has been carried out without any cross-reference. Fragmentation of effort has not helped advance our knowledge of the underlying process.

Perhaps psychologists have been the most guilty in ignoring the related work in engineering and logic. . . .

We shall now pause in the next chapter to consider the molecular aspects of cognition, particularly with reference to the central nervous system.

Summary

This chapter has tried to state the principal features of learning theory without dwelling especially on some of the narrower and more sophisticated discussions that have taken place in the very recent past. It has not been intended for the experimental psychologist in its summarizing detail of such standard behaviour patterns as latent learning, partial reinforcement, as well as in the main discussion of primary and secondary reinforcement; indeed, more detail has been included than would be necessary for him. This extra detail is for the benefit of those other scientists interested in cybernetics but unfamiliar with learning theory.

We have also tried to show in this chapter the connection between logical net models and learning theory, and we have tried to emphasize that our models are capable of reconstructing a whole range of behaviour, and that we are still trying to discover the effective method for reconstructing behaviour that is now fairly well authenticated. The argument is that our method of reconstruction will facilitate our understanding of the material itself, since it is consistently argued that science is *not* merely the collecting of empirical data.

Much of what is stated in this chapter should now be considered from the point of view of the methods of the previous three chapters.

CHAPTER 9

BEHAVIOUR AND THE NERVOUS SYSTEM

So FAR we have discussed the properties of finite automata and their relation to some part of cognition; now we should try to say something of the nervous system and its more directly established properties.

This is where the trail narrows, since automata are essentially conceptual systems, and when we apply them to the task of modelling behaviour, one problem we presumably have to face sooner or later is to make comparisons with the human organism, and this means primarily the nervous system. It should be clearly understood that while this is ultimately necessary if automata theory is to be biologically useful, it could be argued that the maximum utility of automata theory at the moment lies in its application to the modelling of molar behaviour. However, some brief survey of neurophysiology will, in any case, be suggestive for future applications in the subject.

We should emphasize at this point that it is increasingly clear that the gulf between conceptual nervous systems and 'actual nervous systems' is narrowing. It is no coincidence that experimental psychologists have often claimed that they have contributed more to an understanding of the 'actual' human brain than neurologists and neurophysiologists who are directly observing human and other organic brains. The cybernetician, playing here a somewhat similar role to the experimental psychologist, may also claim to have contributed to a greater understanding on grounds of his ability to construct conceptual brains.

The plain fact is, that we can go a very long way to establishing a rigorous picture of what happens in the human brain and central nervous system, knowing the basic functions which this must subserve. It should therefore be borne in mind that one of the main themes of this book is that automata (particularly those in neural net form) can be used as theoretical models of the brain and that these when supplemented by empirical information collected by direct observation, both at the cognitive level and the neural level, should come very close together and ultimately fit together like the pieces of a jigsaw puzzle, providing realistic brain models. It is only the enormous complexity of the human nervous system and our difficulty in observing it in its functional form, that makes it difficult to check our speculations and try to distinguish between various models and theories. Hence understandably many physiologists have felt that the sort of speculation done by psychologists and cyberneticians is idle and a waste of time. The answer is, as so often in science, that different goals are subserved by different people with different motives. A failure to understand this leads to a misunderstanding over the work being attempted.

For the person who believes in firmly establishing empirical facts, it may often seem pointless to develop a large theoretical framework. The author believes this is a fundamental mistake, since the mere accumulation of facts never makes a science. One should add, however, that no neurologist ever does work without some sort of schematic picture of the central nervous system, the only thing is that he does not seem to make it *explicit* or feel the necessity to tie its ends in rigorous logical terms. Whilst it may in some ways be premature to do this, there can be very little doubt that the conceptual frameworks provided by cyberneticians are becoming increasingly useful. Uttley (1966) has made the point that any brain models must satisfy logical, mathematical and behavioural criteria as well as fit the empirical facts and this is exactly what cybernetics is about. It is for this reason that logical or neural nets have played such an important part in the recent development of brain models.

In our logical net models we have talked of elements or cells which clearly could be interpreted as neurons, and for many purposes this is desirable. McCulloch (1959) when challenged as to the use of a two-state switch to represent a neuron, admitted that something like an eighth-order differential equation was necessary to describe a neuron's behaviour. But this is only true at one level of description, and we are happy to model—at least initially—the neuron at an altogether simpler level, while at the same time bearing the more complex levels in mind.

The nervous system, we shall say, is a complex switching system made up of neurons which are special cells for the purpose of quickly reacting to and communicating changes in the environment, both internal and external. Even amoeba and simple multicellular organisms react to environmental change, and in the latter case certain specific cells have been developed for the purpose.

As we go up through the various species, through the invertebrates and vertebrates, it is possible to detect an evolving pattern of complexity. The spinal cord with its increasing modification at the head end, and the developing complexity of the specialized receptors, are indicative of the trend. Then with the primates we have increasing complexity with the development of a highly specialized brain, and different layers in the 'control' centre itself; the cerebral cortex being divided into fairly well localized areas concerned with 'controlling' or 'integrating' specific functions in the body.

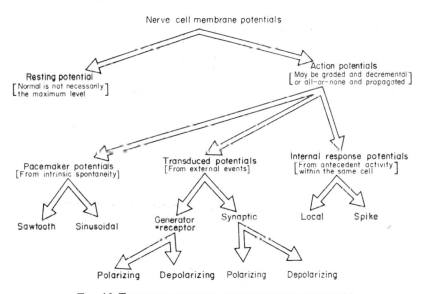

FIG. 46. THE TYPES OF NERVE CELL MEMBRANE POTENTIALS.

A neuron is a specialized cell with an especially high degree of excitability and conductivity. There are, of course, various neurons in the nervous system, motoneurons, short connecting Golgi type II neurons, bipolar neurons in sensory nerves, and so on. These neurons may differ from each other greatly in size and sensitivity, and straight away we can see that our logical nets cannot be identified literally with an actual nervous system, since all the elements of the automaton are basically the same, and this must at least imply a many-one relationship with actual nervous systems (Bullock, 1959).

Whether nerves (elements) have myelin sheaths or not is something that does not enter into automata theory, but neither do any of the particular characteristics of a physio-chemical kind; this matter of the chemistry of the nerves will shortly be discussed, since with the development of chemical-type computers this whole subject is put into fresh relief. This is perhaps of special interest in view of the efforts of Pask (1959) and others to show that a growth process can be mimicked in a manner not wholly different from that involved in the regeneration of nervous tissue.

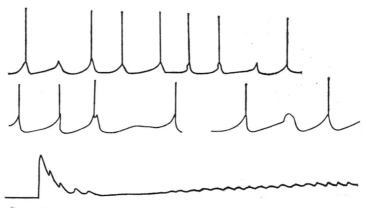

FIG. 47. SPONTANEOUS ACTIVITY IN A GANGLION CELL as revealed by an electrode inside the soma or body of the nerve cell. The spikes are about 10 mV here and are followed by a repolarization, then a gradual depolarization—the pacemaker potential—which at a critical level sets off a local potential. This in turn usually rises high enough to trigger a spike but is seen here several times by itself.

We can think of the gross divisions of the nervous system as: (1) the spinal cord; (2) the myelencephalon, including the medulla; (3) the metencephalon, which includes the cerebellum, pons, and part of the fourth ventricle; (4) the mesencephalon (the midbrain, including the colliculi of the tectum); (5) the diencephalon, which includes the thalamus, hypothalamus, optic tracts, pituitary, mammillary bodies, etc.; and finally, and perhaps most important to an understanding of human behaviour, (6) the telencephalon, which includes cerebral hemi-

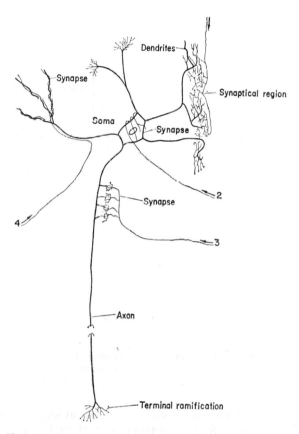

FIG. 48. A NERVE CELL with synaptic connections involving axon and dendrites.

spheres, olfactory bulbs, and tracts and basal ganglia. A schematic diagram is shown in Fig. 49.

The spinal cord itself carries tracts running up and down its length, and these are nerve fibres or white matter, while the cells or grey matter are the core of the spinal cord. Figure 50 shows a typical cross-section of the spinal cord with incoming, or ascending, and outgoing, or descending, nerve fibres at every level, and represents the reflex arc of input–output activity.

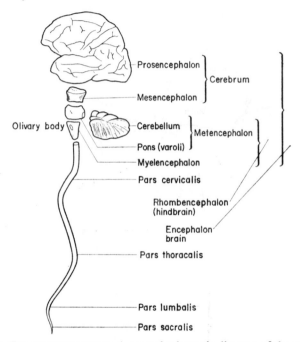

FIG. 49. THE NERVOUS SYSTEM. A general schematic diagram of the principal parts of the nervous system; these are severed to show more clearly where they are in relation to the rest of the system.

Closely associated with the spinal cord is the autonomic nervous system. This is responsible for the control of the internal organs such as the heart, lungs, pancreas, etc., and is made up of two parts called the sympathetic and the parasympathetic systems, the sympathetic chains, so called, lying along the ventro-lateral aspects of the vertebral column. The parasympathetic system emanates from the midbrain, medulla and pelvic nerve, and is complementary to the sympathetic system in its control; they act together like the two reins controlling a horse. The whole autonomic system is represented in the cerebral cortex, and is clearly

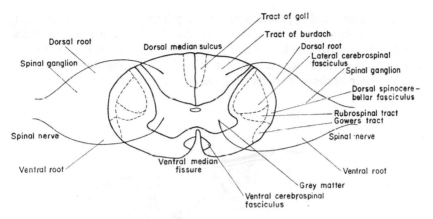

FIG. 50. TRANSVERSE SECTION OF SPINAL CORD. This diagram shows the principal tracts in the white matter of the spinal cord; the grey matter lies in the centre, and the tracts on top (at the back of the cord) travel upwards, while those at the side and at the bottom (at the front of the cord) travel downwards.

closely associated with emotions and motivation. Here, lack of space will not allow us to say very much about this system.

For the benefit of those for whom it is unfamiliar, it is perhaps worth saying that the various divisions of the nervous system, mentioned above, are to be investigated with respect to their function. This means that we are bound to use their names, and these become unwieldy and ugly. It is hoped that, with the aid of the figures shown—and bearing in mind that almost every part of the nervous system is made up of collections of neurons called nuclei—the reader will find it easy to follow. The names of the nuclei will usually illustrate their positions. The thalamus offers a good example for illustrating this point, being sometimes described in terms of its surfaces which are called dorsal (uppermost), ventral (underneath), medial (central) and lateral (sideways), although the nuclei of the thalamus include the anterior nucleus, the medial nucleus, the paraventricular nucleus, the intralaminar nuclei, the lateral nucleus, the posteromedial ventral nucleus, the lateral ventral nucleus, and so on, each part of the thalamus having a specific position relative to the whole and to the closely related structures called the metathalamus, subthalamus, epithalamus and, most important of all, the hypothalamus.

The thalamus and hypothalamus are very important to our behaviour picture, and they have connections with the visual and auditory systems through parts called the lateral and medial geniculate bodies respectively. They are also rather complicated anatomically, being surrounded by various other nuclei and tracts of fibres in a somewhat complex arrange-

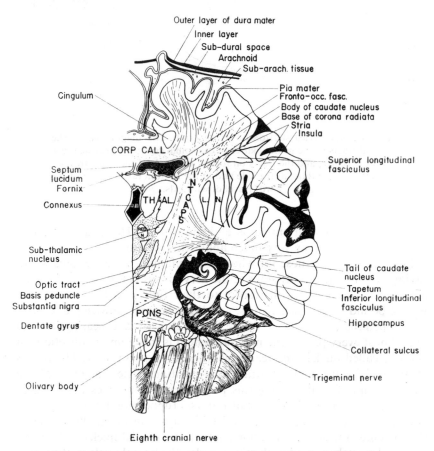

FIG. 51. A CROSS-SECTION OF THE BRAIN. This section is cut in a plane parallel to the plane of the face. It shows the white fibres of the internal capsule (INTCAPS in the figure) spreading out and separating the tail of the caudate nucleus from the central part of the thalamus and the central system. The lenticular nucleus (L.N.) also lies outside the internal capsule.

ment. The main points that might be borne in mind to help the reader new to neurology are: the thalamus is centrally placed, as is the hypothalamus, and surrounds the third ventricle which is part of the canal system of the brain carrying the cerebrospinal fluid in which the brain is bathed.

A large collection of fibre tracts from the spinal cord (called the 'internal capsule') runs up to the cortex outside the thalamus, dividing it off from the ventricular nuclei and caudate nuclei. These two bodies with the amygdaloid nuclei make up a large part of that part referred to as the basal ganglia, and constitute the chief organ between the thalamus and the cerebral cortex.

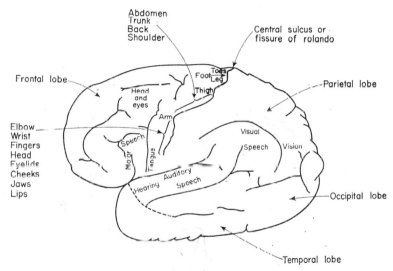

FIG. 52. THE CORTEX. This diagram of the outside of the external surface of the cerebrum shows some of the principal cortical areas with some of the principal functions that are associated with these areas named against them.

Figure 51 shows a transverse section through the brain, Fig. 52 shows the external surface of the left side of the brain, and Fig. 53 shows a 'phantom' of the striatum. It is hoped that this note and these figures will help to orientate those readers unfamiliar with the maze of the nervous system.

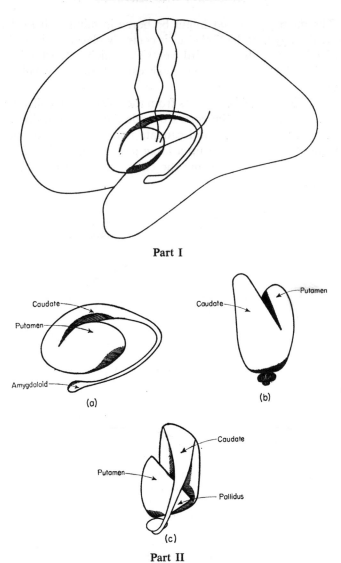

Part I

Part II

FIG. 53. Part I. Phantom of striatum within the cerebral hemisphere.
Part II. Form of striatum of left side. (*a*) Lateral aspect; (*b*) anterior
aspect; (*c*) posterior aspect.

Our problem is to relate these structures to fairly specific functions. We know that this cannot yet be done, but we can say something about the function of the various parts involved, and make some guesses as to how they may be related to our automaton.

But before we try to elucidate this major problem, let us turn again to the basic factors of nervous tissue, particularly the chemistry of nervous function and the synapse.

Chemistry of the nervous system

R. S. Lillie is a name that springs readily to mind when we think of early attempts to construct chemical models of the nervous system. His model was built some years ago, and was a fairly simple one. It consisted of an iron wire which had been immersed first in nitric acid and subsequently in sulphuric acid and water, having the property, if stimulated at one end, of firing off an impulse which travelled along the length of the wire, and destroying the thin film of iron oxide that separated the iron from the acid.

Lillie's model was able to imitate, to some extent, the protoplasm and its surrounding medium, and the special problem of the semi-permeable membrane that divided one from the other. This semi-permeability allows some substances to go through it and not others. On the other hand, from the point of view of physiology it was clearly unsatisfactory, not only in that it was quite different in its chemical action from that of the living nerve, but also in that it lacked one very important property that nervous tissue was known to possess: that of resealing itself after firing, so that a new impulse could follow after the refractory period, which is the short delay following the firing of a neuron, during which time it is either totally or relatively insensitive to further firing.

It has been known for a long time that the train of depolarization that effectively connects one end of a nerve fibre with the other depends upon the characteristics of semi-permeable membranes, and that the nerve's firing of impulses, and the transmission across the synapses, is accompanied by electrical and thermal changes; the details of the chemistry are still elusive, however, and the problem is thought of as existing in a background of great complexity, even though our knowledge of the process has been steadily increasing since the concept of the action current theory of the nerve impulse itself, which is only 100 years old.

Before proceeding to a description of what is now being attempted in the field of nerve chemistry, it is necessary to restate briefly what has become known as the Ionic Hypothesis (see Hodgkin, 1951, 1957; Eccles, 1953). This hypothesis is aimed primarily at giving an account of how nervous functions are chemically explained. The nervous impulse is to be thought of as a wave of electrical negativity that travels without decrement along nerve fibres.

The nerve itself is an extended cylinder of uniform radius, filled by a watery substance called axoplasm, and bathed in an ultrafiltrate of blood. These are separated from each other by a very thin membrane of lipid-protein structure. This membrane has special electrical properties that make it highly resistant to the passage of ions.

It is thought that the resting membrane is readily permeable to chloride and potassium ions which move across the membrane solely by diffusion; yet the reaction of the membrane to sodium is much more selective, at least in that these ions are removed from inside as soon as they appear. What has been called a 'sodium pump', assumed to be incorporated in the membrane itself, is responsible for this. The pump derives energy from metabolic changes within the fibre, and keeps the internal concentration of sodium at a level of about 10 per cent of the external concentration.

Glutamic, aspartic and isethionic acids provide a high internal concentration of impermeable anions which, together with the sodium concentration, make for a potassium gradient of twenty to fifty times more inside than outside the membrane, and about the opposite for chloride ions.

At room temperature the resting membrane potential E is given in terms of potassium and chloride concentrations by the following formula:

$$E = RT/F \log K_i/K_0 = RT/F \log Cl_0/Cl_i$$

This is the potential in Donnan Equilibrium where RT and F are constant and the logarithms are to the base e.

At room temperature this equation can be rewritten in microvolts

$$E = 58 \log_{10} K_i/K_0$$

and the outside would be around 85 mV to the inside; this keeps the gradients for potassium and chlorides in a state of equilibrium.

If the resting potential is now diminished by the application of electric currents, the membrane immediately becomes highly permeable to sodium ions. This is said to be due to a 'sodium carrier mechanism' which has a feedback that proceeds until the potential across the membrane approaches that of a sodium electrode, creating a reversed potential with the inside positive to the outside. As the peak is reached the sodium carrier starts to decline, the process is reversed, and the nerve fibre returns to its resting state.

A large number of experiments have been carried out to confirm the truth of the Ionic Hypothesis, and much confirmatory evidence has been forthcoming, although a certain amount of detail, particularly about the sodium pump, is still lacking. The refractory periods of nerve fibres have been studied and can be shown to be consistent with the above account which, while thought to be basically correct, is still lacking in detail and not effective in a way that is sufficient for cybernetic purposes.

There is much more to be said about this field, and the interested reader should refer to specialist literature on the subject (Eccles, 1953; Beach, 1958; Shanes, 1958; Tower, 1958).

Before leaving the chemistry of nerves altogether, it will be very useful to the cybernetic view to have a short comment on this same work from a different angle.

A new set of experiments has been carried out by a group of chemists with the object of trying to understand the chemistry of cell membrane formation.

Work has been in progress for some years on the nature of organic membranes, and something must be said here about the advance that has been made.

The Ionic Hypothesis had assumed the presence of lipid membranes between the inside and outside of a nerve, and protein or lipid films have been used between two liquids to model this membrane. The problem of studying these interfaces between aqueous liquids depends on being able to study the electrical and optical properties of the surfaces in question.

Saunders (1953, 1957, 1958; Elworthy and Saunders, 1955, 1956) has designed and built an apparatus for studying diffusion processes and photographing them at the membrane. From this work it was discovered that lecithin sols (a complex chemical colloidal substance derived from egg yolk) formed stable membranes between liquids, and that these

T B C 18

membranes could be further strengthened by injections of serum albumen sol at the actual interface between the liquids.

A more sensitive appratus was then built by which it was possible to measure the surface forces that existed at the boundaries of the lecithin sols and water. The next step was to study the effects of various inorganic salts such as potassium and sodium chloride on these surface forces and, as a result, suggestions were made as to the formation of actual cell membranes. With an intracellular fluid sufficiently rich in phosphatides, and with a little calcium and some lecithin, the lecithin was thought to be stabilized to the monovalent metal salts by soaplike substances, probably lysolecithin (also derived from egg yolks). By contact with fluids of higher calcium content, a calcium–lecithin complex film is formed which becomes fixed and relatively insoluble by absorption of proteins and insoluble lipids.

It was later shown that the appearance of the film surface force was related to the stability of the lecithin sol, and that a wide variation of stability to salts can be achieved by altering the ratio of lysolecithins to lecithin in a mixed sol of the two phosphatides.

Various other experiments on the properties of the viscosities, stabilities to salts, and haemolytic activities have been carried out, and there is current research on the electrical properties of lecithin membranes and their permeability to electrolytes.

The results as a whole show that our knowledge of cell membrane formation has taken a large step forward. It is even to be hoped that the next year or two should see the completion of a chemical picture of the membrane formation process, and the diffusion properties that operate in nervous and other organic tissues. In the meantime we have the power to produce artificial cells that could be used in a computer system in the place of relays. This much is clear in principle, and work is afoot now on the practicability of actually carrying through such an undertaking.

This brief account of certain aspects of the chemistry of the nervous system is included for heuristic and orientating purposes, but its importance for cybernetics may be very great indeed, since an effort is now being made to produce what Beer (1959) has called Fungoid Systems, and what may be thought of as chemical or ultimately, it is hoped, chemical-colloidal computers (Pask, 1958).

The main importance of chemical computers for cybernetics lies in the fact that, *unlike the digital computer, they exhibit the properties of growth in direct fashion*, and this is something that was bound to be needed sooner or later in our biological modelling.

In more recent years a great deal of advance has been made in brain chemistry and some attempt has been made to relate it to learning. Not only have the RNA and DNA molecules been the source of a considerable amount of speculation, particularly as they relate to the genetical background of the organism, but also there has been an increasingly large number of hypotheses (Roberts, 1966) which suggest that brain chemistry is involved in quite specific ways in both learning and memory. Three particular aspects of their involvement are: (1) by searching for chemical changes in the brain during and after training has taken place; (2) by studying the effects of centrally active drugs on learning and retention and memory in general; and (3) by attempting to transfer memory by injecting brain extracts from trained naïve animals. So far the evidence is insufficiently clearcut to justify any firm statement.

The effect of antibiotics on learning and retention and other cognitive activities is also being studied in some measure and once again the work tends to be in the in-progress stage, but there is enough general evidence perhaps to draw some conclusions. One conclusion is that the complete connectivity of the central nervous system is aided by chemical changes which may be necessary to synaptic transmission, which may in turn be party to neural growth, certainly of a functional if not a literal and anatomical kind. It may be that the anatomical form of growth occurs at certain stages of maturation while the functional growth is the growth that takes place thereafter.

There is a temptation, of course, to think of the *M*-nets of motivation as being represented by the chemistry of the organism. Thus the *M*-nets which we have drawn showing their relation to the *B*-nets of our automaton are perhaps best thought of as chemical systems and therefore only represented formally or symbolically by a neural net-type of device. This is something which we have always expected to be the case and it does not in any way impair the value of constructing *M*-nets, it being remembered that we are as much concerned in general with synthesis as we are with simulation in the field of cybernetics. Learning itself is mirrored in the growth nets and is subserved by external stimulation as well as internal chemical mediation; the growth nets then become fixed nets after the learning period is over and the 'having learned' period is reached. There are clearly two kinds of learning periods, one is the early learning period during maturation, which is as much dominated by internal control from genetic maps as by external events, whereas later learning is almost entirely dominated by the interaction of external and internal states of a non-genetic kind.

The nervous system

Turning again to the general properties of the nervous system, we must note that the properties of the synapse are very important, and we do not yet know sufficient to enable us to build models with absolute certainty; but the synaptic junction clearly plays a vitally important part in our neurophysiological theory of behaviour, both in the classical sense as a junction station and in the modern sense of Hebb (1949) with the development of synaptic knobs. We should mention here the many attempts to build electrical models of neurons (e.g. Taylor, 1959), but while such a study is useful, it does not come quite within our purview.

Apart from the chemical mediation of the spike potential or nervous impulse, there are other factors which are well known about the neuron; it has a critical intensity that fires it and this property, realized in our logical nets is called the threshold. Another property that is accepted in the logical nets, which is in keeping with the facts, is the all-or-none law, which states that when a nerve fires it fires 'completely' or not at all. The after-potentials (changes of excitation immediately after the main excitation) that follow the spike potential are not mirrored in our model, nor is their physiological function wholly clear.

There are many further properties of neurons, such as their relative and absolute refractory periods, but these will not be discussed further here. It might just be mentioned that the fact that there is some delay (an instant) in the logical nets can be taken to be an analog of the refractory period. But let us turn to the synapses.

The synapse is a functional junction between neurons such that transmission between neurons takes place across the synapse. Transmission between neurons may also occur through ephaptic transmission (Eccles, 1946), which means directly across the membranes of adjacent neurons.

There are two currents, the anodal and cathodal in nervous transmission, and these can cause successive states of inhibition and excitation in ephaptic transmission. However, in synaptic transmission—unlike the ephaptic case—there is no final inhibitory impulse following the excitatory, and thus the resting fibre which is the other side of the synapse can build up a considerable potential. There are local potentials at the synapse which makes the firing of the resting fibre contingent on the relation between the potentials in both neurons in the chain. Sometimes, when an impulse is not itself sufficient to arouse the resting fibre, summation of local impulses from the same source in quick succession, or from two different sources having close contiguity on the synapse, will effect temporal and spatial summation respectively, either of which may then be sufficient to fire the resting fibre.

It is probably because some summation is necessary to fire neurons that the conduction of a nervous impulse will travel in one way only across synaptic junctions. The reasons for this are anatomical in that the synaptic junction is ordered in having many–one and never one–many relations; there are also delays at the synapse.

We can see that spatial summation is easily realized in logical nets, but temporal summation requires that there be at least two elements operating together, and is thus really a contrived kind of spatial summation. However, here there is some evidence that temporal summation in nerves is in fact due to the occurrence of reverberatory circuits, and not merely to the summing of local potentials from the same source, in which case our analogy is a close one. The same argument, somewhat extended, leads to the phenomenon called recruitment.

The inhibitory function of nerves can occur either directly, when two stimuli act antagonistically, or when one follows the other after a delay, a delay which is too long for temporal summation to occur. Again, in our logical net model, inhibitory endings are assumed so that an impulse travelling along a fibre will be specifically inhibitory or specifically excitatory. In Chapman's growth nets (1959) it is possible to have the same nerve fibre carrying either an excitatory or inhibitory impulse, and this seems likely to be even nearer to the physiological facts.

Let us next consider some of the classical work of Sherrington (1906) and his co-workers on the nature of excitation and inhibition in collections of neurons joined together into a network, which is certainly how we wish to view the total organization of the nervous system.

It is well, in the first instance, to regard the central nervous system as a distributed network of more or less specialized tissue, and as working together as-a-whole. The parts will work autonomously under certain circumstances, but the whole system cannot be assumed to be the simple sum of the working of its parts; in fact it may be expected to exhibit characteristics which are both non-additive and non-linear.

The cortex might be regarded as having a controlling influence on sub-cortical and spinal nerve tissue, differentiated in something like hierarchical layers. As Sholl (1956) puts it:

> The cerebral hemispheres of all vertebrates are hollow cylinders of nervous tissue with a ventricle for the cavity. At first they are only associated with impulses arising from the olfactory organs but, in the higher vertebrates, connections are developed so that impulses arising from all the sense organs are transmitted to the forebrain and interact there to control the behaviour of the animal.

Methodologically, we have to make the classical findings (or interpretations) of anatomy, histology and physiology fit with the findings from work on the EEG, the organism-as-a-whole behaviour studies, work on brain injuries, electrical stimulation studies, ablation studies, and so on.

However, Sherrington's approach tells us something like this about the human nervous system: the nervous system has a property of excitability, and it is organized into networks in living organisms in such a way that its behaviour appears to take the form of an interconnected hierarchy of reflexes. The notion of a *reflex*, of a simply connected input–output system, may, of course, be an artefact of our method of isolation. A simple example is that of the spinal reflex. If we stimulate an afferent nerve the impulse travels to the spinal cord and, with a synaptic junction, is transferred to an efferent nerve (here we assume the Bell/Majendie law which distinguishes motor and sensory nerves). The number of internuncial or 'shunt' neurons involved may be quite large. Similarly, specialized receptors may be involved—but we shall not immediately consider the extra complexity this implies. The 'segmental reflex', as it is called, is the simplest reflex of the nervous system that is readily available.

The theoretical terms 'central excitatory state' (c.e.s.) and 'central inhibitory state' (c.i.s.) are at the heart of Sherrington's theory, but before discussing them let us consider some observable data from which these theoretical terms were derived.

We directly observe, in the muscle–nerve preparation, excitability of the nerve and a change of excitability as a result of electrical stimulation. We also observe the properties of relative and absolute refractory period and—due to our ability to measure the velocity of nerve conduction—we can, by arithmetical subtraction, observe a delay in segmental reflex (in the more complicated reflexes called 'reflex latency') which are assumed to represent synaptic delay.

Directly observable also are the properties of 'spatial summation' and 'temporal summation' of nervous impulses, and the 'threshold' of nervous tissue as a way of measuring the sensitivity of nerve cells; all these we have already mentioned.

The notion of spatial summation requires some comment. If two afferent nerves are stimulated, and both play on the same reflex centre, summation takes place, and reflex responses take place which would not occur in response to either stimulations acting alone. An example of this phenomenon is that of *tibialis anticus*. Changes in collections of central neurons may last as long as 15 msec, and Sherrington assumed that a subliminal stimulus set up a c.e.s., and that a further stimulus might then be additive and fire off the efferents. 'c.e.s.' is here playing its role as a theoretical term, and it is interesting to note that it must take care of delays up to 20 msec.

Lorente de Nó's (1938a, 1938b) work on this problem shows that in a single central synapse, summation of subliminal stimuli can be demonstrated over an interval no longer than 0·5 msec. However, de Nó believed that c.e.s. can be taken to mean (operationally) delay involving several internuncial neurons intercalated between sensory fibres and anterior horn cells, thus accounting for the longer delays assumed by Sherrington. This allows of more enduring responses than can be accounted for by this setting up of internal excitatory circuits.

Eccles's work on electrical states at synapses has suggested a model for synaptic delay and summation. To build these synaptic phenomena requires, largely, the ordering or organization and control of systematic detail (see Creed *et al.*, 1932; Erlanger and Gasser, 1937; de Nó, 1947; Eccles, 1953). It will suffice here to add that the majority of synaptic connections considered were of the *boutons terminaux* type, and the development of these may be correlated with states of the organism-as-a-whole. Furthermore, *boutons terminaux* apparently exist in abundance in the cortical areas, though there are histological difficulties with respect to their staining.

Next, the notion of 'central inhibition' must be dealt with. In the decerebrate cat the crossed extensor reflex can be inhibited or blocked entirely. In view of the time relations involved, Fulton has suggested the ventral horn cells as the seat of the inhibition. Sherrington showed that the knee jerk was inhibitable, and it was used as an index of c.i.s. That inhibition (operationally, this is the suppression of normally elicitable reflexes when they are elicited contiguously with certain other reflexes) is observed is clear, but theory is more concerned with the explanation of why it takes place. There are in fact many theories, and we shall take as examples those of Gasser and Eccles. Gasser believes that the internuncial circuits normally involved in the now inhibited reflex have a greatly heightened threshold and become relatively unresponsive. This is not wholly dissimilar in essence to the explanation of Creed *et al.* (1932) when the competition for the final common path led to selective changes of excitability in one centre. By final common path (f.c.p.) we mean simply the final response path that decides the behavioural act. They point out that when an antidromic volley travels up motor nerve fibres to moto-neurons, the excitation is thought to disappear from those neurons, and this accounts for the long duration of inhibitory effects produced by a contralateral volley.

They summarize the properties of inhibition in the following way:

(1) Centripetal volleys in ipsilateral nerves normally excite contrac-tions of flexors and inhibit extensors, while centripetal volleys in contralaterals have the opposite effect.
(2) Inhibitory processes in motoneurons can be graded in intensity.
(3) Summation of inhibition may be produced by successive volleys on one or more afferent nerves.
(4) Inhibition is antagonistic to c.e.s. and may slow down the build-up of the c.e.s.
(5) c.e.s. and c.i.s. are mutually antagonistic.
(6) c.i.s. undergoes a progressive and spontaneous subsidence.

It should be noticed that no evidence was dealt with by these writers for inhibition other than with motoneurons.

In the descriptions of inhibition by most early writers we find little reference to the chemical means by which this is achieved, although Eccles (1953) has something to say by way of summary on this matter.

It is already clear that the notion of the reflex arc in isolation is some-what artificial, and that reflex activities occur together in a very compli-cated manner. In the first place there is the competition for the final common path, the competition that occurs for the control of motoneurons and thus of all movement patterns.

Direct inhibition is explained in terms of hyper-polarization of the neuronal surface membrane. Indeed it is now thought that during a period of hyper-polarization there is the need for a larger post-synaptic potential to activate the self-regenerating sodium carrier, and there is much evidence to support such a view.

Eccles goes further than this, and explains more complicated and more prolonged inhibition in terms of hyper-polarization, and the theory has been developed that this inhibitory synaptic activity is a function of a specific transmitter substance liberated from inhibitory synaptic knobs.

However, we have agreed to leave the development of the chemical aspects of nervous function outside our range, and it must suffice to say that there is an increasing awareness of the workings of the inhibitory activity which is so necessary to account for the gross activity of the nervous system, and that it is possible to guess at a plausible form of explanation of 'central inhibition', whether it be direct or indirect. The really important point is that it does take place.

Before leaving the subject of inhibition we might consider its relation to logical nets. It will be remembered that we assumed merely two sorts of nerve terminations, served by identical fibres carrying identical impulses, except of course for the individual differences among fibres, which is something we have not considered in our logical nets. This can be met in many ways by using many pathways together to make up a volley of impulses, or by changing the idealized nets to fit the facts more closely. From the behavioural point of view this last demand is not obviously necessary.

Inhibition is therefore brought about in a logical net by direct stimulation of a neuron (we shall now use the word neuron, as we are placing the nerve interpretation on these models), or by altering the effective threshold of a neuron by retaining the record of some previous firing. This means that something very like a classical neurological picture is really subsumed in the construction of nerve nets. What perhaps is more interesting is the manner in which the differences between the two can subsequently be met. It would be easy to show in logical nets two neural chains carrying impulses for a final common path, and the manner in which these chains can be regarded as antagonistic, so that the path is given to only one chain at any particular time.

The next stage in the classical theory involves the types of reflex which are elicitable in the central nervous system, e.g. postural, flexor, extensor, intersegmental, etc. For illustrative purposes the classical experiments by Sherrington on the spinal cat should be sufficient. As a result of this work we have explanations given in terms of convergence, final common pathway (f.c.p.), occlusion, after-discharge, reflex centre, etc.

It is assumed that the co-ordinated activity of muscular action is the result of overlap in reflex fields, made possible by the convergence of afferent and internuncial paths on to one efferent f.c.p. Occlusion, in particular, takes place as a special case of this overlap when two afferent nerves, simultaneously stimulated, fire off a high percentage of the same motoneurons. After-discharge is regarded as a function of internuncial delay paths. The discussion of the remainder of the reflexes introduces no essentially new idea: they may all be explained in terms of the principles already referred to.

So far we have built up a conceptual picture of the nervous system as a complicated network like a telephone exchange, in which reflex activity is the element we have inherited, and the selectivity of the reflexes is made dependent on the inhibition of these networks at synaptic junctions. Both excitation and inhibition are summable, and they may interact in complex ways which are partly determined by the anatomical organization of the nervous system.

In modern neurology, more and more, the concept of the reflex is being replaced by the simple graded servo or feedback system (neural homeostats), but while we shall review some of the grosser evidence, it must be remembered throughout how little we know of the more intimate and detailed connections in the nervous system.

Information theory and nervous impulses

It is well known that information theory is used to describe possible nervous activities, and the appropriateness of such descriptive means is obvious enough.

The most evident point about the nervous system and its transmission is that the code is, basically, a simple one, being of the same pulse–no-pulse kind that is used by computers. It is a Morse code with dots only, and thus of a binary form, based on the all-or-nothing principle of nerve transmission.

It is also easy enough to guess that the intensity of stimulation—clearly a necessary variable—is correlated with frequency of discharge of impulse along afferent fibres, and such a factor automatically suggests the occurrence of summation, where relative economy of fibres occurs entailing many–one and one–many relations from cells to fibres and fibres back to cells. It is partly because of this that temporal and spatial summation are such essential features of nervous activity, and the thought follows naturally that inhibition will be included in the means by which integration takes place.

Rapoport (1955), Sutherland (1959) and Barlow (1959), among many others, have considered the problem of coding with respect to the visual system, and their work will be discussed further in Chapter 11.

The implication that all parts of the nervous sytem, as well as the whole organism, could be studied from the point of view of an information system is clear, for the brain is indubitably an information-receiving, transmitting and storing system; but these facts, apart from being useful in the construction of *molar* models of organic behaviour, do not help substantially in unravelling the intricacies of the function of complex

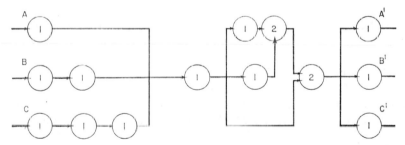

Fig. 54. Logical net for firing through a constriction. The figure shows one simple way in which an input can be fired through a channel which has less fibres than there are inputs and yet an input event can still be reproduced correctly as an output.

nervous tissue. What it achieves, in conjunction with other cybernetic methods, is an almost ideal behavioural model as a basis for neurophysiological comparison.

A further point should be made with respect to the importance of many–one relations mentioned above. This seems to occur commonly in the nervous system, and involves a mapping of a set of impulses from a set of neurons on to many fewer nerve fibres and vice versa. This is well known to occur in the visual system, among many other parts of the nervous system, and leads to the firing through the restriction of the visual pathways. Figure 54 shows the fairly straightforward logical net principle that could be used to mirror just this sort of thing.

What is important about this is that the splitting up of nerve impulses into a sequential train of pulses makes it necessary to reaccumulate that train in part or whole at some later time, and this requires precisely the operation of *summation*.

Broadbent (1954) has shown that the operation of the ear, in accepting different items of information simultaneously presented to it, is itself sequential. The implication is that the auditory system is able to store information prior to its being dealt with centrally, and this is precisely what is implied by passing information through a constraint.

So far we have only dealt with the elements and their simple organization into a network, we must now look for a while at what has been discovered about the brain itself. Here we shall simply select certain relevant features from various points of view, and indicate in each case what sort of equivalent logical net organization would be possible and plausible. In this next section, it will be borne in mind that we can think of the logical nets originally described in Chapter 5 as being very high speed in their function and thus being influenced by whole volleys of impulses rather than single ones alone. This implies a statistical type of description for a large network, and such statistical models have already been discussed to some extent (Beurle, 1954; Rapoport, 1950a, 1950b, 1950c, 1950d, 1955; Sholl, 1956). In any case they will become essential as our logical nets increase in size, as indeed they must if they are to mimic in any useful way the human brain.

We shall also bear in mind that as the search for neurological models becomes more urgent, our problem will be to discover how the nervous system *is actually wired*. There is no reason to doubt the ease with which nets can be drawn that will perform the necessary behavioural functions, but in order that they may be scientifically useful ultimately, we shall wish to draw the nets with only particular information flow, which have the right dimensions as regards numbers of elements used, and which can also perform the necessary function in the same manner as the nervous system.

With these ideas clearly before us, let us look at some of our information on brain analysis.

Our subject-matter is so vast that the best that we can hope to do here is to give a brief summary of relevant work. This means that the more detailed analysis of neural transmission, and detailed work on certain chemical aspects of neurology, will not be further considered; but even after putting these aside, there remains an immense bulk of neurological data which would fill many volumes, and we can discuss here only selected aspects, selected always with one eye on the ultimate interests and needs of the cybernetician.

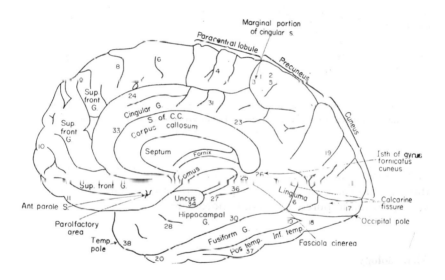

FIG. 55. CENTRAL SECTION OF CEREBRUM. The section is cut in a plane at right angles to that of the eyes and approximately bisecting a line joining the two eyes. The numbers refer to Brodman's areas (see text).

Before discussing the rest of the nervous system let us look at some more diagrams that will help in our terminological problem. Figures 55 and 56 show the inner and outer surface of a cerebral hemisphere with names *and also numbers* (Brodman, 1909) that indicate its general topog-

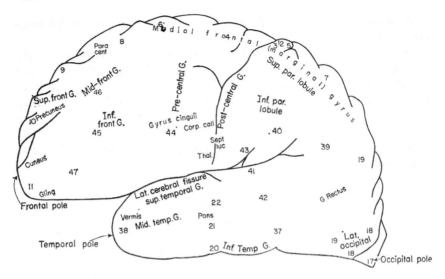

FIG. 56. EXTERNAL SURFACE OF CEREBRUM. This figure shows more of the names for features of the cortex and also gives some of the numbers for Brodman areas mentioned in the text.

raphy. Brodman's numbers were based on histological distinctions, and these are now known to be inadequate on these grounds, but are convenient to retain purely as spatial coordinates.

Methodology

The first question of importance is that of methodology in neuro-anatomy and neurophysiology, and this will be discussed immediately. The anatomist can contribute an enormous amount to our knowledge of neurological function, as has been pointed out by Le Gros Clark (1950). But there are certain limitations that need to be observed; the general topography of the nervous system may not in itself be a good guide to function. The histological staining techniques, used on mapping fibre connections in the brain, have also had considerable doubts attached to them.

The mapping of the cortex, however, is now considerably advanced, thanks to specialized silver techniques, intravital methylene blue neurography, electrical stimulation, and the methods involving experimental lesions and accidental brain damage. Le Gros Clark has noted that the blood vessels, and their mapping, is especially important to neurology since it supplies a clue to the degree of metabolism, and hence to function. It is interesting to note, in this respect, that the cortical arteries, being confined to the cortex and immediately subadjacent to the white matter, can serve the purpose of cerebral lesion; for example, if the pia mater is stripped from the area to be studied, a lesion is effected.

For an account of the histological features of the brain, reference should be made to Ramon y Cajal (1952) and Sholl (1956).

The method of neuronography, devised by Dusser de Barenne, and used by him and McCulloch (Dusser de Barenne and McCulloch, 1937, 1938, 1939; Dusser de Barenne, Garol and McCulloch, 1941; et al.) has been very useful in the mapping of direct neural connections. The application of filter paper soaked in strychnine sulphate to one cortical locus leads to 'strychnine spikes' occurring at certain other loci.

The central assumption of neuronography is that there exist direct connections, without synapses, between the two areas involved. There is a high correlation between anatomical detail and neuronographical records, where corroboration has been possible, but against this must be stated the evidence of Frankenhauser (1951). As Frankenhauser points out, the above work in neuronography implies that the absence of spikes in a given region excludes the existence of direct pathways. He strychninized the olfactory bulb, but was unable to find any spikes in regions where many direct pathways from the olfactory bulb are known to exist. He feels, therefore, that the negative implications of neuronography are unjustified.

Electrical techniques

The method of electrical stimulation of nerve tissue has also been critized from time to time, especially with respect to spreading effects on the surface of the cortex; other workers in this field (Gellhorn and Johnson, 1951), however, have defended the method with some cogency.

Another source of information with seemingly enormous potentialities is the electroencephalogram (EEG), and an assessment of the various methods adopted here is far more complicated than in the case of anatomical localization, histology, neuronography, or electrical stimulation.

Darrow (1947) inferred that the relative failure of the EEG to contribute much to the field of psychology may be from one of two reasons: either the code of the EEG is simply not understood, or the EEG gives, not an integrated cortical record, but a record of subsidiary homeostatic processes. This failure would appear to be—certainly partially—due to the first cause, although from a physiological viewpoint some guesses have now been made at the code. For the second point, it may be true that the EEG does give a homeostatic picture, and homeostasis is to be thought of as a fundamental characteristic of neural activity.

Hill (1950) has given an assessment of the EEG in its relationship to psychiatry, in which he points to the fact that EEG characteristics are as typical of an individual as, say, his fingerprints, or his I.Q. What is of special interest is that many of the individual differences exhibitable on the EEG may disappear on suitable chemical, or physiological, stimulation.

Burns (1950, 1951, 1958) has studied carefully the levels of response from electrical stimulation, and his results are consistent with those found by Albino (1960) in ablation experiments. It is clear that different strengths of stimuli do in fact elicit quite different sorts (or levels) of response.

Burn's work was on isolated cortex, and his results were thought to be caused by chains of neurons which, when they all become fired under strong stimulation, become refractory. Similarily, he found that repeated strong stimulation of cortex gave rise to bursts of responses which may last for as long as an hour after cessation of stimulation.

Some of the summarizing characteristics of the EEG work noted by Hill are:

(1) Attention and increased cerebral activity are associated with low voltage and fast activity, while relaxation and decreased cerebral activity are correlated with high voltage and slow activity.
(2) 'Emotional tension' changes EEG patterns.
(3) Hypothalamic activity influences cortical rhythms.
(4) Amplitude of waves in a rhythm is a rough measure of the number of cellular units taking part in its production.

(5) Hill thinks, more speculatively, that the constant pattern of the EEG reflects maturation of the brain in terms of functional organization.

With respect to (3), Henry and Scoville (1952), in a discussion of suppressor bursts from isolated pieces of cortex (they were considering patients who had had frontal lobotomy performed, which also involved undercutting of areas 9 and 10, and the orbital gyri), considered that the fundamental rhythms of the brain emanated from the hypothalamus.

The whole question of the value of the EEG as a research technique is of immense complication and demands specialist consideration. The volume of work already produced on the EEG is enormous, nevertheless it is probable that nothing has yet been discovered which critically affects the behavioural picture.

All afferent volleys to the cortex set up an initial surface positive wave (Eccles, 1953) which is restricted to the cortical region in which the volley terminates; the wave form may be complex, although this is not true for single afferent impulses. It has been suggested that the initial positive wave is caused by the synaptic excitatory action of afferent impulses generating post-synaptic potentials on the deeper parts of the apical dendrites and the bodies of pyramidal cells.

It should be added that there is some evidence that reverberatory circuits from the thalamus contribute to the later stages of the responses to afferent stimulation in the cortex.

In such terms it is worth considering the nature of the α-rhythm. It is thought to be due to impulses travelling in closed, self-exciting chains.

More recently, Eccles has suggested that the α-rhythm is due to circulation of impulses in closed self-re-exciting chains, the idea being that it is due to the low intensity bombardment during states of attention.

Stewart (1959), taking a more cybernetic view of the problem, has suggested that the α-rhythm and the other brain rhythms are due to the inevitable periodicity of a finite automaton, and that it is something we might expect from the very construction of any finite automata. Kennedy (1959) has proposed that the α-rhythm may arise from mechanical oscillation of the gel of the living brain and not from the synchronization of neural activity, except very indirectly.

Certainly it must be admitted that this whole matter requires further investigation, especially since it offers clues of a fairly definite kind for the designers of artificial brains.

In the last decade a tremendous amount of detail has been added to our models of the nervous system as a result of studies by EEG. We now have a much better idea of the correlation which exists between different wave forms and combinations of different wave forms and different sorts of cognitive activity. However, in spite of this, there is nothing that can be substantially added at the level of brain models that affects our overall picture as of yet.

Sensory deprivation

A very large number of studies have been done in recent years on sensory deprivation and Riesen (1966) has extensively reviewed the literature. Animals reared in darkness have cellular changes and a greatly reduced thickness of visual cortex and lateral genyptic body and decreased cortical vascularity among other things. It has even been suggested that cats reared in darkness develop fewer higher-order branches in the dendrites of neurons in the visual cortex than do visually experienced cats. This is not entirely surprising and confirms a very general view which has been held for a long time that sensory stimulation plays an essential role in the maturation of connections in the central nervous system.

Hubel and Wiesel (1959, 1962, 1963) together and Hubel (1967) have reported an interesting series of studies indicating that connections necessary for binocular interaction can occur even without any visual experience. They also say that this integration can be disrupted by independent activities of the eyes. It may therefore be that in something like the visual system which is laterally symmetrical and the same with coordination of hands and legs and hearing, etc., it is the integration which may suffer from lack of sensory stimulation as much as the individual capacity of the organ.

We must now say something of the functions associated with gross anatomical divisions of the brain.

The myelencephalon

The myelencephalon or *medulla* is relatively simple; it is simply the joining point of the spinal cord to the higher brain levels. It is composed of groups of cells or nuclei, and is the point of exit and entrance for many of the pairs of cranial nerves.

It is probable that the medulla is a relay station for the autonomic nervous system since it contains certain nuclei which directly affect autonomic function, and yet there is evidence of cortical representation of autonomic function, and therefore its role is probably an integrative one allowing partial classification. The words 'relay station' which we will use from time to time are meant to suggest little more than the fact that certain locations are on the direct paths between different parts of the brain, although the presence of nuclei suggests that there is some switching function to be performed there.

The metencephalon

The metencephalon, which consists of the *cerebellum, pons* and a part of the fourth ventricle, is something like the cerebrum in that it consists of grey matter on the surface with white underneath, the rest being largely nuclei. Problems of cerebral localization also occur (Fulton, 1949), but for the purpose of our précis it is sufficient to indicate its principal areas, which may be called ventral, dorsal, anterior and posterior respectively.

The semicircular canals, utricle and sacule, send fibres to the ventral portion, while the spinal cord supplies fibres to the anterior and posterior portion. The dorsal portion, or neocerebellum, as it is sometimes called, has connections with the pons and the frontal lobes of the cerebral cortex.

The pons itself forms the ventral part of the metencephalon, and is composed of fibres that leave the cerebellum and return to it, after crossing the ventral surface of the hindbrain. Other nuclei and fibre tracts—both ascending and descending—make up the rest of the pons.

The cerebellum is almost certainly concerned with co-ordinating motor activities, and it is known that injuries to the cerebellum will destroy muscular co-ordination. The pons is probably concerned with the association of motor activities, and since the trigeminal nerve has its nuclei in the pons, it may be supposed it is closely concerned with the sense of touch, and movement of the face and mouth.

The mesencephalon

The mesencephalon or *midbrain* connects the forebrain and hindbrain. This is probably a motor reflex centre in part, with ascending and descending tracts. The *tectum*, which forms part of the midbrain, has a sensory function involving the four colliculi, so called. The superior colliculi have already been thought of by Pitts and McCulloch (1947) as a possible feedback centre for the operation of visual scanning.

The inferior colliculi are concerned with hearing, and the colliculi generally again qualify for the vague description of relay centres.

The reticular system

This is perhaps an appropriate moment to describe the non-specific neural mechanisms, especially the system called the ascending reticular system.

If the central reticular core of the brain stem is stimulated then there is a change of cortical electrical activity which is closely associated with attention. Jasper (1958) has given a fairly loose definition of the reticular system in the following terms:

> ... the reticular formation, extending from the thalamus down into the medulla, is represented by all those neuronal structures which are not included in the specific afferent and efferent pathways.

The development of our knowledge of the reticular system is extremely relevant to our understanding of the problem of attention and alertness, and also perhaps of consciousness.

These studies have developed from an interest in spinal reflexes (Magoun, 1958), and to an interest in the allied function of non-specific brain mechanisms.

Olds and Milner (1954) have shown that direct stimulation of the central reticular core of the brain stem exhibited some of the same electrical changes in the cortex as occur in waking from sleep, or on the sudden alerting of an individual. This leads to the replacement of high voltage slow waves and spindle bursts in the EEG record by low voltage fast discharges (Moruzzi and Magoun, 1949).

Lesions of the ascending reticular system caused sleepiness in animals, and stimulation caused wakefulness.

As well as peripheral sources of input to the reticular system there are also projection fibres from the cortex to the central brain stem (Jasper *et al.*). Also projecting to the central brain stem, are the associated areas of frontal, cingulate, parieto-occipital and temporal cortex, and the sensory and motor cortical areas.

One implication of this work is that the excitation of cortical sensory areas is insufficient by itself to induce arousal or cause sensation.

A further set of results shows that afferent transmission is also affected by these non-specific central states.

Morrell and Jasper (1955) have been able to demonstrate, in terms of conditioning, that the blocking of the α-rhythm as a conditioned response is a method for the study of temporary connection formation in the brain. At the beginning of conditioning, a generalized blocking reaction occurs which, with repeated conditioning, becomes more specific, and restricted to some local cortical area. There is a general activation and blocking prior to any learning operation.

Consciousness can perhaps be seen to be emerging from this sort of work, although as Jasper (1958) puts it:

> The stream of our consciousness is only a minute sampling of the multitude of simultaneously active cells and circuits in the complex machinery of the mind.

Much, even most, of the function of the reticular system is probably still unconscious, and it is the ascending reticular system that is probably primarily concerned with consciousness. Attention is probably a further differentiation of the generalized arousal mechanism, where there is little doubt that generalized arousal is dependent on activity within the mesencephalic and caudal portions of the diencephalic reticular system. As far as attention is concerned Jasper (1958) says:

> The fact that the thalamic reticular system seems to possess a certain degree of topographical organization relative to its cortical projections may provide a neurophysiological basis for the direction of attention.

It is interesting that the most important cortico-fugal projections seem to arise from areas not primarily sensory in function. They are the frontal, cingulate, temporal and parietal areas and area 19.

The implication is perhaps that these elaboration areas are the places where consciousness enters the picture; and the integrative process of the brain is possibly to be regarded as a multistage process, and one in which the reticular system may be thought to play a central part.

It has been noticed (Delafresnaye, 1954) that moderate activity in the reticular formation of the brain stem is correlated with fast asynchronous EEG recordings, and also correlated with alertness and attention. Lesions of the reticular formation lead to slow synchronous EEG recordings, and unconsciousness or somnolence.

Lindsley (1951) has actually suggested a theory of excitation based on activation of the reticular system, and more generally, it has been concluded that the reticular system was vital to skilled voluntary acts, and to memory and intelligence. The effect of stimulating the reticular areas at increasing intensities has been to lead through a progression from *alerting* to *searching*, and then to *flight*.

The limits of variability of cortical organization (Lashley, 1947) are a matter of 'individual differences', 'species differences', etc., and therefore the generalized suggestions made here must necessarily be particularized for different species, and ultimately for a particular individual.

Much current work is going on in the field of the reticular system, much of which must be taken to modify the neuropsychological theories of Hebb, Lashley and others. From the point of view of our own approach, we should seek to give interpretation to the reticular system as bearing closely on the *M*-system or motivational system and the closely related *E*-system or emotional system, and the relation of both these to the *C*-system.

Further evidence that the reticular formation is a homeostatically controlled one has been given recently by Dell. He suggests that the final common path on the motor side are selectively placed at the disposal of one of the various afferent systems or cortical spinal projections capable of activating them. He goes on to argue that in the waking animal a whole pattern of reciprocal associations of non-specific systems and sensory motor mechanisms of high specific function determine the fine adjustments of activity and the differentiation of motor responses. What he is suggesting, of course, is a critical adaptive reaction, homeostatically controlled which once again must refer to the hierarchical type of model that we have in mind and links in directly with the notion of a partial adaptive classification system.

The diencephalon

The thalamus and hypothalamus, the optic tracts and retinae, the pituitary, mammillary bodies and third ventricle make up the diencephalon.

The main interest for behaviour theory, with the exception of visual perception (see Chapter 11) lies in the thalamus and hypothalamus.

The thalamus is thought of as another relay station, the principal one in the brain, and it is made up of various nuclei.

Thalamus and hypothalamus

The thalamus is embryologically old compared with the cerebral cortex, which has been modified in a series of extensive ramifications. The thalamus (Fulton, 1943) appears to be best viewed as an end station in the forebrain of sensory systems of the body. The geniculate bodies appear to be connected with the special senses. Its associative functions are cortico-diencephalic and intradiencephalic. It has seven principal afferent tracts, and is connected with the adjacent mass of the hypothalamus. Anatomically, the thalamus may be divided into three groups of nuclei with (1) subcortical connections, (2) cortical relay nuclei which transmit impulses from somatic sensory systems and the special senses, and (3) its association nuclei.

Lesions of the posterior third of the ventral nucleus cause transient cutaneous impairment, and rupture of the thalamogeniculate artery 'causes' paresthesia and hyperesthesia. Starzl and Magoun (1951) suggest, as a result of studying the cat's thalamic projection system, that it is organized for mass thalamic influence on the association cortex.

It has been generally assumed that the hypothalamus is connected with the emotional aspects of behaviour. However, the anatomy and physiology of the hypothalamus is, like the thalamus, closely associated with cortical areas. Its main divisions are: (1) periventricular region,

(2) pre-optic region, (3) lateral region, (4) rostral or supraoptic middle region, (5) tuberal, infundibular middle region, (5) caudal, or mammillary region. The existing knowledge of the hypothalamus is somewhat mixed but, as Le Gros Clark (1950) has said, much of the most recent development on 'psychosomatic' medicine has surrounded a study of the hypothalamus. The work of Philip Bard (1934) and Masserman (1943) on 'sham rage' is now well known, and needs no further comment here; Le Gros Clark's survey continues the same line of thought. Lesions of the hypothalamus are still considered to be closely related to the 'emotional' aspects of behaviour, as well as to the autonomic nervous system. The hypothalamus is probably central to any 'total' theory of behaviour, but does not contact the more restricted aspects of 'learning' to quite the same extent.

However, a few words in summary on the hypothalamus may be suggestive for purposes of general development (Le Gros Clark, 1950);

(1) The hypothalamus is situated in the base of the brain, and has the cerebral peduncles immediately behind, and the optic chiasma in front; it is also, of course, close to the pituitary which is an outgrowth of the hypothalamus.

(2) Its considerable blood supply suggests high metabolic acitivity, and the hypothalamic–pituitary connections are again emphasized.

(3) In submammalian vertebrates, the supraoptic and paraventricular nucleus is fused in a single mass which suggests a close functional connection.

(4) The hypothalamus has a motor pathway from the posterior and lateral hypothalamus into the brain system (possibly autonomic).

(5) The medial thalamic nucleus projecting to the granular cortex of the frontal lobe might suggest a railway station function.

(6) The Mammillo-thalamic tract (bundle of Vicq d'Azur) connects the thalamus and hypothalamus.

(7) There are fibres derived from the globus pallidus running from the subthalamus to the hypothalamus, and this, perhaps, implies partial basal ganglionic control of the hypothalamus.

(8) The frontal cortex has (possibly autonomic) fibres direct to the hypothalamus.

(9) The fornix, en route from the hippocampus to the mammillary bodies, is a large afferent tract to the hypothalamus. The fibres

from the Mammillo-thalamic tract to the anterior nucleus of the thalamus, and to the cingulate cortex, form a closed circuit. It may be that the hippocampus is not only olfactory (as will be emphasized later; Scoville and Milner, 1957), and the mammillary bodies are probably relay stations. This last is of special interest in the now well-known possible role of cerebral prolongation at cortical level.

(10) The frontal lobe is a projection area for the hypothalamus.

(11) It can be tentatively restated that the hypothalamus is to be regarded as a relay station under cortical (and striatal) control. This is especially related to autonomic function, and also plays an integrated part in normal cerebral function; it is, indeed, probably connected closely with reverberatory circuits.

(12) Recent work on the thalamus (Albe-Fessard and Fessard, 1963) suggests further evidence for believing that whereas the cortex is still the main site for the integration of sensory messages, there is a great deal of this type of activity taking place within the thalamus or even at lower levels of the central nervous system. Albe-Fessard and Fessard have designated this process 'projected convergence' and have assumed the point of convergence is at whatever level is appropriate to the type of activity being integrated. It is natural to think in terms of our cybernetic models that the thalamus is part of the hierarchical classification system and that any of the functions performed at the highest level can be performed at any of the lower levels, only that the ratio of integrated classification must go up as the level of integration goes up in the classification system.

The telencephalon

Under this term we subsume the olfactory bulb and tracts, the lateral ventricles and basal ganglia and, rather especially, the cerebral cortex.

Very generally we can divide the cerebral cortex into the four areas which are duplicated, one in each hemisphere. These areas are called: (1) Frontal (especially areas 4, 6, 8–11, 44 and 45), (2) Parietal (especially areas 2, 3, 5 and 7), (3) Temporal (especially areas 38, 39, 40, 41 and 42) and (4) Occipital (areas 17, 18 and 19). It has been suggested that the broad function of these areas is that the frontal lobes are integrative and the posterior portions concerned with relatively specific motor functions and also motor elaboration functions, the speech areas, areas 44 and 45, being specialized regions. The parietal lobe is concerned with sensory control and sensory elaboration, the temporal with speech recognition, musical recognition and generally with memory, while the occipital areas are specialized for vision and visual elaboration.

Within the compass of this very general statement there are problems about the relation between the two cerebral hemispheres which are by no means fully understood, and this makes all subsequent analysis of the function of specific areas somewhat tentative. The notion of cerebral dominance is of the first importance neurologically, and although there is some evidence that left-handed people are right hemisphere dominant, the whole problem is much more complex than this suggests. This matter is very important for comparative neurology since animal experiments seem to show that bilateral ablation is often necessary to produce impairment of specific function whereas in human beings this may often be produced by unilateral ablation. Clearly the human brain is more specialized and their equivalent cerebral areas are not merely mirror images of each other.

The cerebral cortex

We must now turn to a more detailed study of the cerebral cortex and, of course, the closely related neural structures of the immediately lower levels. In this discussion it is the cerebral hemisphere, particularly the cerebral cortex, the study of the Brodman areas and their function, cytoarchitectonics, the alleged suppressor areas, and the reticular system, etc., which are of the first importance. This involves the basal ganglia and other parts of the nervous system viewed as functions of the control of the cerebral mantle.

In discussing the cortex we should note the recent terminology that has been suggested by Pribram, Jasper and others (1958).

The Paleocortex or allocortex is phylogenetically older, and includes the hippocampus (Ammon's Horn and the dentate nucleus), the pyriform lobe, and the olfactory bulb and tubercle. The Juxtallocortex includes the cingulate gyrus, presubiculum and fronto-temporal cortex. The non-cortical tissue of first importance includes the amygdaloid complex, the septal region, thalamic and hypothalamic nuclei, as well as the caudate

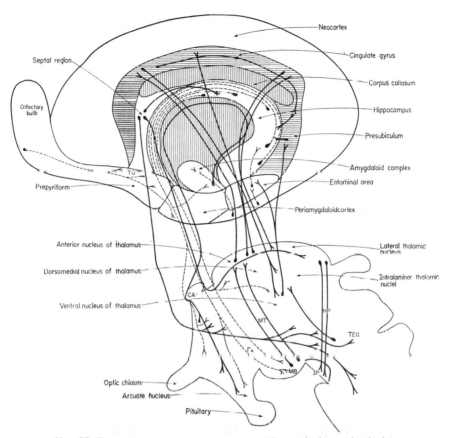

FIG. 57. THE FIGURE SHOWS THE CORTEX and its extrinsic and intrinsic thalamic connections. *Fx* is Fornix, *HP* the Habenulo-interpeduncular tract, *IP* the Interpeduncular nucleus, *MB* the Mammillary bodies, *MT* the Mammillo-thalamic tract to the olfactory tubercle, *TEG* the midbrain Tegmentum and *CA* the Anterior Commissure.

and midbrain reticular formulation. The isocortex, or neocortex, is further divided into Extrinsic and Intrinsic areas. The extrinsic have projective fibres from the thalamic relay nuclei and fibres from outside the thalamus, while the intrinsic project solely from the thalamic relay nuclei to the isocortex.

There is some evidence that the extrinsic fibres are closely connected with the different behaviour functions of peripheral receptor mechanisms, and the intrinsic are concerned with discrimination, which is known to be affected by removal of posterior intrinsic cortical areas.

It is necessary now to select carefully our analysis of the structure and function of the cortex with an eye to behaviour theory and automata construction. We shall first consider the function of the frontal lobes (Stanley and Jaynes, 1949; Hebb, 1945, 1949; Fulton, 1943, 1949; Sholl, 1956).

Cytoarchitectonically, the frontal lobes are part of the isocortex and are stratified in five layers. An outstanding feature is the presence of giant pyramidal cells in area 4. Furthermore, it is interesting to compare the smaller pyramidal cells of 6 with those of 4, and also with 7 in the temporal lobe. Campbell (1905), it may be noted, did not differentiate areas 6 and 7. Area 4 is usually regarded as a motor area, with giant pyramidal, (or Betz) cells in layer V. It may be subdivided into 4A (leg), 4B (arm), 4C (face), for superior, middle, and inferior parts (Vogt, 1919). Variation is only apparent in the size of the pyramidal cells, and it is noteworthy that, in man, area 4 is largely concealed in the central sulcus. For a comparative study reference should be made to Bucy (1944).

It is probable that the motor areas of the frontal lobe are not immediately vital to the behaviour picture; what, however, may be of importance is the strip region between areas 4 and 6 which is known as 4S, a suppressor area (Marion Hines, 1936). Area 6 is similar to area 4, without the pyramidal cells in layer V.

The subdivisions of 6 refer to buccal and respiratory musculature. Area 8 is also motor in function (transitional cortex which has extensive extrapyramidal projections to the striatum, thalamus (latero-ventral nucleus), subthalamus and tegmentum. It also possesses another suppressor area, 8S. Areas 9, 10, 11 and 12 (orbito-frontal cortex) are sometimes referred to collectively as the frontal association areas.

Cytoarchitectonically these are vastly different from areas 4 and 6. There are, for example, no motor cells in layer V. As regards function, 13 and 14, in the near orbital region, have been earmarked as respiratory and olfactory areas by Walker (1938).

Generally it is probably true to say that cytoarchitectonic analysis, with its extensive staining methods, has not yet reached its limits, and its contribution has been largely in its divisions of cortical areas in terms of cellular structure. One needs to supplement this knowledge with knowledge of the frontal areas derived from psychological experiments, neuronography, and so on. Here one must draw on the work of Fulton, Stanley and Jaynes, and many others.

(1) The frontal lobes may be divided into the orbito-frontal cortex (projection area of dorso-medial nucleus of the thalamus), 9, 10, 11, 12, as well as 13 and 14 on the orbital surface.
(2) The cingulate gyrus (24); the projection area of the antero-medial nucleus of the thalamus.
(3) Broca's speech area 44 and 45.

Area 24 has an antero-medial connection which, in turn, has a projection from the mammillary bodies, thus the hypothalamus is linked with the cortex. The antero-ventral and antero-dorsal nuclei project to areas 25 and 29. The dorso-medial nuclei are stationed on hypothalamic, and orbito-frontal, projections.

The hypothalamic-frontal connections imply a connection between autonomic function and the cerebral cortex, and the methods of neuronography have well illustrated this. The integration of autonomic responses probably takes place in the frontal, particularly in the orbital, surfaces. Evidence on these points comes from leuchotomy cases, as well as from neuronography. There appears, indeed, to be considerable overlap (Fulton, 1949) of autonomic and somatic function in cortical areas in the frontal lobe.

It is necessary now to pass on to the consideration of the behavioural aspects of the frontal lobes, and the correlation between somatic function and behaviour, and one is forced to concede straight away that there are serious problems to be faced.

(1) There are, as yet, insufficient behavioural checks on neurological findings, and contrariwise, neurological methods are not yet sufficient.
(2) The difficulty of finding homologous areas in different species.
(3) The difficulty of individual variation within the species.
(4) The complex problem of individual differences in learning. This may dominate the actual neural model with respect to neural patterns.

(2) and (3) have been built up to a great degree by the work of Clark and Lashley (1947), and bear on matters of localization.

The function of suppressor areas, as described by Stanley and Jaynes is to relax all striate musculature, raise the threshold of the precentral cortex, and reduce, or disrupt, after-discharge of the motor cortex. It is also of immediate interest that all the suppressor bands connect directly to the caudate nucleus, although it must be admitted that the very existence of suppressor areas is open to some doubt and, in view of this, they will not be discussed further.

Kluver's classical experiment, involving bilateral frontal ablation in a monkey, is concerned with the monkey's reaction to the stimulus of the sight of a grape. He will pick up the grape and begin to move it towards his mouth, but if he is then shown a second grape he will drop the first one and pick up the second. This process may go on until the monkey is surrounded by grapes, having eaten none (Kluver, 1933). It need hardly be added that this cannot be reproduced in the normal monkey. One is reminded, parenthetically, of the behaviour of very young children.

A large number of such experiments are quoted and compared both by Fulton (1949) and Stanley and Jaynes (1949), and mentioned by Hebb (1949), and we shall now gather together their results on the effect of frontal ablation.

(1) The increased food intake factor (Hyperphagia).

(2) Alternations in emotional and social behaviour as exemplified by the experiment of Jacobson, Wolfe, and Jackson, who found that two previously excitable chimpanzees were persistent, and benign, in a delayed reaction test, even in the face of repeated failure. Both had bilateral ablation of the frontal region. Ward (1948) found that unilateral or bilateral ablation of area 24 (cingulate gyrus) in four monkeys led to a profound change in the animals' emotional and social behaviour, while other workers have been able to observe no such changes.

Arnot (1949), in presenting his theory of frontal lobe function, re-emphasized the now well-established fact that changes in social behaviour take place. Arnot saw the frontal lobe function as one involving the persistence of emotional states, chains of thought, motor activities and motor inhibitions. This will certainly be seen to fit some of the facts well.

(4) Thirdly, there is the fact of hypermobility (sometimes also inertness is observed) following on bilateral ablation of the frontal region. This has been specifically demonstrated by Ruch and Shenkin (1943) on bilateral ablation of area 13 of Walker, and on no other part of the frontal

cortex, and has been confirmed by Fulton, Livingstone and Davis (1947); Mettler (1944), however, failed to confirm it. He found that hypermobility follows bilateral ablation of area 9, or the pre-motor areas. It is also interesting to note that vision apparently plays a major role in the sensory control of hypermobility. Kennard, Spencer and Fountain (1941) found that enucleation of the eyes, occipital lesions, or even darkness, reduced the total amount of activity in monkeys.

(4) According to Settlage, Zable and Harlow (1948), there is a difficulty in 'habit reversal' in an 'either–or' test, which is subsequently reversed for the correct response. In the view of these workers there is a marked difference between the reversal patterns of the frontal animal, as opposed to the normal. There exists a perseverance of the non-reinforced habit shift in the normal monkey.

(5) There is intellectual loss sometimes observed, and finally

(6) We should mention that there is normally a general change in motivation.

In another report, Harlow, Meyer and Settlage (1951) discuss a study they carried out on the effects of extensive unilateral lesions in a group of monkeys. They also used another group of monkeys (there were four in each group) who had both unilateral lesions and destructions of lateral surface of contralateral pre-frontal region. A control group of four was also used. They found that there was almost complete loss of function in the 'delayed response' situation, even though medial and orbital surfaces of the frontal lobe were intact. They also found that generalized response was affected in the pre-frontal monkey.

Some interesting comparable results were found by Blum, Chow and Blum (1951) on the *Macaca mulatta*, in the auditory dicrimination habit and the delayed reaction test (auditory and visual clues used). Blum noted that the mid-lateral destruction caused serious impairment, whereas ventro-lateral or dorsal destruction caused only slight impairment. It was noticeable, too, that the total amount of destruction seemed important in the mid-lateral case.

(5) Seriatim problems involve poor performances in 'frontal' monkeys. Jacobson's experiments (1931, 1935, 1936; Jacobson and Elder, 1936; Jacobson and Haslernd, 1936; Jacobson, Wolfe and Jackson, 1935) are illustrative of this. He had two chimpanzees and gave them 6 months' training in (a) delayed reaction tests, (b) problem boxes, and (c) stick and

platform problems. The problem boxes, of which there were two types, involved in the first instance a simple, single operation, such as pulling a rope or rod. The second operation had a more complex combination box, in which a rope, rod and crank had to be operated in a particular order to open the box. Both animals were operated on, and at first one frontal area was removed in each, the areas involved being 9, 10, 11 and 12. The animals were subsequently tested for three months, and then the second frontal area was removed, with apparently no change in behaviour. However, between the first and second operations there were, in fact, certain not easily observable changes that Jacobson (1931, 1936) described as 'frustrational behaviour' (e.g. when unrewarded in discrimination or delayed reaction tests if the wrong choice was made), and the presence of 'temper tantrums'. After the second operation three was a complete lack of emotional expression, and the chimpanzees appeared to be un-worried by failure. After the bilateral ablation, the chimpanzees failed the double stick and platform test. In Jacobson's work it appears that the anterior parts of area 24 were destroyed, and that the orbital surfaces, on the other hand, were left intact.

The next experiment is concerned with Lashley's conditioned reaction problem, a type of discrimination problem in which two stimuli are pre-sented, and one is conditioned with respect to some other feature of the environment, e.g. black and white cards were presented, and food was given for response to the black card. Normal animals learnt this easily, but the 'frontals' failed in a thousand trials. The delayed reaction prob-lems are of various forms and reference should be made to the original work for further details (Jacobson, 1931, etc.). The results are fairly con-sistent. Jacobson found delays up to 2 min in normal monkeys, and also found that the responses were, at worst, destroyed by bilateral ablation; at best, delays of some 3 or 4 sec were obtained. Campbell and Harlow (1945) have found that by certain devices, such as increasing the time inter-val after operation, and time intervals between trials, longer delays could be obtained.

One confirmatory experiment was carried out by Chow, Blum and Blum (1951) in which they used monkeys (*Macaca mulatta*) with bilateral parieto-temporo-preoccipital ablations. Subsequently there was removal of the frontal granular cortex. Tests and observations of sensory states and abilities in discrimination (vision, somesthesis, audition) were made before and after the frontal operation, and the conditioned reactions and delayed reponses in the monkeys were listed. The effects of additional pre-frontal ablation on the four monkeys were, as interpreted by the experiments: (1) Decrease in visual activity in one monkey, and restriction of visual field in another; the other two were apparently unaffected with respect to sensory defects. (2) Deficient retention was observable in two monkeys, and deficient discrimination with respect to temperature and roughness in two. There appeared to be no failure in visual discrimination. (3) There was a decrement on the conditioned reaction problem. (4) Three of the monkeys failed completely on the delayed response, and the fourth was considerably poorer. (5) There was a general increase of activity in all the animals.

One further inference made by these workers is of interest. They discuss the occurrence of 'fringe activity' in the cortex, and imply that a model of cortical activity must include the notion of dominant and recessive controlling factors overlapping. Such cortical overlap is very suggestive and consistent with a conception of the cortex as a functional mosaic, which may account for the variable results so often found after repeated stimulation of the same cortical 'point' even without differences of strength of stimulation.

Sholl (1956) believes the frontal lobes are the seat of co-ordination and fusion of the incoming and outgoing products of the several sensory and motor areas of the cortex and we may guess that the frontal lobes are probably simply storage areas, from the computer point of view, and although these storage areas are probably primarily concerned with the higher level integrative activity, it is also likely that they participate in the networks of the cortex, having effects of a variety of kinds on other particular activities such as autonomic function and emotional changes. The speech areas, of course, are specific but can still be regarded as storage registers. This sounds ridiculously simple, but it is a fact that, from the whole vast amount of experimentation so far performed, little more could be said in a general way as a pointer to frontal lobe function.

Cortical stimulation

Penfield and Rasmussen (1950) have carried out extensive research in the cerebral cortex in the course of cranial operations on a number of patients suffering from epilepsy. One of the important reminders they give is with respect to the facts discovered initially by Sherrington and Graham Brown on reversal of response, and the allied problem of facilitation. These are worth stating in operational form.

If point A on the precentral gyrus is stimulated and produces finger flexion, then the same response may be elicited considerably anterior to A, say at B, whereas direct stimulation of B would not in fact produce finger flexion. Reversal of response can be elicited similarly by stimulating a point B to elicit *extension*, then stimulating A, producing flexion, and continuing to stimulate in turn points at short intervals downward along the precentral gyrus. Flexion will follow each stimulus up to and including point B. Anomalous results of the same kind may be found in the motor cortex when a point C, say, apparently changes its function to a wrist movement instead of a finger movement.

Summation, after-discharge, inhibition, etc., were all elicited by cortical stimulation, and it is of interest that Sherrington and Brown regarded inhibition as more characteristic of the cortex than excitation.

Temporal and parietal areas and motor-sensory cortical areas

Information on the cortical areas other than the frontal lobe are of some considerable interest. The areas 17 and 18 of the occipital lobe are rather especially connected with visual function, and these will receive further consideration in the next chapter. The temporal and parietal lobes will now be briefly discussed.

Penfield (1947) associates the 'dream states' of Hughlings Jackson (1931) with the temporo-parietal areas under the name 'psychical seizures'. Penfield and Rasmussen (1950) consider that the temporal area, while including auditory and vestibular representation, is primarily devoted to 'memory' and 'sensory perception'. As far as perception is concerned it is assumed to depend on memory; but with epileptic discharge in only one temporal area and the resulting confused hallucinations, a 'false memory' becomes involved. Thus perceptual illusion results in part from disturbance in one temporal area. If, as Penfield and Rasmussen have pointed out, a patient had epileptic discharge in a single remaining lobe, then the faulty 'perceptions' could not be corrected. Faulty perceptions, it should be added, are not always corrected when there is another healthy lobe available.

It is emphasized that the temporal areas are not distinct, or clearly delimited, from their surround, so that there appear to be involved: hearing, vestibular function, speech and hand skills, visual and smell function. Temporal lobectomy (involving only the lobe) does not *normally* involve *serious* memory defects (Penfield and Rasmussen, 1950), although sometimes interference with the optic radiations affects the patient's vision. Indeed more recently, Milner (1958) has shown some specific memory loss depending on the side of the lobectomy.

Marsan and Stoll (1951) report that the temporal pole is frequently the focus of epileptic discharge; using neuronography, conduction of electrically induced after-discharge, and evoked potentials, they investigated subcortical structures in monkeys and found the pulvinar-lateral nucleus, septal-fornix, hypothalamus, basal ganglia and thalamic reticular system all had thalamic connections.

Especially interesting from the behavioural point of view are the studies of temporal lobectomy (Riopelle *et al.*, 1953; Chow, 1952, 1954; Meyer, 1951 and 1958) on learning sets (Harlow, 1949).

The simple problem confronting a monkey, say, is to discover which of two covers is concealing food; they can transfer then to other such covers in a single trial. Meyer describes this in terms of freeing the monkey from trial-and-error behaviour—we shall, of course, be tending to think of this in terms of the transfer from one store to another (Chapter 4), but let us see what the connection with the temporal lobes is. Very briefly, the normal monkey accumulates knowledge (generalizations) while the temporal monkey seems to find each problem a new one, indeed he does not form learning sets.

From the cybernetic point of view this last is one of the most interesting results since it suggests the possibility, at least, that the temporal areas contain precisely the storage registers associated with material that *has been learned*, mostly in the form of generalizations. Other experiments have been carried out confirming these results (Meyer, 1958) and aimed to distinguish the factors of retention and acquisition, both of which were found to be affected. Scoville and Milner (1957) showed that in human, bilateral medial temporal lobe resection extensive enough to damage the anterior hippocampus and hippocampal gyrus results in persistent impairment of recent memory. On the other hand neither the bilateral removal of the uncus and amygdaloid nucleus nor unilateral temporal lobe removal affects recent memory. It may be concluded that the hippocampus and hippocampal gyrus are therefore important features in recent memory. At the same time it would be rash to say they were actually the registers directly concerned yet they may supply a source of registers concerned with recently acquired data which are essential to the learning process, and thus of course vital to the formation of learning sets.

Milner and Penfield (1955) performed partial temporal lobectomy on two human epileptics. They extirpated the hippocampus, hippocampal gyrus, uncus and amygdaloidal nuclei in the dominant hemisphere .

There was evidence of damage to the opposite hippocampal area; there was also a deficit in recent memory but without any change in I.Q., reasoning, etc. Tests given showed that immediate recall was unaffected, but that there was a total loss of information after 5 min, and this also obtained for recognition and recall, for verbal and non-verbal material.

A third patient without non-dominant hippocampal damage did not show these memory effects.

There is further evidence to substantiate these findings. Lashley was apparently influenced by Hughlings Jackson in a fairly extreme way when he showed, in a series of experiments, the surprising ability of the cerebral cortex to recover from all sorts of insult, and as a result he moved away from the older concepts of cortical localization to a much more functional view.

General conclusions on the temporal lobe must include Penfield's (1947) work on temporal stimulation, which generally elicited relatively precise, familiar, visual scenes in the patient. Penfield and Rasmussen are quoted:

> It would seem, also, that the original formation of the memory pattern must be carried out from a high level of neural integration, for a man remembers the things of which he was conscious and especially the substance of his own reaction to them. The same was true of memories evoked by stimulation. They were usually composed of familiar elements, at least to the same extent as dreams are.

The general conclusion on the temporal lobe at this stage is that it involves a fairly high degree of neural organization in the form, presumably, of some sort of synaptic patterns. Naturally these relatively stable patterns (whatever their detailed form may take) are primarily associated with memory and perception.

The parietal area appears (Penfield and Rasmussen, 1950) to be, largely, an area involving elaboration of certain functions; for instance, the superior parietal area may be associated with hand and foot movements, and the inferior parietal area with speech 'elaboration'. The parietal area here referred to lies directly behind the postcentral gyrus. The arguments are, generally, inductions made from operative surgical cases of parietal removal, from both the dominant and non-dominant hemispheres. One example concerns a patient who had a large cortical removal from the non-dominant parietal lobe. He had no sensory disturbances in the opposite arm, but found difficulty in manipulating this hand in tasks set him. He also had difficulty in dressing himself, as the left arm was to a large extent ignored.

Lashley (1950), in dicussing memory in terms of nervous function, drew the following conclusions:

(1) It seems certain that the theory of well-defined conditioned reflex paths from sense organs via association areas to the motor cortex is false. The motor areas are not necessary for the retention of sensori-motor habit, nor even of skilled manipulative patterns.

(2) It is not possible to demonstrate the isolated localization of a memory trace engram anywhere within the nervous system. Limited regions may be essential for learning or retention of a particular activity, but within such regions the parts are functionally equivalent. The 'engram' is represented throughout the region.

(3) The so-called associative areas are not storehouses for specific memories. They seem to be concerned with modes of organization and with general facilitation or maintenance of the level of vigilance. The defects which occur after their destruction are not amnesias but difficulties in the performance of tasks which involve abstraction and generalization, or conflict of purposes. It is not possible as yet to describe these defects in the present psychological terminology. Goldstein (1939) has expressed them in part as a shift from the abstract to the concrete attitude, but this characterization is too vague and general to give a picture of the functional disturbance. For our present purpose the important point is that the defects are not fundamentally those of memory.

(4) The trace of any activity is not an isolated connection between sensory and motor elements. It is tied in with the whole complex of spatial and temporal axes which forms a constant substratum of behaviour. Each association is orientated with respect to space and time. Only by long practice under varying conditions does it become generalized or

dissociated from these specific co-ordinates. The space and time co-ordinates in orientation can, I believe, only be maintained by some sort of polarization of activity, and by rhythmic discharges which pervade the entire brain, influencing the organization of activity everywhere. The position and direction of motion in the visual field, for example, continuously modifies the spinal postural adjustments, but—a fact which is more frequently overlooked—the postural adjustments also determine the orientation of the visual field, so that upright objects continue to appear upright in spite of changes in the inclination of the head.* This substratum of postural and tonic activity is constantly present, and is integrated with the memory trace (Lashley, 1949).

I have mentioned evidence that new associations are tied-in spontaneously with a great mass of related associations. This conception is fundamental to the problem of attention and interest. There are no neurological data bearing directly upon these problems, but a good guess is that the phenomena which we designate as attention and interest are the results of partial, sub-threshold activation of systems of related associations which have a mutual facilitative action. It seems impossible to account for many of the characters of organic amnesias except in such general terms as reduced vigilance or reduced facilitation.

(5) The equivalence of different regions of the cortex for retention of memories points to multiple representation. Somehow, equivalent races are established throughout the functional area. Analysis of the sensory and motor aspects of habits shows that they are reducible among components which have no constant position with respect to structural elements. This means, I believe, that within a functional area the cells throughout the area acquire the capacity to react in certain definite patterns which may have any distribution within the area. I have elsewhere proposed a possible mechanism to account for this multiple representation. Briefly, the characteristics of the nervous network are such that, when it is subjected to any pattern of excitation, it may develop a pattern of activity, reduplicated throughout an entire functional area by spread of excitations, much as the surface of a liquid develops an interference pattern of spreading waves when it is disturbed at several points (Lashley, 1942). This means that within a functional area, the neurons must be sensitized

---

* It has been drawn to my attention that in fact mistakes in orientation will in fact occur under certain circumstances with a change of inclination of the head.

to react in certain combinations, perhaps in complex patterns of rever-beratory circuits, reduplicated throughout the area.

(6) Considerations of the numerical relations of sensory and other cells in the brain make it certain, I believe, that all of the cells of the brain must be in almost constant activity, either firing or actively inhibit-ed. There is no great excess of cells which can be reserved as the seat of special memories. The complexity of the functions involved in reproduc-tive memory implies that every instance of recall requires the activity of literally millions of neurons. The same neurons which retain the memory traces of one experience must also participate in countless other activities.

Recall involves the synergic action of some sort of resonance among a very large number of neurons. The learning process must consist of the attunement of the elements of a complex system in such a way that a particular combination or pattern of cells responds more readily than before the experience. The particular mechanism by which this is brought about remains unknown. From the numerical relations involved, I believe that even the reservation of individual synapses for special associative reactions is impossible. The alternative is, perhaps, that the dendrites and cell body may be locally modified in such a manner that the cell responds differentially, at least in the timing of its firing, according to the pattern of combination of axon feet through which excitation is received.

This statement, by one of the greatest authorities on the neurological foundations of behaviour, seems worthy of mention in this context even though it is being used here mainly to underline the intrinsic complexities of the nervous system.

The above statement of Lashley's could have been made more compre-hensive if it had not been for the lack of an adequate background model; for example, the search for a memory, in the above terms, shows a compartmentalized attitude to a theoretical term that is incompatible with the sort of philosophical analysis and cybernetic model required. As a result, although it is not possible to accept wholeheartedly Lashley's conclusions—at any rate at all levels—the neurophysiological evidence put forward by Lashley remains vital. The six points he makes are largely consistent with the notion of a logical network whose reverberatory activity may be short-circuited by cells from any particular area without destruction of the network.

The principal implication, from this, is to drop the notion of a cortical area whose function is controlling *only*, and of the circuit that can *only* be controlled from a particular localized area. It *may* be controlled, normally from one cortical area, but it may be amenable to control from any point in the network. Looking back over the reports made by Lashley and his associates on their extensive neurosurgical experiments, it seems that if one assumes a network that involves many anatomical layers, and which fires off circuitously, and in more than one way, then the sort of destruction carried out by Lashley would produce precisely the results that he found.

If the existing neurosurgical results are coupled with those of Penfield and Rasmussen, Milner, Scoville, and Milner *et al.*, on stimulation of the temporal areas, they complete the suggested picture of a network, where the 'elaboration' areas may be assumed to play an important part in the integration of networks.

It can well be seen that the age-old argument about movement-patterns and musculature and their cortical representation is partly a verbal problem and partly an organizational one. What is represented is some part of a network which is directly a function of all the body musculature. In short, the cortical neuron is not in control of a particular muscle, but may be connected with one or more networks which initiate specific muscular activity. Thus cortical localization takes on a rather new significance.

The programming of computers to learn suggests that information may be changing fairly quickly in the central nervous system. At least, if it is true for the nervous system that the continuous recording of information is necessary—as it seems to be in a computer program—then this, too, would account for the results derived by Lashley.

We must also ask at this stage how the nervous system represents information if it can be moved quickly from location to location, as it does from register to register. We shall leave the answer to this question until the end of the next chapter.

Aphasia

We cannot complete even a cursory survey of neurology and its relation to behaviour without a brief mention of the very extensive field of language and speech disorders. We can at least outline the terminology used:

There is a certain specific set of complaints concerned with loss of recognition. This is collectively called 'agnosia', and it may be visual, auditory and tactile. On the motor side the name 'apraxia' is given to loss of ability to do things—this implies loss of habits like tying a necktie and so on, even though no paralysis may be involved.

Aphasia is used to describe language disorders in the brain, both sensory and motor, and a wealth of different sorts of problems are involved.

To take one typical example, a patient may have motor aphasia, and he may know what he wants to say, and be able to write this, but be quite unable to say it. The implication being that transfer into the output has somehow been destroyed. From the point of view of neurophysiology the problem is one of strict localization versus non-localization (Goldstein, 1939), although it seems likely, as Head and Jackson have suggested, that it is actually a matter of 'degree of localization'. Visual recognition has been connected with area 18 and visual reminiscence with 19; area 39 for reading language; area 7 for tactile recognition; Wernich's area in the temporal lobe for speech recognition; area 38 for musical recognition; and so on.

From the cybernetic point of view it looks as if one would get a series of similar effects in an ordinary digital computer if particular instructions were obliterated; e.g. if the transfer to output 1 instruction were missing, the information could only be put out through output 2 say, and this parallels motor aphasia. The same effect might be achieved by cutting the wire carrying the information to output 1. These analogies are natural ones to adopt and suggest, perhaps, not so much a crucially high degree of localization—since a computer can place the same information in different registers, and can be multiplexed in order to offset the effects of destruction—but a measure of localization with effects brought about by partial destruction of a fairly specific kind. This seems to mean, in view of the neurophysiological evidence, a fair measure of localization as far as 'area' is concerned, if not actual 'points'.

Evidence on conditioned reflexes

Conditioned reflexes have been the basis for much neurological investigation. Doty (1965) showed that electrical stimulation of brains in macaques provides systematic results of significance. He used 0·2–1·0-msec pulses as conditioned stimuli and these evoked lever-pressing conditioned responses. He found that if a particular point of the striatal cortex was stimulated, then the lever pressing started. He also found that this conditioned response could be elicited by stimulation of other points in the striatal cortex, even when stimulated from the contralateral area, suggesting a rather more complex picture than merely that of a simple stimulus response.

Spinelli and Pribram (1970) though have shown that in all probability at least a functional connection is effected between the visual and motor cortex, where they used monkeys to make panel-pressing discrimination responses. They studied the wave forms by electrodes planted in the visual and motor cortex and showed that after ablation the signs of functional connections were greatly diminished.

In a series of experiments which were not concerned directly with conditioned responses, Buchwald and Hull (1967) have shown that low-frequency electric stimulation of the caudate, ventral or ventral anterior nuclei of the thalamus inhibits the performance of learned behaviour. A new afferent stimulus can disinhibit this effect: such a stimulus can either inhibit or disinhibit (presumably) as a function of the existing internal state of the nervous system.

It has been shown that cats could be trained to discriminate differences between sequences of tones (Sharlock et al., 1965). Sharlock and his associates then carried out bilateral ablation of the auditory cortex and followed it with a retention test. They worked out a map showing that certain areas of the cortex, when destroyed, not only destroyed the retention but stopped relearning.

Semmes and Mishkin (1965) studied the effect of ablation of the sensory motor region on monkeys. The monkeys were tested on a tactile discrimination test. When using the ipsilateral hand, they found their learning of difficult form discrimination was retarded; they were also less sensitive to rough surfaces, although not to different sizes of object.

Another approach to the conditioning type of model has been offered by Stein (1966) who has suggested in his general model of habituation that this depends on the classical conditioning of inhibitory processes. In fact he suggests that a conditioned response is determined by a dual system consisting of both excitatory and inhibitory components, and it is easy enough to imagine this being integrated into our general picture.

It has been suggested (Olds and Olds, 1965) that there are four main central mechanisms operating in operant conditioning behaviour. The first is a sort of homing mechanism of a stimulus–stimulus kind which tends to be closely related to the basic senses such as that of the olfactory system. The second one is a periventricular mechanism which is connected to the somesthetic system. Then there is the final common pathway of goal-seeking behaviour, and this is really another word for operant, located neurologically primarily at the thalamus and perhaps having cortical representation. And finally the extra-pyramidal system consisting of collections of neurons which control the gross directional pattern of skeletal behaviour.

Olds and Olds reckon that these four mechanisms work together in fairly close harmony, and it has been suggested that they collectively work to provide motivational reinforcement to the association system which is primarily an S–S activity.

Spinelli and Weingarten (1966) have noted auditorily elicited activity in the optic tract which they regard as the neural response of fibres which terminate in the retina. This is illustrative of the cross-fertilizing of different sensory modalities and in terms of our neural net models, it suggests that in the partial partitioned hierarchical model there are a certain number of 'cross checks' which alert alternative sensory systems particularly under conditions of events of great 'value' or urgency, which are happening in one sensory modality and which are going to directly affect others.

Further experimental evidence

An example of another development is that of Adey (1961) who implanted electrodes in the temporal lobes of cats and analysed records of their changes on a computer. He discovered certain characteristic wave patterns—one he called an 'approach rhythm' which he associated with learning. Adey has suggested that learning is associated with spatial pattern changes in neuronal currents, which is reminiscent of the models of Hebb and Milner.

The relation between the behavioural state of man, the state of awareness, and the electro-encephalographic record (Schade and Ford, 1965) is now known to some extent. For example, in a state of alert attentiveness, where the subject describes himself as concentrating, there is an associated

EEG record of characteristic partially synchronized low-amplitude waves. In deep sleep, on the other hand, where there is no consciousness, there is an EEG record of large and very slow waves, with random irregular patterns. Such results have a direct bearing on the picture we are gradually building up of the structure and function of the nervous system. In a state of strong emotions which can, of course, be artificially stimulated, there are variously described states of confusion, divided 'attention', etc., with an associated EEG record of a desynchronized kind and of a low to moderate amplitude. There are also fast mixed frequencies which accompany these highly emotional states.

The concept of drive has been thought of by Stellar (1960) for response patterns. But he also assumes that the degree of motivated behaviour varies directly with the activity of certain excitatory centres in the hypothalamus. Stell arassumes the interaction of inhibitory and excitatory hypothalamic centres. The external world can, of course, modify this hypothalamic state through sensory stimuli, and external states influence this hypothalamic state through the vascular system. It is also assumed that cortical and thalamic influences exert further excitatory and inhibitory influence on the hypothalamus.

In some recent work, based on histological studies, Braitenberg (1967a, 1967b) has described some brain models and has described them and other such models in cybernetic terms. He was especially concerned with 'nervous integration' and is persuaded that there is scope here for neural net modelling. But he accepts the fact that such models are rather generalized and should perhaps be more clearly integrated with models which are strictly special purpose such as that mathematical model used to stimulate lateral inhibition in the eye of Limulus, the wiring model to stimulate the perception in insects, and the various models drawn from histological experiments.

Braitenberg has quite rightly made the point that we can have all sorts of models at all sorts of levels, and one of our problems is to be able to translate between such modelling procedures and be able to integrate various sets of models. The integration needed here will always be a function of the particular problem in the particular context.

It is known that there are certain changes in neurophysiological states which are correlated with learning. Thinking too is related to neurological changes in the temporal, parietal and frontal areas. Furthermore, as Schade and Ford put it: 'In general one can say that the speech mechanisms probably form a condition for certain kinds of thinking processes and provide a special way for handling of information'. Thinking and problem solving are known to be related to each other but perhaps it is not reasonable to expect that it is yet possible to distinguish one from the other at the neurological level.

It is impossible to spare space to discuss any further experimental evidences from either cognition or neurology. Indeed, it is not possible to consider many aspects of the subject at all, but only to draw some brief conclusion about the present state of brain models. We shall be continuing this discussion in the next chapter.

Summary

In this chapter we have attempted to give some idea of the range of knowledge of neurophysiology, and sufficient anatomy to follow the argument. It has not been intended as a chapter for the neurophysiologist, but rather for the experimental psychologist with a fair knowledge of the nervous system. We have also tried to fill in enough extra explanatory detail to make it intelligible to the reader interested in cybernetics, but with little or no knowledge of the workings of the nervous system.

It is clear that the nervous system divides into sections or units that can be broadly correlated with behavioural function, and we have now arrived at a stage where the correlation has to be made much more detailed. The way we are advocating that this should be done is through the development of a series of models in paper-and-pencil and hardware which will help us to gain a clearer idea of nervous function.

It should be added that this chapter should be read in especial conjunction with the next chapter, since one of the later sections of that chapter summarizes the recent views on neurophysiological function as outlined by Pribram. This could well have come at the end of this chapter, where it would certainly be relevant; nevertheless it seems reasonable, in the light of other considerations, to defer it.

CHAPTER 10

THEORIES AND MODELS OF
THE NERVOUS SYSTEM

IN THIS chapter we turn our attention to more general ('molar') models of the nervous system. We start with what are explicitly theories, but which are perhaps best regarded as models, or at least preliminary blueprints for models.

This chapter attempts to form a sort of link between the physiological evidence of the previous chapter and the idealized or conceptual system dealt with earlier.

It may appear inadequate and even inept to the physiologist that cyberneticians and other model builders should proceed by steps to the reconstruction of physiological models for human behaviour, but it seems to be the fact that it is quite impossible to effect the transformation in one step, and this means that we must make the most of every analogy and clue that offers itself in what will undoubtedly prove to be a slow and lengthy process.

We shall start within the realm of neurophysiology, with the *ad hoc* model suggested by Pavlov. This is built around the notion of a conditioned reflex (see Chapter 8, page 174).

Fundamental to Pavlov's neurophysiological theory comes the notion of 'excitation' and 'inhibition', but his use of these terms, particularly 'inhibition', is different from that of Sherrington and most of classical neurophysiology; here it is made to refer to actual cortical processes of a gross kind, without reference to the state of individual synapses. He further assumes that the cortex is an analyser upon which the whole of the muscular, etc., systems of the organism are mapped.

The cortex, and probably also the subcortial ganglia, are assumed to have the property of plasticity, which refers to relatively permanent neural changes.

It is as well to remember that the Pavlovian neurophysiological theory is essentially a mirror of classical conditioned response theory, and the conditioned response is assumed to be the fundamental unit of nervous activity. The actual formation of the conditioned response involves the establishment in the cerebral cortex of a connection between the centre of the conditioned stimulus and the centre of the unconditioned stimulus.

The actual cortical processes pictured by Pavlov took place in phases. Afferent stimulation set up an excitatory process at a definite point of the cortex, diminishing with the distance from the point of origin. The second phase is one of recession and concentration at the initial point. The picture is then supplemented by a further series of theoretical terms which try to make for consistency between theory and observation, and we find introduced the notion of (neural) induction. As the cortical process subsides at any point, it may be succeeded by the opposite process which is called 'induction'. *Negative induction* intensifies inhibition under the influence of preceding excitation (induction comes about in a relative way, due to relative change of threshold, in a manner analogous to the fatigue theory of after-images); *positive induction* intensifies excitation following inhibition.

The conditioned reflex is assumed to be set up in the following way: excitation set up by neural stimulus at A irradiates from A and will be concentrated at some other point B which is the focal point of the unconditioned stimulus. Thus, to speak metaphorically, a sort of channel is set up between A and B in such a way that drainage takes place from a 'weak' to a 'strong' centre.

Generalization next follows, from the fact that excitation at B will be aroused by A, or excitation at some near centres A', A'', A''', etc., all very similar to A. *Inhibition* arises if B is extinguished by presentation of stimulus without reinforcement. *Internal inhibition* is really the name for this last process, as opposed to *external inhibition* which involves the contemporaneous eliciting of a different unconditioned response with the conditioned stimulus. Other manifestations of inhibition are in the form of *inhibitory after-effect* and *disinhibition*. Inhibitory after-effect is generalization of inhibition. Furthermore, inhibition can be removed temporarily under the influence of foreign stimuli, and this is disinhibition.

The presence of generalization in the theory implies the presence of *differentiation* and of conditioned inhibition, which is a particular case of differentiation. There is also one further kind of internal inhibition, known as *inhibition of delay*, which involves a conditioned response followed after an interval of the unusually long time of 2 or 3 min by an unconditioned response.

Following some concentrated experimental work by Krasnagorsky there exist some experimental generalizations which we shall call the *Krasnagorsky generalizations:*

(1) The more the conditioned stimulus resembles the stimulus originally inhibited (extinguished or differentiated), the more lasting is the inhibitory after-effect.

(2) The more the conditioned stimulus resembles the inhibitory stimulus, the stronger is the inhibitory after-effect, granted equal time intervals.

(3) Secondary inhibition of all conditioned stimuli applied after inhibitory stimuli increase gradually, achieves its maximum after a dozen or so seconds, and then diminishes.

(4) The more times the inhibitory stimulus is repeated, the stronger and more lasting is the inhibitory after-effect.

(5) Secondary inhibition of active conditioned stimuli impinging upon the same analyser as the inhibitory stimuli is stronger and more prolonged than the inhibition of stimuli impinging upon other analysers.

With all that has gone before there exist some further assumptions about the nature of the cortex itself. The cortex, in fact, becomes viewed as a mosaic of points in states of relative inhibition or excitation, and this introduces one or two more notions.

Capability is the term used to denote the fact that different cells have different degrees of excitability, and the application of more than top excitation brings out protecting inhibition.

The *phase of equalization* is defined as the condition when both strong and weak conditioned stimuli evoke an identical conditioned response.

This brief summary of the rather vague Pavlovian model illustrates the principal points made and the general methods adopted, which should be sufficient for our present purpose.

Let us now consider some criticisms of the Pavlovian theory.

(1) First it should be said that the cortical picture is generally vague, idealized, and somewhat removed from experimental fact. Pavlovian

excitation and inhibition are essentially inferential processes, and should be broken down into their constituents. Much of the model is also *remotely* metaphorical, e.g. the notion of drainage.

(2) More specifically, irradiation is non-demonstrable in the simple form suggested by Pavlov. Neuronography techniques (de Barenne *et al.*) have demonstrated great variability in spread of excitation; Brodman areas 5, 17, 18 and 19 show virtually no spread, while spreading effects in other areas are by no means as simple or symmetrical as is suggested by Pavlov.

(3) Pavlov assumed that conditioning was an explicitly cortical process, and the apparent conditioning of de-corticate animals (even though difficult to obtain) by Ten Cate (1923), Culler and Mettler (1934), and others suggests a revision of the idea that cortical integrity is essential.

(4) For Pavlov, the term 'inhibition' is at least different from the term 'inhibition' which implies synaptic inhibition in the classical neurophysiological theories. From comments 2 and 3 it is clear that Pavlovian inhibition, which refers to a quasi-permanent state of the cortex, is not a model with much empirical support, although it is not alone in this respect.

(5) In the classical theory we have action by contact in the sense that neurons fire neurons in a more or less precise manner. Neither Pavlovian irradiation of excitation or inhibition behaves quite in this manner, although they could perhaps be made to conform to this extra constraint, particularly by using the Lorente de Nó hypothesis of closed chains of cortical activity; but again this might be difficult to reconcile with the specific usages of Pavlovian terms.

(6) From Konorski's (1948) viewpoint the most important error of a fundamental kind is the assumption, deep-rooted in Pavlov, that excitation and inhibition are not only essentially cortical processes, but that both the excitatory state evoked by application of an active conditioned stimulus, and inhibition evoked by application of an inhibitory conditioned stimulus, are localized in the cortical centre of the stimulus. This leads to the total omission of the reflex arc (not necessarily a bad thing) and, more dubiously, it leads to concentration on unspecified states of excitation and inhibition which irradiate or concentrate, summating or restricting, etc., and above all, it is not committed to particular neuron chains.

The point made by Konorski is that different states can be introduced at a cortical centre merely on the grounds of whether or not a stimulus is reinforced.

(7) Another difficulty remarked upon by Konorski is that of making sense of the notion of 'indifference states' that exist between centres of excitation and inhibition.

Now we shall summarize the further developments of Konorski's arguments against the background of the internal inconsistencies in the Pavlovian model:

Firstly, there is the vagueness in the distinction between excitation and positive excitability, as there also is between inhibition and negative excitability. The notions of positive and negative excitability refer to states (more or less permanent) of cells, as opposed to the processes of excitation and inhibition. An example of the confusing manner in which these terms have been used is the establishment of differentiation which may be followed by an increased conditioned response, thanks to the permanent influence of positive induction from the inhibitory focus, in spite of the fact that it is also said that positive induction can be brought about only by inhibition. Another example of the confusion appears in the proposition that the administration of bromides increases the size of the conditioned response and of the positive induction evoked by the concentration of inhibition. When we go on to read that a wave of excitation caused by an extraneous stimulus may summate with the excitation of a conditioned stimulus, whereas a wave of excitation may 'wash away' the inhibitory excitability of a given point and leave a temporary state of positive excitability, the confusion increases, and the versatility of these theoretical terms becomes embarrassing.

A further assertion of the theory, which is attributable to Pietrova and Podkopayez (see Pavlov, 1927), is that which says that irradiation is immediate with very strong or very weak stimuli, and is delayed until the stimulus has ceased with medium stimuli. This assumption is not verified, and (particularly if we add the Pavlovian notion of top inhibition) it leads ultimately to an explanation of internal inhibition by two quite separate mechanisms: concentration of excitation and negative induction, *or* irradiation of excitation and top inhibition, and these processes appear to be opposed. Here again the theory is confused.

There are many other details of internal inconsistency, for example, the problem of sleep as explained by internal inhibition is open to criticism. Furthermore, other writers before Konorski, such as Beritoff (1932), have noted defects in the Pavlovian model. But probably enough has been said here to show that, at the best, it is not adequate, for although it has indeed been of considerable service in the past, it is no longer sufficiently useful as a model for cybernetics or behaviour theory.

Konorski's model

We will now consider what appears to be a useful integrative step, the Konorskian model (1948), which represents the Pavlovian theory in a Sherringtonian guise.

Konorski's first point is that plasticity is a concept central to all neurology and behaviour theory, and he suggests that it is a property of the intact organism-as-a-whole. He gives some interesting examples of the properties of plasticity; for example:

(1) The application of a certain combination of stimuli (here we include an individual stimulus in the term combination) tends to give rise to a definite plastic change, the repetition of the combination leads to 'cumulation' (i.e. an increase in this change), and this cumulation, like the law of effect, has certain limiting properties.

(2) If the combination of stimuli, which is the cause of the plastic change, is not applied, this change suffers regression, etc.

These propositions represent, of course, generalizations from observations of behaviour in the organism-as-a-whole, and it is not easy to demonstrate the neurological correlates. The best-known theory of neural growth is probably that of Ariens Kappers (Kappers, Huby and Crosby, 1936). He proposes that new neural connections are established by growth of neural processes. They grow after stimulation in such a way that if two cells are simultaneously excited, the resulting ionization is assumed to direct the growth of axons towards the cathode, and dendrites towards the anode, and thus sets up new synaptic connections. This idea has been used by Holt (1931), and Hebb (1949) has restated the position that a Kappers-growth is morphologically impossible, and has not, in fact, been observed over any large distance, but remains a possibility over small distances which, in Hebb's own treatment, is all that would be necessary.

Konorski's integration starts from the assumption that the simplest and best-known type of plasticity is the conditioned reflex, which involves the setting up of new functional relationships between concurrently excited groups of nerve cells. Konorski calls the centre of the conditioned stimulus the 'conditioned centre', and the centre of the reinforcing unconditioned stimulus is called the 'unconditioned centre'. These centres may or may not be cortical, but they will normally involve the cortex. The connection between these centres, unlike the Pavlovian centres, is assumed to be extremely complex, and involves a number of intermediary stations or internuncial centres. Konorski substitutes for the 'top capability' of cortical cells the classical notion of occlusion. The occlusion, which involves the diminution of the strength of two stimuli, say, when their sum is far too strong for the effector system, is assumed to occur in the unconditioned centre. This form of modification has been extensively carried out throughout Pavlov's work, with the aim of increasing internal consistency.

Now there is one important extension of the Pavlov theory that needs to be considered before we can adequately summarize the Konorskian revision. With respect to plasticity, the classical conditioned response is not considered to be the only mechanism. The classical response, or conditioned responses of the first type, must be supplemented by conditioned responses of the second type; this has been referred to as 'instrumental conditioning' in some of the psychological literature. The data, which are well known to psychologists, need not be repeated here. The various examples of type II conditioning were enumerated in Chapter 8: (1) reward, (2) escape, (3) avoidance, and (4) secondary reward, involving us (Hilgard and Marquis, 1938) in the principles of substitution, effect, expectancy, etc.

Konorski takes a type II experiment and infers from it that unconditional stimuli can be divided into two categories: those which by reinforcing the animal's movement cause it to perform the movement spontaneously, and those which by reinforcing the movement cause it to perform an antagonistic movement. He calls these *positive unconditioned stimuli* and *negative unconditioned stimuli*, respectively.

It should be said in the first place, with regard to the changes suggested by Konorski, that there is at least a doubt as to whether the conditioning terminology is usefully taken over to describe the whole of nervous activity. It seems that the classical conditioned response is a special case of the general associative processes involved in the central nervous system, and that whether or not we regard type II conditioning as a type of conditioned response is purely a matter of terminology, and therefore not one of the greatest importance to our *cybernetic modelling*.

There are certainly some aspects of the changes in notation made by Konorski that seem to fit the facts better, in that a definite gain appears to have been made in breaking down some of the theoretical terms by our increased observation. The phenomenon of generalization of excitatory conditioned reflex seems perhaps better accounted for by the notion of partial cortical overlap, for which there is some evidence (Liddell and Phillips, 1951; Lilly, 1958).

The notion of 'occlusion', which acts as a limiting mechanism in the top value of conditioned reflexes, seems a more satisfactory theoretical term than the 'top capability' of cortical cells, if only in so far as we thereby attain an integration with classical theory.

This last remark, of course, is generally applicable to the Konorski revision, which is to be commended on the grounds of integration in scientific theory, and the achievement of the use of the same theoretical terms and formulations as classical theory. Much, also, of the internal inconsistency of Pavlov has been remedied, with the result that the confusion over inhibition, negative excitability, etc., has now largely gone. The new statement about the formation of the inhibitory conditioned response is now explained in terms of the contemporaneous excitation of the conditioned centre, with fall of excitation in the unconditioned centre. Also, the observable fact of increase of the excitatory conditioned reflex concurrently with the inhibitory reflex seems more adequately explained by summation of the excitatory conditioned response and the excitato-inhibitory response, with facilitation predominating.

But whereas Konorski has supplied a necessary criterion for conditioning—and thus, perhaps, for all learning—in the notion of plasticity, his particular idea of how this may take place is perhaps, in the light of the latest neurophysiological work, not wholly plausible.

He assumes that there is an emitting centre where the stimulus to be conditioned is centred, and a receiving centre for the unconditioned stimulus, and potential connections between these centres which involve growth and the multiplication of synapses.

This bears a relation to the theory proposed by Hebb, but with this difference, that it seems to fall foul of the evidence on cortical localization from experiments in cortical ablation by Lashley and others, evidence which suggests something a little more subtle in the actual organization of these cortical centres. This model, as well as Hebb's, at least lacks experimental verification as it stands.

Eccles (1953) assumed, in his explanation, that two knobs were necessary for the synaptic excitation necessary to generate an impulse. He also assumed that the same neurons could contribute to different patterns of nervous activity involved with a concept of cortical overlap, for which there is some empirical evidence.

In his explanation of conditioning Eccles starts from the reflex arc, and then assumes that the conditioned stimulus causes the discharge of afferent impulses along a particular pathway, where they converge on neurons also excited by the impulses in the collaterals from the afferent pathways of the unconditioned stimulus. Synaptic facilitation is caused by the post-synaptic potential, and leads to impulses being set up in otherwise unaffected neurons, and there is an increased sensitivity of those synaptic knobs that are most used. Here we see a close parallel to Hebb's basic assumption of the development of neural connections.

From this area so affected we generate a spatio-temporal pattern of impulses that link the conditioned and the unconditioned stimulus. And for this purpose Eccles draws a particular 'neuronal' net, as he calls it, which shows just how this interaction could take place (Eccles, 1953, pp. 221 *et seq.*).

The models that are considered here are all rather generalized, and neglect the more recent and more detailed analysis of particular nervous areas; especially, they neglect the work on the reticular system, and the latest research of an electrical kind. This is no defect in the theories considered, since their value lies in the fact that they were built as descriptions, however elementary, of the nervous system, and they *can* be translated into cybernetic terms.

It is of interest that the building of cybernetic models to mirror these models of nervous activity depends on making the model precise, and at the same time acts as a check on its functional accuracy.

From what has already been said in earlier chapters it is clear that a finite automaton can easily be constructed to carry out the activity of a Konorski or Eccles type model, but equally it seems certain, for reasons which are partly based on the economy of cells and partly on further neurophysiological evidence, that these models are still nothing like a precise model of what occurs in the actual human brain.

The ethologists

Ethology is closely bound up with behaviour and with the models for that behaviour and—rather like much of molar experimental psychology—has tended to construct theories and models using any available analog whatever (Thorpe, 1956; Lorenz, 1950; Tinbergen, 1951; *et al.*). Ethology is the study of animal behaviour, carried out in the main by zoologists and primarily from a comparative point of view.

We shall not here attempt to summarize the various fields of ethological modelling and experimental activity, since much of it overlaps what has been said in this and the previous chapter. Pavlov and Konorski have been reviewed, and although Pavlov's theory is now largely rejected, Konorski's grew from it, and this in turn has led to many other theories such as those of Hebb (1949), Pringle (1951) and Eccles (1953), which have received careful consideration in ethological circles.

Indeed, it is increasingly realized that cybernetics is a source of models for theorizing in neurophysiology. Pringle's model, involving the coupling of oscillators which show properties of locking and synchronization, is typical of the cybernetic approach, even though not carried out under that particular name.

Hebb will be considered more fully later in this chapter and in the next, in the background of perception, but his theory, too, tends towards the cybernetic, and falls short of being so classified only in the degree to which it is *effective*. It is not mathematical as are those of Shimbel (1949, 1952), McCulloch and Pitts (1943), Minsky (1954) and many more that have been constructed, and by the same token it is not wholly precise. Also, it depends upon the concept of closed active circuits of the kind suggested by Lorente de Nó, as well as the idea of neurophysiological growth suggested by Kappers and others, and both these suggestions, especially the first, are open to some doubt, even though it is difficult to imagine how learning in the nervous system would be possible without at least one of the two concepts.

Lashley's theory

There is a theory of nervous function that has been proposed by Lashley (1929b). Some indication of Lashley's ideas was given in the previous chapter, and here we shall simply append some of the principles that Lashley regarded as important—even necessary—to any models of the nervous system.

In the first place, generalization is thought to be an essential basic property of neurons, and one dependent on the integrity of the cerebral cortex, without which the organism loses the necessary capacity to adapt to a changing environment.

Such generalizations, according to Lashley, must occur in the visual system where the fixation of points varies, and thus occasion stimulation of many different retinal cells, although we are aware of a single object only. This is assumed to involve a memory trace which is a property of the whole nervous system.

The cortex was regarded by Lashley as being a set of resonators. He further assumed the interference of different sensory excitations which would lead to modification of ordinary, isolated, sensory stimuli.

He also believed that cortical neurons were in constant activity, and that complex patterns of interaction were the basis of integration. This view is, of course, intended to be in opposition to one that regards external events as mirrored in the nervous system by specific, and relatively isolated, pathways.

This particular conclusion is one we should bear in mind when trying to construct economical finite automata, since it seems certain that such a view is fundamentally correct; in fact it may not be inconsistent (Hebb, 1949) with the concept of specific pathways and neuron circuits being connected with different learned items.

Lashley proposes four types of integration in the cerebral cortex: (1) the selective patterning of excitation, (2) sensitization to pattern anticipation, (3) stimulus equivalence, and (4) convertibility between temporal and spatial patterns. Some of these matters directly affect perception, and they will be discussed later in Chapters 11 and 12; in the meantime we shall consider a specific problem of learning and the nervous system; one that was dealt with especially by Hebb. This is the problem of early and late injuries.

Early and late brain injuries

This is doubtless a matter of considerable importance both to the behaviour-theorists and to the neurologists, and the evidence will be summarized briefly.

Penfield and Rasmussen (1950) are of the opinion that there is a marked difference between cortical destruction in youth, and cortical destruction later in life (see their work on the use of speech 'elaboration' areas, p. 222). Hebb's summary states the essential points (1949, pp. 289 *et seq.*). I.Q. is generally far more affected by brain injury early in life than by equivalent injury in adulthood. One interesting point, made by Hebb, is that the 'Binet' type test shows least well any change in I.Q. after brain injury (except for the relatively specialized speech areas) since the nature of such tests is not sufficiently fine a probe. Obviously a great deal of the argument here depends on the nature of the term 'intelligence', and this term, as used in most test situations (especially Binet-type), includes much that depends on memory function, general experience, etc. If the injury occurs early in life, the necessary generalized functions will not be sufficiently developed; if later, then the logical (neural) nets set up will by-pass the injured areas. The inference is that much cortex may be needed initially for making the network which, later, can be retained by far less cortex. The implications for automata construction are very significant, and suggest an important distinction between *learning* and *having learned*. However, there may well be two factors (the hereditary and the experiential) which contribute towards 'intelligence', and the problem here is to guess what light it throws on neurophysiological function. It could be that a certain set of neurons may be included in a network, all the cells of which are necessary to the initial assembly, and that destruction of a part may, in general, lead to a by-passing of the missing parts, but not to the destruction of the network. This is, roughly, the Hebb view, and it has the ring of credibility.

Of the hosts of further experiments on different cortical areas and their total or partial destruction, we would mention here Sperry, Stamm and Miner (1956), who showed that the corpus callosum was necessary in cats for the transfer of training of a tactile discrimination from the left paw to the right. Since the work of Olds and Milner (1954), Bursten and Delgado (1958) and others have done a great deal of work showing that direct stimulation of the cortical areas had a reinforcing effect on behaviour. There has also been some work on the function of the lateral and medial geniculate bodies.

Adding to the enormous amount of work already done, each new publication in this subject brings more enlightenment; even while this is being written some new evidence may have taken us a step further. But in the whole body of the knowledge we have acquired in this field there is still nothing which denies the very general view that the brain is an extremely complex switching system, the details of which will take us many years to unravel.

In absolute terms, the sum total of our present information is indeed large, but it is small relative to what we wish to know. We can see, however, the possibility of applying the principles of classification and conditional probability to what we know.

The visual cortex could certainly be viewed as a visual classification system; other areas could also be regarded as classification areas (association areas) with respect to input information from the other special senses. This means that the greater part of the brain could feasibly be thought of as being made up of a set of storage registers. Information is clearly transferred in complex fashion from point to point, and the system as a whole is sufficiently 'multiplexed' to make it fairly certain that loss of particular neurons does not necessarily stop the activity normally associated with particular cortical areas.

It would seem unreasonable to regard the cortex as being *wholly* pre-wired, as is a finite automaton, in terms of logical nets; but when viewed in terms of growth nets, or growth processes, we can see the possibility of formulating an appropriate blueprint.

Consciousness even (Culbertson, 1950) has been analysed in logical net terms, and this is a significant indication of the range of cybernetics. Even if we reconsider the problem of human activities in terms of their nervous systems, we can still supply models appropriate to the task, at least in principle. From this point of view the complexity of electrical and chemical-colloidal changes is unimportant, although to neglect such evidence would ultimately prove to have been extremely foolish.

There is nothing by way of evidence in this or the previous chapter which goes against the idea that the brain is appropriately viewed as an enormously complicated computer system even if *both digital and analog*. Indeed, when viewed in this light, there are no results of electroencephalography, cortical destruction, or electrical stimulation that should occasion any surprise whatever. All that is derived from neurophysiology is a series of clues to the blueprint we are looking for. At the moment, the scent can hardly be called warm, but already we can see the sort of results that might be expected from a cybernetic point of view.

In the digital computer, we think of the routine behaviour as being carried out in terms of a program that places the instructions inside the storage and then automatically operates on the data—usually numerical—according to the nature of the instructions.

This could equally mirror the human activity, except of course that the human is not generally operating on a fixed set of special instructions; in certain cases, though, he may be, such as where he is following an exact set of instructions in his job. But generally he will be told the desired end-result, without being given an explicit method for reaching that end-result, and then he must scan his storage system for information that allows him to proceed to the end state. He will also be subjected to further inputs while working on a programme, which means that he has to have storage space for future programmes necessitated by these inputs, which may also modify present programmes. Obviously the human differs from the digital computer—*as normally used*—in this respect.

It is for the above reason that we tend to think of our computer analog with a functionally interdependent input tape and output tape. These tapes work in one direction, and are associated with instants of time. In such an automaton it is, of course, now essential to have a storage system, and the store we would envisage is precisely the sort of general storage arrangement described in Chapters 5 and 7. The problem of human organization is thus the same as the problem of organization of stored information, apart of course from showing how the concepts, etc., are built up inside the storage system in the first place.

The implication is clear that the human brain is primarily a storage system, and it is connected with the immediate processing of input data from the main sensory sources. This still leaves a variety of questions about the manner in which the storage is effected, and this is the great problem for future physiological psychologists.

Let us now consider some of the other approaches to our problem. Incidentally, in so doing we shall be led back to the problem of conceptual models.

Beurle's model

Beurle (1954, 1954b) has suggested a theoretical model for aspects of neural nets (Sholl, 1956), for which he considers a whole set of units with the following properties: (1) they are connected in a non-specific manner which can be described statistically; (2) active units can excite inactive units by means of immediate connections; (3) over a period of time, summation of excitation occurs; (4) when the summated excitation exceeds a certain 'threshold' value, the unit becomes active; (5) there is a 'refractory period' after firing before a unit takes any further part in neural activity.

Beurle predicted many interesting properties from these assumptions, and he used a further assumption similar to that of Chapman, in supposing that a threshold is slightly diminished with each firing.

The assumption of random connectivity is one that can be introduced into logical nets, from which starting point, by growth, or by the non-use of pre-wired connections, the specific logical nets can be derived. Beurle's block of units is thought to be similar in some respects to the cerebral cortex, and there is little doubt that some extension of this kind is necessary to bring the Uttley type of model into line with the neurological facts; such an extension could be easily achieved.

A somewhat similar viewpoint to Beurle's was expressed by Turing in an unpublished paper on 'Intelligent machinery', in which he was able to show that a randomly connected network with experience could take on a specific and well-organized form.

Ashby's model

In returning to Ashby (1947, 1948, 1950, 1952, 1956a, 1956b) we are coming full circle with respect to cybernetic models which purport to bear some resemblance to the brain.

The Homeostat has already been discussed in Chapter 4. Ashby has also set down his design for a brain in a separate book; the theory, being essentially mathematical, proposes that step functions are appropriate descriptions of a feedback system which has the necessary property of ultrastability.

Stewart (1959) has pointed out a difficulty in the application of such 'homeostatic' principles to the brain:

> The number of moves needed as a stable field is achieved increases as a roughly exponential function of the number of degrees of freedom of the system. For large systems, it is therefore essential to increase the probability of stability by some means.

This difficulty may be overcome by having a number of ultrastable systems—a 'multistable' system—and Ashby has designed such a model.

More recently, Ashby has proposed a theory of cybernetics which depends on the notion of transformation and permutation groups. This represents a form of description that has some advantages at a purely functional level, and indeed such a description could be regarded as an alternative to a logical net description, since logical nets can easily be dealt with as a branch of matrix algebra, as we have seen, and such sets of matrices have, *in certain cases*, group properties which bear a similarity to the suggestions made by Ashby. But here we are heading right away from the neurological, and are back wholly in the realm of finite automata.

Hebb's cell assembly and Milner's Mark II cell assembly

Hebb's (1949) cell assembly is a hypothetical structure obviously intended to be understood as a conceptual nervous system. It is made up of a collection of cells which are closely associated as a result of learning. The learning involves the firing of a set of cells which may be originally in a fairly randomly organized state. Cells excited in the visual cortex (area 18) are actuated by some visual stimulus A, say, and this set will have many cells in common with the assembly activated by other visual stimuli $B, C, D, \ldots$ These cell assemblies, through fractionation and recruitment, or growth, become differentiated and highly organized. In the future, sequences (a 'Phase Sequence') of cell assemblies occur, mirroring the activities of perception and learning.

Hebb's system will not be discussed here; for a detailed discussion reference should be made to Hebb's writing. Some mention of Hebb's system is also made in the next chapter, but the main point is that his system is too versatile as it stands, and although it is similar in many ways to the sort of logical nets we have been describing, it has needed a good deal of modification.

In Hebb's cell assembly four factors determine whether or not a cortical neuron fires. These four factors are: (1) the number of impulses bombarding the neuron from all sources for the few milliseconds during which temporal summation is assumed to take place; (2) the strength of the synapses, which is a function of recurrent firing; (3) whether or not the neuron is refractory, and (4) neural fatigue.

Hebb's system starts in random form but learns much too quickly to be a realistic model of learning in organisms; but this rate of learning can be brought into line with the facts by use of inhibition (cf. Chapman's model).

Milner (1957) assumes that cell assemblies and phase sequences occur subject to the neural postulate as suggested by Hebb. Figure 58 shows the Milner assumptions in network form.

He first assumes that there are neurons with long axons with cortico–cortico connections, and neurons with short axons with local inhibitory connections. Through facilitation from the non-specific projection system cortico–cortico transmission is made possible, and thus one neuron may fire some ten or more neurons, and then these may themselves each fire

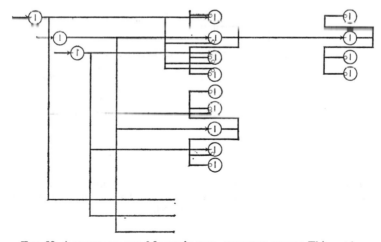

Fig. 58. A network for Milner's cell assembly system. This net has the simple property of exciting one element and at the same time inhibiting the neighbouring cells (see text).

ten or more. The idea is that neurons with long axons fire the neurons with short axons in their neighbourhood and, as more of the short axon cells fire, more inhibitory neighbourhoods come into being.

Figure 59 demonstrates the next point, which is that recurrent inhibitory connections are assumed to occur whereby a cell *A* fires and inhibits *B*, *C* and *D*, but not itself. This means that by firing *A* we are protecting it from inhibition, and this will affect equilibrium activity in the cortex by the setting up of re-exciting pathways. Eventually adaptation brings about a lowering of firing.

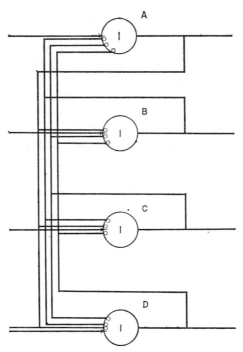

FIG. 59. A NETWORK FOR MILNER'S CELL ASSEMBLY. This net shows cells which when fired inhibit their neighbouring cells. This figure is closely comparable to Fig. 58.

In these terms we can undertake to look again at the manner in which a stimulus *A* leads to a response *C* and to a further stimulus *B*. (These letters do not apply to the letter names for the cells in Fig. 59.) Milner says that a cell assembly, after being under direct control, is under indirect control for some minutes, and A has either latent or active trace associations with B and C. The word 'priming' is used to describe the lowering of threshold that follows the stimulation of a cortical cell by an afferent impulse; the effect is supposed to last only a few seconds. The sensory projection areas of the cortex are final distribution centres for sensory impulses, and the organism ignores stimulation if the cortex is already very active. But if the cortex is not very active, and the stimulus is very strong, then the activity of the cortex will be significantly changed.

Learning is presumed to occur because sets of neurons once fired together are assumed to refire together. Selective excitation occurs much as in the original cell assembly; however, there is assumed to be a fringe of uncertainty, which means that the total pattern of cortical activity is not determined by a single stimulus. Phase sequences may be fired by internal as well as sensory means.

Finally, Milner assumes that recruitment comes from priming, and that perceptual overlearning implies ease of linking assemblies.

Now motivation affects learning and rate of responding, and it is assumed that arousal systems are cholinergic, that motivation and emotion are correlated, and that novel stimuli are more potent than ordinary stimuli in arousing activity.

This model of Milner's is ingenious and is not lacking in physiological plausibility; we shall see that the basic ideas, or some of them, are incorporated into the Pribram model which is described in the next section.

It should be added that a number of recent investigators (Barondes and Cohen, 1966) have superseded the dual trace hypothesis, which is the essence of Hebb's view, and suggested that there are three or more stages involved in memory storage. There is an initial phase, which is chemically influenced, a second phase which is involved in further chemical effects but particularly involves the temporal lobes and inhibition and this could be a lengthy process operating over any number of days not minutes, and a third stage beyond these, which involves the diffuse intercerebral interactions; again one is reminded of the stages of a hierarchical classification model. Furthermore, it has been suggested that the final stage is dependent on DNA-directed synthesis of protein and therefore is itself also a chemical process or at least a chemically influenced process.

McGaugh (1966) has speculated that immediate memory store may be composed of three independent systems. One such system would be for short-term memory only, the second for intermediate memory and the third for long-term memory, and this parallel mechanism is offered as an alternative to the sequential mechanism suggested by Barondes and Cohen and others.

There are a number of experiments which can be cited which support both points of view and certainly the latter is consistent with the view that a filter operates at the input end of cerebral activities and such factors as frequency, recency and 'value' will influence which of the three stages of memory information was filtered. However, is seems more likely that some information may not appear 'valuable' when it first enters the brain and it becomes valuable afterwards and therefore is transferred from one stage to the other. For this reason, it is suggested that the stages of memory while being multiphasic are capable of being both sequential and parallel in their operations.

One thing we should say about the Hebb type of theory, which in automata terms is a growth type of theory, and that is that there is increased and ever-accumulating evidence that the brain can change anatomically as the person interacts with his environment (Rosenzweig and Leiman, 1968). There is much evidence, for example, from lesions in the cerebral cortex of rabbits that new branches occur in the injured area and new fibre connections represented growth of central nervous tissue rather then regeneration of fibres.

Kruger (1965) was also able to show the same effect as growth while pointing out that the radiation technique which has been used in these sort of experiments does not completely interrupt the fibres passing through the area, hence once again creating the doubt that perhaps one is dealing with functional growth rather than anatomical growth as a primary source of connectivity in the cerebral cortex.

Pribram's brain model

The penultimate section of this chapter will be devoted to a summary by Pribram (1960) of the world of neurophysiology. His most interesting summary is selective, and really amounts to the outline of a theory—almost of a model. It is of special interest to us because of its strong cybernetic leanings.

Pribram's first point is that brain tissue has intrinsic rhythms, and although the cerebral cortex may be said to be quiescent without input, it is easily aroused to prolonged activity, and this may be taken to imply a complex memory process. In the intact organism, the spontaneous discharge of receptors maintains a certain level of cortical activity.

In recent years, of course, this spontaneous activity has been increasingly thought of as occurring in the reticular system.

The second, and perhaps the main point of Pribram's view is that the reflex arc is increasingly being thought to be replaced by the closed loop circuit elements, feedback units or homeostats, and indeed evidence for the feedback unit is now growing rapidly. Granit (1955) and Galambos (1956) have shown that the optic and otic systems respectively have efferent activities originating in the receptors that can be directly modified by the central nervous system. Thus, the assumption of sensory and motor nerves made at the beginning of the previous chapter must, like the concept of the reflex arc, be modified to some extent by these new ideas.

To generalize, the stimulus–response or reflex arc is now the problem, and Miller, Galanter and Pribram (1959) have suggested a unit they call a TOTE. The letters T O T E stand for test-operate-test-exit. The tote sequence is a basic neurological unit; it represents a sort of servo-operation, and one which suggests graded responses in organization, in opposition to the all-or-none law of nervous function.

Steps taken in the direction of graded response mechanisms are exhibited by the recent discovery of graded dendritic potentials (Li, Culler and Jasper, 1956; Bishop and Clare, 1952).

It is of interest that these graded response mechanisms were discovered during an attempt to establish the source of potentials recorded on the EEG. Their significance is by no means fully understood, but Pribram himself has suggested that they play some part in the test of the TOTE sequence. Somewhat similar graded responses are also observed in the interaction between the cortex and the reticular system.

Pribram describes the work on the reticular system and the diencephalic structures as leading to a new concept of what he calls the 'concentric nervous system', the system built from the inside outwards. The system, which contains further homeostats in the form of respiratory control, food intake control, and so on, is near the midline of the ventricular system.

Hebb (1955) and Olds (1959), among others, have emphasized the

22*

drive-regulating aspect of the reticular system, but drive itself is now thought to be composed of many components, such as: (1) selection, (2) activation and (3) equilibration. The resemblance here to a servo-control system is obvious, and of course the implication is clear that the type of need-reduction theory of motivation suggested by Hull is only a part, in reality, of the total motivational process, and that at this level the motivational system can act by 'conceptual' means—which is something that we had anticipated on other grounds.

The limbic system, which is the name for the structures on the inner-most edge of the cerebral hemispheres, have been closely associated with motivational and emotional behaviour, and there have been suggestions that this system has associations with memory.

One of Pribram's main hypotheses is that the limbic system regulates the disposition of organisms, and this it does by the use of neural homeo-stats.

The frontal intrinsic mechanism, he believes, is like the posterior intrinsic mechanism in being loci sensitive to and partly determinated by experience in their representations, the big problem being the timing of the pattern of firing. The intrinsic representational process is hierarchi-cally organized, and is sensitive to variations in circumstances, provided that these variations are not overly abrupt. The posterior systems are primarily related to the major projective systems, and are organized to select the invariant properties of receptor stimulation.

The frontal mechanism is primarily related to the limbic formations of the endbrain, which are organized to enhance constancies of state which, in turn, are dependent on the biased homeostats of the brain stem core.

The posterior intrinsic mechanism is reinforced completely when the organism is fully informed, and the frontal intrinsic mechanism is rein-forced completely when the organism is fully instructed. Pribram sug-gests that attention is given to instructions until conditions are met. The first reinforcement is through the identification of the similarities among the range of differences, and the second is through the fulfilment of inten-tions. This seems, as Pribram says, very different from Hull's need-reduc-tion principle, but it could be that only a slight modification is necessary to make the two come together, and indications of the sort of changes we are looking for are not far to seek. In the first place, we are fairly sure that need-reduction is not a simple or linear process, and that conceptuali-zation comes into the picture. There is also the strong probability that curiosity may be acceptable as a drive that is to be reduced, and by virtue of which generalizations and classifications, both perceptual and conceptual, take place. All this is built upon Hull's admittedly oversimple, but very useful, concept of need-reduction.

In summary, Pribram suggests that a hierarchical process in the nervous system is necessary and sufficient for reinforcement to occur and, using Mackay's (1956) idea, it is suggested that selective modification interacts with representation. A unique match will stop the searching process, which has proceeded by successive probabilities.

There are two stages to problem solving. The first stage is to gain information, and the second is to order and utilize that information. The posterior and frontal intrinsic systems are thought to be responsible, and are concerned, in the first case, with differences between past and present invariance in stimulation. The frontal intrinsic areas, through the limbic system, are sensitive to differences between past and present and dispositional states of the organism.

All this is achieved by multi-linked homeostats attempting to attain ultrastable dispositional states; these connect directly with the limbic system of the endbrain, and so control the biases of the central core of the brain stem, while others control the ordering of the behavioural processes and sequences of actions.

Homeostats are assumed to abound in the internal core of the brain stem, and there is a modality non-specific activating system that is directional, with drive components in a generalized, specific sensory and hedonistic form. Changes in the activating system, through graded response mechanisms, modify homeostats in their area. The graded response shows a change in excitation in the nervous system and this, with signal transmission, suggests to Pribram the usefulness of the models of Kohler, Lashley and Beurle. In Pribram's own words:

> Reinforcement by cognition, based on a mechanism of hierarchically organized representatives, dispositions and drives regulated by multi-linked and biased homeostats; representational organization by virtue of graded, as well as all-or-nothing, neural responses; spontaneously generated, long-lasting intrinsic neural rhythms; organisms thus conceived are actively engaged, not only in the manipulation of artifacts, but in the organization of their perceptions, satisfactions and gratifications.

This quotation reminds us again that the gulf between empirical descriptions and conceptual analyses is very narrow indeed. We are not to be thought of as either stating facts or as theorizing, for the two go together; and Pribram's ideas, when clarified by semantic and cybernetic analysis, will be found to be very close to those that are being put forward in this book.

One more thing should be said before leaving Pribram: the particular emphasis on Lashley and Kohler is indicative of the link between the cruder mechanisms of the past and the better integrated mechanisms of today. This does not, of course, mean that materialistic thinking was wrong—even assuming the present trends are correct—but rather that models have become more sophisticated and slightly less simple.

Cybernetic models in general

The brain is clearly a vastly complicated system, and there is an obvious naïvety—doubtless irritating to a neurophysiologist—in such statements as, 'just a switching device', 'the eyes are like a television scanning system', 'the brain is a complex digital (and analog) computer', and so on. Let us, then, put the whole matter in another way.

A great deal of progress has been made in neurophysiology and neuro-anatomy by thinking of the brain and the nervous system as a telephone exchange system; and although a great many objections have been made to this analogy, it has had its uses. However, without pressing analogies into literal descriptions, we may say that the concept of computers is also a useful one for, of course, through finite automata, we can make our computer any way we like. Growth nets (Chapman, 1959) may eventually be the appropriate description of models which would serve as bases for descriptions of the nervous system. For the moment, it would be a considerable step if we could see some relation between the particular finite automata outlined in Chapter 4, and what has been said of the actual nervous system.

The principles involved were classification, stochastic storage, conditional probabilities, generalization, and of course the existence of built-in systems. Feedback is taken to be implied by the organization, which is essentially an elaboration of an input–output system with complex storage, and with modification of response-tendencies through experience. At the highest level we have the problems concerned with symbolic representation of input–output events. This problem of language represents without doubt one of the big challenges for the future.

While emphasizing once more that finite automata—even those in logical net form—are not necessarily to be interpreted as actual nervous systems, it is clear that such a relation would be desirable.

Von Neumann (1952) has hazarded the guess that 'neural pools' may occur in the nervous system which are similar in form to the restoring organs which he has described; these might be used for maintaining accuracy in those parts of the nervous system where analog principles apply.

Kleene (1951) makes our purpose clear when he describes his own neural nets in the following manner:

> These assumptions are an abstraction from the data which neurophysiology provides. The abstraction gives a model, in terms of which it becomes an exact mathematical problem to see what kinds of behaviour the model can explain. The question is left open how closely the model describes the activity of actual nerve nets. Neurophysiology does not currently say which of these models is most nearly correct...

Rashevsky (1938), Householder and Landahl (1945), and others of the school of mathematical biology, have tried to apply the methods of mathematical physics directly to biology, and therefore represent yet a further attempt in the direction of cybernetics.

Sholl (1956) has discussed the quantification of neuronal connectivity, as has Uttley (1955, 1966) and other writers since.

A different approach to the problem has been made by Coburn (1951, 1952) in what he describes as the 'Brain Analogy', in seventeen postulates. This model keeps close to the facts of conditioning, and has the advantage of being precise in form, and capable of being translated into logical nets. The relation to actual neurology is slight, but nevertheless it has the advantage of being in keeping with some of the facts. As a model it is a step in the direction of the mathematical models of learning mentioned earlier.

Automata theory and brain models

The main point about the field of finite automata, certainly in its tape and scanner form (such as was used by Turing in the Turing machine (1937)), is that it is primarily concerned with mathematics and meta-mathematics and not with behaviour of brain function. This means it is primarily concerned with what is computable, provable, and the like. Secondly, the primary search in this field is for an effective procedure or algorithm and not with heuristics; but it does place some limit on what is possible in brain structures. Thirdly, the neural net form of automata is a convenient device for making explicit the properties of particular brain models, as we have already discussed in some detail. We shall now turn to consider automata briefly, primarily from the tape point of view.

Arbib (1965) has summarized the relevance of mathematics and automata to brain models as follows:

> I do not believe that the application of mathematics will solve all our physiological problems. What I do believe, though, is that the mathematico-deductive method must take an important place beside the experiments and clinical studies of the neurophysiologist and the psychologist in our drive to understand brains, just as it has already helped the electrical engineer to build the electronic computers which, though many, many degrees of magnitude less sophisticated than biological organisms, still represent our closest man-made analog to brains.

McNaughton (1961) has summarized the field of automata, and makes a number of distinctions which it is helpful to follow. Growth automata can become arbitrarily large, but some (partial) *growth automata* are limited in the upper limit to which they can grow and turn out to be no more powerful than a *fixed automaton*. It is possible to think of growth automata as being *potentially infinite* in that they can always add on more tape indefinitely as and when they need it, even though at any time t, the amount of tape they possess is clearly finite.

It is clearly possible to accept the obvious meaning of synchronous and non-synchronous, deterministic and probabilistic as modifying the noun 'automata' and accept, as a starting point, McNaughton's definitions of an automaton:

> An automaton is a device of finite size at any time with certain parts specified as inputs and outputs, such that what happens at the outputs at any time is determined by what has happened at the inputs.

McNaughton accepts this as both broad and vague as a definition and proceeds to refine as follows:

> A finite automaton is an ordered quintuple S, I, U, f, g where S, I and U are elements, f is a function mapping $S \times I$ into S, and g is a function mapping $S \times I$ into U. Then for every element s in S and i in I, $f(s, i)$ is an element of S, and $g(s, i)$ is an element of u.

It is intended that this definiton be interpreted so that S, I, U, f and g are the set of states, set of input values, set of output values, the transition function, and the output function respectively.

One specific question of interest that follows from the study of automata is the relative power of a probabilistic and deterministic automaton. It has proved difficult to make precise comparisons, but in at least one case it has been shown that a probabilistic automaton can do no more than a deterministic automaton (de Leeuw *et al.*, 1956).

However, this book is concerned primarily with brain models. And although, as McNaughton says, in a broad sense, probabilistic automata can do more than deterministic ones, it is possible to accept, for brain models, the idea that probabilistic automata are automata that approximate to deterministic ones.

It is always important to bear in mind that the search for a mathematically interesting problem is by no means the same as the search for scientifically interesting facts which may be expressed succinctly in mathematical form. A failure to understand this difference has led in the past to a lot of wholly irrelevant criticism from both parties.

A good illustration of the importance of the context of operation is the use of multi-tape Turing machines. Mathematically, it can be shown that no problem is solvable in a multi-tape Turing machine that is not solvable on a single-tape Turing machine. This may take mathematical interest away from multi-tape Turing machines, but not cybernetic interest. The cybernetic interest here is in the methods of proof and solution which may be quite different in the two cases: thus as a brain modelling system, the multi-tape machine is of great interest.

Neural nets as automata

Since the pioneer work in neural nets of McCulloch and Pitts (1943) and the further developments supplied by Kleene (1951), von Neumann (1952), Culbertson (1950), Stewart (1959) and others, there has been a lot of research activity connected with the neural net version of automata.

The work on reliability of automata has some measure of importance. Moore and Shannon (1956), Blum (1962), Cowan (1962), Verbeek (1962), Lofgren (1962a, 1962b) and others have all written on this subject and they have provided a variety of different approaches to the problem of how to ensure a high degree of reliability in a system with some unreliability in the component parts; this is much the same as asking about the degree of confidence one should have in the application of heuristic methods.

Von Neumann (1953) carried out the pioneer work in unreliability. He assumed through the existence of better components than the brain is likely to possess, and the recognition of this has led to a reconsideration of the whole problem of unreliable nets. It has, in fact, raised the specific question of whether an arbitrarily high reliability can be achieved in a neural net that uses unreliable components and where the nets are not necessarily completely redundant.

One other aspect of neural nets that has received some degree of attention is that of reproduction and self-repair. Lofgren's results seem to suggest a finite lifetime for any such system. Indeed, he shows that a species can survive longer than an individual member, and that a member can survive longer than all its components, and that a self-repairing organism can survive indefinitely if some of the automata's normal input-output conditions are relaxed. E. F. Moore purports to have shown that if a machine can grow to only a *finite* maximum size, and if each of its components has a probabilistic rate of decay, then such a system must be 'mortal'. But this is again, in view of Lofgren's work, a discovery apparently without serious biological significance, since biological systems are never *isolated* in the manner of the Moore type of automata, i.e. they do not need to be self-repairing, but can depend on external 'repairing stimuli'.

One of the next most important questions that now arises is as to whether the automata or neural nets which are adequate for the purpose of modelling humanlike brain activities need to be *growth* automata, or can still be fixed and pre-wired. It has been argued that automata that grow are representative of organic and other biological processes and are hence essential to models of behaviour. However, it has also been shown that growth automata which do not have unlimited and indefinitely fast growth may be even more restricted in their' capacities 'than 'fixed automata. Whichever is the case, the capacity to stimulate growth on fixed automata suggests that herein lies the greatest potential for the immediate future as far as brain modelling is concerned.

Landahl and Runge (1956), among others, have shown how neural nets can be represented by matrices and thus, of course, may easily be computerized: this appears to hold out one of the major hopes for the future of this approach. The reason for this state of affairs is simply that unless neural nets can be computerized they cannot generate sufficiently large models to make essential tests realistic. A slightly different approach to these same, or similar, matters has come through abstract sequential automata (Glushkov, 1961; Ginsberg, 1962; Rosen, 1965) and these hold out promise that perhaps a further set of principles might be so demonstrated. George (1962, 1966) has demonstrated that induction can be achieved by conditional probability computing and in essence this is a further result derived from the field of sequential automata.

The most important feature that neural nets have to offer, however, is that they make models such as Hebb's, Uttley's and Lashley's explicit and testable, at least as far as it is possible to test a model which purports to represent a more complex system for which the blueprint is not possessed.

General hardware and software models

More general models, both in software and hardware, are numerous in cybernetics and only a few will be mentioned. Farley and Clark (1961) have demonstrated some of the electrical characteristics of the nervous system by suitably programming a computer. This is an attempt to increase our understanding of the functional picture of sets of neurons or nets.

Beurle (1962) has studied these same functional characteristics rather differently and has studied random nets of actual neurons. There is again some progress from such a standpoint, and Beurle is able to show a great deal of humanlike trial-and-error and learning behaviour, and even more speculative behaviour.

Turing (1951, 1952) also developed a theory of network brainlike structures starting from a random organization and went on to study the chemical features of brain structures: he developed a theory of morphogenesis which has been followed up by Apter (1966) and others.

We (George, 1957, 1958, 1959, 1960) may now summarize a few of the tentative interpretations that are implied by our own investigations. Broadly speaking, our C-system is to be identified with the cerebral cortex and basal ganglia; the input is identified with the special senses, merging into the cortex and the C-system. The M-system is surely to be identified with the effects of the internal organism, making use of the reticular system, on the thalamus and hypothalamus. The E-system is identified with the hypothalamus and the autonomic system. These ideas are, of course, crude, and need to be refined.

In the first place we must regard the nervous system as having special purpose and analog systems (both built-in and chemical), to which our logical nets are only an approximation.

The storage systems make up the bulk of the cerebral cortex, and the problems are largely of the special function of particular sets of registers and their mode of operation. It is not difficult for the reader to take the next step and envisage the range of possible models which might next be described with an eye to experiment. However, more will be said on this matter in the final chapter of the book.

We shall turn in the next chapter to an analysis of perception, and we shall perform the analysis from a cybernetic, a molar psychological, and a neurophysiological point of view, together.

Summary

In this chapter we have taken our neurophysiological discussion one stage further. Apart from Pribram's summary of the contemporary neurophysiological situation, the chapter is largely concerned with more conceptual models of the nervous system which are not intended to have anything like complete and immediate verisimilitude. This in itself brings out clearly, and yet again, that in science, models and theories that mirror precisely, or make precise predictions of events, cannot always be immediately built; and this is the reason why conceptual and logical models are so useful, even necessary, to our theory construction programme.

Although we have not explicitly discussed Hebb's cell-assembly theory, we have mentioned many aspects of it. It is, in any case, one of the best known of neurophysiological theories, and it is hoped that Milner's modification of the cell-assembly theory as described in this chapter has been found intelligible.

The work of Pavlov and Konorski is not always easy to read, because of the rather ugly nomenclature, but nevertheless it was thought important that their views should be summarized.

We have given little more than a mention to the work of the ethologists, and readers interested in the work of Tinbergen, Lorenz, Thorpe and others may feel that we have hardly done them justice. The reason for this, as for the brevity of comment on many other closely related topics, is simply that this book has to be kept to a reasonable length; no biologist, at any rate, will be ignorant of the very useful work in this field done by ethologists.

CHAPTER 11

PERCEPTION

CHAPTER 8 dealt with some of the traditional problems of what has been called 'cognition', with special emphasis on learning as well as thinking and problem solving, and while it is necessary to 'break-down' our analysis of behaviour into such terms as 'learning' and 'perception', we must bear in mind that we are doing so with some measure of arbitrariness. A precise definition of either term is very difficult to phrase, and since we may assume that the reader is fairly familiar with what occurs between the covers of books on *perception*, we shall not attempt anything approaching a careful analysis or formalization of the term. In the meantime we can at least say that 'to perceive' is something more than 'to sense' and something less than 'to know'.

The majority of psychologists have given approval to the position taken up by Hebb (1949), who believes that one of the big problems of modern psychology is to find large-scale relations between psychology and physiology.

In perception, this attitude led directly to Hebb's efforts to initiate the job of reinterpreting physiologically the evidence collected within psychology; indeed, Hebb's evidence has helped to demolish the arguments—stemming partly from Lashley's work—that the behavioural facts of *perception* cannot be represented by any sort of *specific* neurophysiological processes. There is, in fact, no evidence to support a denial of the possibility of specific behavioural acts being directly correlated with specific states of the nervous system, neither is there any evidence to support a field theory of neurology of the type suggested by Kohler (1940). At the same time we have seen that too narrow a mechanistic view has had its particular difficulties. The writer has no wish to minimize the value of the Gestalt theory, but it must be said that it never was a complete theory, and useful concepts such as 'wholeness' that it has formulated have now been more or less incorporated into the body of scientific behaviour theory.

Osgood and Heyer (1952) have done much, as did Marshall and Talbot before them, to suggest a more satisfactory link between physiological states and introspectively-given *perceptual* data, and this connection will be followed up. These present tendencies are of importance to a general account of the visual system in its perceptual as well as in its sensory aspects; the figural after-effect has been of special interest in this respect.

The figural after-effect is simply the effect of one perceptual configuration on another. If you look at an open line circle on a piece of paper, and then look at a square on another piece of paper, where the square falls on roughly the same area of the retina, then the square is liable to be severely distorted. This distortion is fairly systematic in character, and has been extensively studied (Köhler and Wallach, 1944).

The use of the optic chiasma, which is the point in the optic system where the nerve fibres from the left eye cross over to the right visual cortex, and vice versa, has been a standard method of distinguishing *central* from *peripheral* visual phenomena. With this method, after-effects of the after-image kind can be shown to be primarily peripheral and thus, presumably, a function of physiological correlates in the retina, or eyeball, itself.

The non-peripheral effects such as the figural after-effect, and the closely related plateau spiral effect, are of interest since they involve the 'higher interpretative' levels of the central nervous system. The lateral geniculate body has an uncertain status in these matters, but the main problems are thought to be cortical.

The Plateau spiral should be rotated with the subject fixating its centre, and as a result it may seem to unwind towards or away from the subject. If it is stopped, there follows an apparent movement in the opposite direction.

In the closely connected problems of perception of movement, *apparent* and *real* movement are intimately associated with each other, as is the pendulum effect, which is immediately related to apparent movement (Hall, Earle and Crookes, 1952) where the form of the apparent movement observed was directly dependent upon the extra clues, which were auditory, in the form of rhythmical clicking. Most of those subjected to these conditions formed the impression that they were observing the movement of a pendulum.

Kendon Smith (1952) has pointed to some of the difficulties that are involved for Osgood and Heyer's (1952) theory in explicating some of the more dynamic central visual effects, and Deutsch (1954) has also raised objections to the theory. These will be discussed more fully in the next chapter.

Deutsch's (1953) work on the spiral is also relevant. He found that intermittent illumination of a static spiral gave an effect of 'apparent rotation', and also (often) gave after-effects similar to those associated with an actual rotation. Of course, it is not difficult to imagine that our sensory apparatus records certain external events and, if certain cues or clues are suppressed, that it cannot distinguish different situations that depend solely on observing those certain suppressed cues. Thus 'apparent' and 'real' movement are *visually* the same, and only contextual clues would distinguish them, through inference. This leaves open the question of central after-effects, but the writer believes that here is a case where an explanation of the effects depends, in the first instance, on giving a physiological account in terms of the eye, the lateral geniculate body, and the visual cortex, and leaving the obviously interpretive effects (e.g. the rotational aspect of the recorded after-effect) to the other cortical areas.

This is surely where *central interpretations* are a function of *experience* in the form of beliefs and expectancies.

Throughout this kind of interpretative work the problem is to deal with different levels of neural tissue as well as different levels of explanation, although the process is in fact a function of the organism-as-a-whole. It does not seem possible to talk of uninterpreted recordings (and their manifold effects) in the visual system alone, and then of their interpretations in various cortical areas, such as area 17 alone, the occipital areas alone, or the cortex-as-a-whole. However, in some respects we can reconstruct a set of models and theories with these crude distinctions in mind.

There are many problems in perception yet to be solved, and it will surely be a most fruitful field for amalgamated work by perception-psychologists, sensory-physiologists, neurologists, etc., for their experimental results are of extreme relevance to each other. We have already summarized briefly the very considerable (but still very inadequate) evidence that has been collected by neurophysiologists and other biologists in general, but the molecular approach to *perception* as such has been only lightly touched upon. Nevertheless, it will be more useful at this point to turn to the molar approach.

Boring (1952) holds a view that regards perception as related to the constructed space of science on the one hand, and the subjective space of the observer on the other. Boring is interested in invariance among the variables that range over both sorts of space. He restates some of the well authenticated data, e.g. that perceived size is positively correlated with change of distance in free binocular vision, sufficient of the normal clues being present. If these normal clues are inadequate, perceptual size depends more and more on retinal size, and less and less on 'object-size'. This sort of relationship, which has been emphasized by Thouless (1931) in his work on phenomenal regression, poses no serious problem, since it is the way one would expect an inference-making organism to respond under such circumstances. Similarly, reduction-screens are simply a means of reducing some or all the *cues* to the holding of a correct *belief* with respect to some object, or more generally, some stimulus.

Boring sees the problem as partly a semantic one when he says that a 6-foot pole close at hand and one 100 yards away are such that the far pole 'looks just as big although it looks smaller'. There is no paradox here; it simply reflects the ambiguity of the word 'looks', which may mean either 'look in the sense of by-literal-retinal-equation', or 'look in the sense of believe'.

One problem left untouched by Boring is that of the relation of size and distance when celestial distances are involved. Here, no doubt, we need the same sort of generalization as was effected by König and Brodhun on the Weber–Fechner law (see p. 357). The relation between size and distance is approximately linear up to some limits, but over a sufficient range it would seem to have a much more general relation where phenomenal size falls off much less quickly with distance.

The question of constancy has made the perception of the moon a matter of special interest, and writers have used data on it for and against both empiricism and nativism. There is also the interesting relation between the degree of size-constancy and the angle of viewing (Holway and Boring, 1941) which is characterized by the well-known case of the 'horizontal moon'.

The moon near the horizon appears much larger than the moon at the zenith, and Holway and Boring seem to show that this depends on the elevation of eyes in the head. This may be a function of non-Euclidean dimensions of *perceived* space, or it may be a function of *experience*, either in the central or the non-central sense, or it may even be a function of these factors together.

The vast number of experiments on the constancies (see, for example, Woodworth, 1938) have, of course, their own intrinsic interest, but apart from that, they seem to the writer to support the empiricist view of *perception* and should therefore themselves be explained in terms of *experience*. This is not, quite obviously, to deny their immediate and essential dependence on the organization of the visual system, but it does seem unlikely that the visual system works independently of the inferential (probably cortical) processes. The general evidence is surely against such a wholeheartedly nativist interpretation.

The general emphasis must be placed on the organism-as-a-whole, and ordered, experimentally determined, theoretical processes, such as the phase-sequences of Hebb, which are near to the best perceptual reconstructions available in molar psychological theory.

To return, though for a moment only, to the question of size-perception, which serves to illustrate the scientific problem of perception, Gibson (1950) has suggested some conclusions that place him on the side which views objects as primary, and sensations as secondary.

This dualism, which both Boring and Gibson accept, has certain difficulties, but the question of the primacy of the object or the sensation is one to which it is difficult to ascribe any significance. It is a matter of theory-construction technique and not of empirical fact.

One of the dangers we have to face in the piecemeal reconstruction of perception is the fact that these various problems of size-perception, apparent movement, and so on, are not sufficiently independent. There can be little doubt, for example, that *motivation* modifies perception, and the danger is that we seek explanations for part processes that are only explicable when the organism is treated as a whole.

The distinction between appearance and reality is better made as a continuous series, or degrees, of interpretation rather than as a dichotomy. The difference emphasized is that between *seeing* (with a high degree of interpretation) and *seeing* (with the minimum interpretation). This is useful, and doubtless on the right lines, but inadequate for some of our more subtle purposes.

Cybernetics and perception

Now we must describe some of the general principles that have been adduced as a result of regarding certain biological systems from the point of view of cybernetics.

It was Hayek (1952) who first suggested that the method of human perception was dependent upon a classification system. This suggestion was followed up by Uttley (1954, 1955), who built, as mentioned earlier, a model of a classification system wherein he assumed a certain set of primitive properties, a, b, ..., n, which could be partitioned into subsets of these properties 1, 2, ..., n at a time. This is the same essential principle on which the input of the digital computer operates, and it seems to be essential to the human visual system (as well as to the other special senses) in one form or another.

Such a classifying system is consistent with our knowledge of the empirical world, which we divide up into classes and properties, and which is precisely a reversal of the process ascribed by us to the special senses. Later, we shall give some account of the human visual system, and our account will rely from the start on the concept of classification. From this starting point we must consider the need for more specific perceptual structures.

A human nervous system must obviously include a storage system in some form. It is clear that without the ability to record previous experience no human being could behave in an intelligent manner, and that part of perception called recognition must depend upon a comparison with what has already been stored. This question has been analysed by Culbertson (1956), who showed that memoryless automata could, in fact, exhibit what seems to be intelligent behaviour but this does not change our view, quite apart from the evidence from introspective (or retrospective) events which we can 'consciously remember'.

Many different methods of storage have been constructed in hardware, including chemical storage systems. These different systems can be utilized to produce certain sorts of results in conjunction with certain types of input, and a direct investigation can thus be made of the central nervous system with the idea of discovering which methods are most plausible, neurophysiologically. There is some neurophysicological and behavioural evidence on this point that suggests the use of at least two different sorts of storage, perhaps in a primarily chemical form, and operating in a manner similar to the registers of a computer. At the very least, a short-term and a long-term storage must exist.

Uttley's conditional probability machine (1955) has some of the inductive capacities required for recognition, and in Bristol a computer has been built capable of exhibiting the same properties (George, 1958; Chapman, 1959). But before we discuss these sorts of systems further, let us return for a moment to the more general molar questions.

We must ask ourselves the cybernetic question: Are the problems of perceiving size and movement and the problem of constancy made clearer by recourse to our models, whether in hardware or, more especially, in logical net form?

We have already started to outline our approach to problems of perception, where we think initially of perceiving as occurring on the basis of classification. To proceed with the argument to the next stage we must further develop the basic assumption of classification.

It is clear that the normal human being receives information from his environment which is of a continuously varying kind, involving considerable redundancy (Rapoport, 1955; Barlow, 1959), and also coming from a wide variety of sources. This stream of information, coupled with the organism's responses, are the events that represent behaviour in an environment, where each event has a certain specifiable probability relation with every other event.

We shall say, then, that the occurrence of a *sign* will give a definite expectancy with respect to other signs or stimuli that will influence the process of recognition or perception. Further to this, there are differently weighted probabilities that will be applicable to certain combinations of stimuli at any instant, in terms of which the process of recognition will operate. These probabilities are weighted not only by frequency and recency but also with respect to their *value* for the organism, both in urgency and extent. But let us start from a consideration of the peripheral elements.

Different sensory endings account for different sorts of classified inputs, since nerve transmission, while varying with strength of stimulus, remains qualitively the same for varying sensations. Thus it seems likely that nerve endings are each specifically sensitive to some sort of definite effect, such as heat and cold. This indeed grants, in part, the argument by Sutherland (1959) which points to the need for specific stimulus analysers.

Similarly, the process of hearing seems to depend on peripheral analysers, with recognition depending on the terminal areas of the cortex
becoming specifically associated with different parts of the cochlea.
To take another example, the retina is specifically related to different
points of area 17 by some set of transformations through the restriction
of the optic nerve, which makes temporal and spatial summation necessary, and thus sets up a correspondence between points of the retina and
points of area 17.

We are not at present concerned with peripheral mechanisms which
mediate the sensory process, nor with the precise mechanisms at the
central nervous level which distinguish between, say, the length of a
contour line and its shape; this matter will be discussed later. Many theories and models are already in existence, but we are primarily concerned
with the handling of the signals as a key to the perceptual act, on the
assumption that the process of classification is somehow possible.

The fundamental process of visual perception can now be said to be
that of recording patterns of discriminable inputs in area 17, using certain
unspecified devices, such as the time interval between the onset and
cessation of streams of stimuli, and so on. But let us now give some consideration to the nature of classification in machines.

The machine design

The idea of photoelectric cells, cathode-ray oscillographs, radio trans-
mitters and receivers, etc., naturally occurs to the builders of sensory
equipment for machines. Uttley (1954) has shown that we can have a
display of photosensitive cells so that any particular shape interposed
between them and the light playing on them will fire whatever cells are
placed in the shadow. This, and many other methods, could be used to
record shapes, and the proper recording of the particular cells so fired,
against the previous experience of the machine, will lead to appropriate
responses in terms of a general classification and control system (George,
1956b, 1957d).

There is no doubt that any system of pattern recognition will have the
difficult job of accounting for that recognition even when the pattern in
question is transformed in various ways. As Selfridge has pointed out
(Selfridge, 1956), '...faces as visual patterns are subject to magnification,

translation, intensification, blurring, and rotation, and they remain the same faces still.'

It is the search for a system that preserves certain invariances under transformations that will model accurately the recognition process. Such recognition is clearly dependent on learning, since we can only classify the details in terms of information already acquired, or possibly previously built in.

Selfridge describes a visual model made up of photosensitive elements that are clustered towards the centre, and which record 1's where inputs occur and 0's where they do not occur. The machine then maximizes its 1-count and this causes a movement of the system in such a way that the objects tend to fall on the greatest density of photosensitive elements; this is obviously a type of retinal model we should bear in mind.

A more general theory along similar lines was designed by Pitts and McCulloch (1947), in which they pictured the recognition system as being made up of two mechanisms that preserve the appearance of an object by pattern, in spite of transformations, by achieving an invariance in terms of a process of averaging.

Neurologically, the group transformation is centred at the superior colliculus, and the general theory depends on the extension of the idea of reverberatory circuits. Perhaps the most obvious field of investigation to suggest itself to the mathematician is that of transformation groups and conformal representation, where retinal figures are transposed from one coordinate system to another, and the question remains as to the nature of the appropriate transformation.

All this is about the nature of the retinal recording and the transference of that record to the area 17, or some higher visual centre, but our chief concern at the moment is with what happens after that, even though the two stages cannot be wholly separable.

Some attempt to separate the two processes occurs in Price's writings (1953), where he distinguishes primary from secondary recognition. Most discussions of pattern recognition have been with respect to primary recognition; in this section, however, our analysis is mainly directed at secondary recognition, with the idea of showing its influence on primary recognition. The whole relationship is certainly relevant to semantic difficulties over the word 'perception', and to the disputes between nativism and empiricism.

Primary recognition is, roughly, the process of recording a shape or property, such as redness, or roundness, while secondary recognition is the process of classifying it, or of putting an interpretation on it. Price says:

> When one sees a red object in a good light, one recognizes the redness of it directly or not at all. Familiar colours, shapes, sounds, tastes, smells and tactual qualities are recognized immediately or intuitively, when one observes instances of them. But when I see a grey lump and recognize it as a piece of lead, this recognition is indirect...

This distinguishes the primary (direct) from the secondary (indirect) process. It seems, though, that they differ in degree rather than absolutely, and in our model we shall suggest that one process grades over into the other.

We have already suggested a brief terminology dealing with the sort of situation that involves perception and learning. We acquire *beliefs* about the nature of reality, and we act on these beliefs when, for our model, we mean the word 'belief' to be understood as a theoretical term linking the input to the output; it is at least some part of that link where the output may not be in fact enacted. Thus the process of perception is one of interpreting, in the light of the organism's experience (making use of its storage system), the stimuli that are selected from all of the potential stimuli. The resulting response to this classificatory act becomes the stimulus for a resulting action, if such action is necessary. This means that the arousal of a perceptual belief leads to the awareness of some object or event in the immediate environment, and this itself may be party to a whole series of events that have previously been associated in a temporal pattern.

It is in this way that selection of stimuli takes place, since the occurrence of one event, correctly perceived, will lead the organism to ascribe some probability to the next event likely to be perceived, in the light of its knowledge of its own response, and the probabilities of such sequential relations, inductively collected from previous experience. This is surely directly responsible for what is called *set* in psychological literature.

Let us return to the actual identification of such objects or events as occur in the neighbourhood of the organism.

We have partitioned sets of receptors

$$\mathop{X}_{i=1}^{n} a_i \mathop{X}_{j=1}^{m} b_j, \ldots \tag{1}$$

such that at any instant there are collections of receptors, generally from each partitioned set, that will be firing. At any instant, therefore, we shall record a finite string of symbols, say:

$$a_1 a_4 a_7 b_2 c_8 c_9 d_1 \qquad (2)$$

and this means that counters of the classification system (that record every possible combination of all the inputs—or so we shall assume for the time being) will alter with each instant. Thus all combinations of the subsets of the string (2) will have 1 added to their count, and then the machine itself will respond by some classification in terms of what this count implies in terms of its experience. More precisely, we shall say that physical objects, for example, are never recognized by all their characteristics at once, and we shall argue that the probability of some physical object A, with respect to the existence of some subset of its characteristics, has a definite probability value to be ascribed to it.

We are saying that a, b, c, ... are the elements of *primary recognition*, and that lengthy combinations of these strings are to be called, for simplicity, A, B, C, ... where A, for example, might stand for (2), and where A, B, C, ... are the elements of *secondary recognition*.

Empirical classification in terms of classes or properties

The above system can now be given a more precise treatment, and to avoid typographical complications we shall talk of a, b, c, ... and A, B, C, ... without the use of suffices, as sufficient for demonstration purposes.

The machine has a classification system wherein the world is divided up into classes of properties, and these properties can be subdivided into indefinitely many subsets. Some classes will be those of colour, size, shape, brightness, noisiness, etc., and size, for example, can be further divided into length, width, height, and so on, whereby a particular object may be classified by reference to its impression: X classifies Y as short; or by reference to an actual measurement: Y is 5 feet 4 inches tall.

Under this general procedure we have subsumed different visual recognition processes, from a momentary exposure under a tachistoscope at one end of a sort of continuum, to a lengthy and detailed analysis, including the measuring of its dimensions, at the other end, here perhaps involving tactile as well as visual recognition.

To recognize an object, we have to recognize its properties—it may be said that an object *is* its full set of properties—and normally we will recognize some subset at any instant; we shall therefore, *whenever it is possible*, take as many instants to perform the recognition as is *necessary* for us to be reasonably sure of its success, ascribing the object to our classification according to its height, weight, colour, shape, and so on. In any instant the probability of its being one object rather than another will be computed purely on the basis of frequency.

At the moment we are not considering the effect of temporal context. If, then, we classify properties *adghjk*, there may be two different physical objects that have these properties, such as *adeghijklnp* and *abdghjklo*, and we can decide the matter in probability terms by reference to the past count. So if we call the first string B and the second C, we can say that the probability of B, given *adghjk*, is p_1, and the probability of C on the same basis is q_1, and now $p_1 > q_1$ implies B, whereas $q_1 > p_1$ implies C.

If we now take the next instant and add the property 1 alone, we shall change the absolute but not the relative probability. The further addition of properties *enp* will decide against C and strengthen the probability of B against all other possibilities, giving it a value p_3, say. Theoretically, this process can go on until a value p_n is achieved, carrying all the properties of B, and thus having the value 1. So we have the possibility of a series of probabilities $p_1, p_2, \ldots, p_n$ with respect to some object which tends towards the limiting value of certainty. We shall call these steps 'categorizing responses' of which the last is called the 'final categorizing response' (F.C.R.). In fact, we are normally content with something far less than a p-value of 1 for an F.C.R., and indeed we have to be, either because we simply are not permitted by time (or space) to see all the properties, or—which is more usual—because we are fairly sure, knowing only a few properties, that we know what the object is, due to the temporal and spatial context of the situation. In effect, this means the weighting of the set-theoretic conditional probabilities by the probabilities of temporal expectancy.

The counting system

The counting system has already been described in Chapter 5, where it depended (although it need not have) on the use of closed-loop elements that fire themselves and continue to fire until stopped by some inhibitory input. A chain of conjunction-counters can be built that will record the frequency of occurrence of any combination of inputs, or properties, whatsoever; and disjunction-counters that will fire when some part of a combination fires but not all of it. Thus, the counters for a and b fire conjunctively if a and b occur together, and disjunctively if a or b occurs alone. In fact events of any length, either positive, negative or mixed can easily be counted by a simple logical net, using a classifying system.

Motivation is clearly a vital condition for the firing of counters, and this is assumed to be occurring in the perceptual process. Combinations have not only to occur but must satisfy, in some sense, the organism—or at least be connected to satisfactions—for the process of counting to take place. Satisfactory associations are broken down by this disjunction-counting when a certain response leads no longer to satisfaction, but instead, to pain. This all depends on certain stimulus–response connections being already built into the machine. Taken in terms of isolated instants, we can use the calculus of empirical relations (see Chapter 3 and Chapter 12) for that seems to describe adequately the perceptual process as a Markov process, in effect, although other relations besides temporal ones could be involved.

The temporal order

So far, in any classification system we have discussed, we have only been concerned with the case of the instantaneous classification of sub-properties to some total set of properties. We have mentioned, though, that it will not generally be necessary to make categorizations, or classifications, in terms of such instantaneous states alone. This is so because there is a temporal order of things such that when a stimulus S_1 occurs, we may respond with response R_2 when the expectation is that S_3 will follow. Indeed, our counter systems for the cognitive process, built on the same principle as for perception alone (George, 1956b), predict precisely the probability of one event following a particular response, in the same manner as some subset of properties is the basis for predicting the total set of properties. Thus if S_1 has occurred 100 times and has been followed by S_3 85 times when the response R_2 has been made, we only need a record, by the use of counters, to tell us the probability of S_3 following S_1, granted that the response R_2 was made. Clearly $p = 85/100$ in this particular case.

The calculus of empirical relations is a method of computation of beliefs that the organism holds merely on the basis of classifying and counting. It is an interpretation of the inductive formula $c(h, e) = p$. Here c means the degree of confirmation, which is given by the probability p, in favour of hypothesis h, by evidence e.

The sequential categorizing responses of a set of instants in the process of perception $p_1, p_2, \ldots, p_n$ includes as a particular case the tests to confirm a scientific theory or hypothesis, e.g. the perceptual process can be thought of as all or as a part of the series.

$$c_1(h_1, e_1), \; c_2(h_2, e_2), \; \ldots, \; c_n(h_n, e_n). \tag{3}$$

Such a system, we shall remember, can be represented by nets, and may in fact be considerably weighted for recency as well as frequency, apart from the fundamental requirement of value through reinforcement.

This very brief account of an inductive logical machine is addressed here primarily to the problem of perception and the central role of secondary recognition. It is felt by the writer that this approach to the problem is one that should be made prior to attacking primary recognition.

By now we should have seen enough, peripheral receptors apart, to ask ourselves the basic question: would a system built on the lines we suggest exhibit all the properties we want?

It is evident that there is no problem for simple differences in size. Granted that we have a receptor mechanism that is able to record anything at all, it may be expected to show differences in the area recorded, and the simplest manner in which this might be expected to occur would be by counting. The problem here seems to be primarily peripheral, and we shall return to it in more detail later.

The real problem is that of size and distance. Is our machine going to say, 'A 6-foot pole close at hand and one 100 yards away are such that the far pole looks just as big although it looks smaller'? If we assume that we have some peripheral receptor which registers a 'retinal size', then it is easy, by simple geometrical considerations, to show that such retinal sizes are quite different for the two poles. Obviously, therefore, two factors enter into the second part of the apparent 'paradox' that suggests that they look the same. It is the context of the process, and our previous experience as represented in our storage system, or in the storage system of the machine, which allow the equivalence. The recognition that it is a pole is said to evoke a particular pattern $a_1a_2a_3a_4$, say, and the peripheral mechanism gives a difference of size, but other cues which the classification mechanism will record are cues in the form of lines of perspective, other objects, and so on, all recognized and with a stored knowledge of their sizes and their 'significance' for size. This again encourages a belief in the empiricist's interpretation of perception.

One group of experimentalists working primarily in the field of perception and called the Transactionalists (Kilpatrick, 1953) are strongly empiricist in bias. They have been able to show that the interpositioning of stimuli between the stimulus under consideration and the eye, will alter the interpretation placed in the size of the distant object. This is so if the nearer object bears (size apart) a relation to the further object that supplies a clue (usually false) as to the further object's distance.

They were also able to show that the relative brightness of an object has an influence upon its apparent size; the reason is to be found in the experiential fact that brighter objects are generally nearer to the observer. The transactionalist arguments for a perceptual theory have not sufficient definiteness to suggest an immediate model, but their general findings are very suggestive for the sort of cybernetic model we have in mind.

Any object, according to transactionalist theory, derives at least a part of its nature and comprehensibility from its participation in a total situation. Such a present transaction—which constitutes the essence of perception—has its roots in the past experience of the individual, and its implications necessarily extend into the future. The world of phenomenological experience is a world of significances provided by such transactions. These significances, resulting from past transactions, are 'externalized' by the perceiver as the basis of his present and future action. The philosophical theory of transactions will incidentally be found in Dewey and Bentley (1949). A brief statement, and a discussion of its application to perception, are given in a series of articles by Cantril et al. (1949). See also Ittelson and Cantril (1954). For a more general application to the phenomena of the Ames demonstrations see Lawrence (1949a, 1949b).

The problem of the context and the transaction of perception is clear in terms of our set-theoretic model, though of course this does not of itself guarantee the correctness of that model. However, this matter will be pursued later, and for the moment we will return to our more general understanding of perceptual problems—indeed, to our *particular* perceptual problems—and ask, as an example, why the 'moon illusion' occurs.

The answer seems to be that the conditions for perceiving the moon as enormously large are lacking, both in our immediate perception of it (there are no cues) and in our previous experience (there are no clues). (We shall use the words 'cue 'and 'clue' throughout in these senses.) The fact that primitive people had no conception of astronomical sizes and distances, and that Anaxagoras was cruelly persecuted for saying that the moon was larger than the Peloponnesus, is an indication that perception here does not follow the form of perception in our immediate vicinity.

Let us next consider movement in perception. Since successive retinal patterns occur somewhat displaced from each other, relative to a retinal datum and a conceptual datum which will allow for eye movements and head movements, we may expect to record a 'moving object', and indeed our idea of a moving object depends precisely on this sensory (not visual alone) fact of successive stimulation of a pattern which retains its identity. This is to be explained in terms of the peripheral receptors, and we can thus concentrate immediately on the difference between apparent and real movement.

We may expect that, subject to certain restrictions in the form of cues that allow the classification system to infer 'apparent movement', such a system alone will be unable to distinguish apparent from real movement. This implies that it is the clues from storage, and inferences made in terms of the subject's knowledge of the overall position in which he is placed, that make the distinction possible. Confirmation of the above argument may be found in the *Pendulum Effect*.

It is perhaps clear by now that the machine system, as thought of in the precise designs of finite automata, will be almost wholly committed to an empiricist form of explanation, where the cues and their immediate bearing on objects in the instantaneous sensory field, although often supplying information for recognition, are themselves dependent for their efficacy on previous associations.

Further to the above, we can see that we should seek to explain *constancy* by the same sort of explanatory process as that already suggested. The co-operative working of the sensory classification and the control system is certainly the source of such effects, and the main interest for us must lie in showing the more precise nature of the models suggested as a result of the more detailed experimental data.

We say, then, that constancy is concerned with the contextual situation where our stored knowledge directly influences the results achieved by our classification system. Again we see the need to specify more precisely the range of possible workings involved. We also have words like 'attitude' which represent the influence of the store in an anticipatory way (possibly with contamination from emotions) on the anticipated occurrence. In ordinary language we might say, 'I had an attitude of suspicion because I had been duped that way before. Instead of $A \rightarrow B$, A was presented and yielded C, so now I am uncertain (suspicious) of the outcome with respect to the stimulus A, and so on.'

We shall be careful to distinguish between constancy in this contextual sense, and the continuous identity of a physical object moving through space, where the identity *might* be dependent upon characteristics in the peripheral receptors; or both these and the storage's interaction with the sensory classification systems.

The effective stimulus in perception

Another problem of importance in perception is that of the nature of effective stimulus variables. Boring (1952) takes up the point raised by Dewey as to what constitutes an effective stimulus—a matter which has also been emphasized by transactionalists. The problem of any stimulus–response system is to identify the stimulus. Boring says of this:

> He (Dewey) was right, for the effective stimulus is not an object but a property of the stimulus-object; some crucial property that cannot be altered without changing the response, some property that remains invariant, for a given response, in the face of transformations of other characteristics.

This problem can be treated in many ways; indeed, the whole question of an appropriate language for descriptive purposes is brought back at this point. There is a certain vagueness over the words 'object' and 'property of the stimulus-object' in the above quotation that calls for further discussion. It seems that both *objects* and *properties of objects* may act as stimuli, and what, for that matter, is an object but the total set of its properties? Certainly, though, it is often the case that the stimulus is a relation (perhaps usually an invariance relation), and certainly it is a distinct problem to establish the identity of an effective stimulus. It is often the case that, in an environment of potential stimuli, one has to wait for the response in order to make a deduction about the nature of the stimulus. Our search for a (public) science is conducted partly by laying down laws such that, given all the potential stimuli and the state of the organism, we shall be able to say which will be effective stimuli, in terms of either the contemporaneous state of the organism (which includes all its experiences in the form of an end-product or resultant vector), or by knowledge of the experience of the organism. For theoretical purposes this matter is a sophisticated end-product rather than a relatively crude initial problem.

Our method of discussing properties of stimulus variables must be in terms of the *objective properties* of the stimuli; the process of making a stimulus effective is *the* problem of behaviour. The study of these objective characteristics is not of special relevance to the present discussion, although it is vital to the nature of the perceptual theory one arrives at, and therefore to the sort of models we shall construct. The objective properties are those of physical distance, size, shape (or form), brightness, colour (certain refractive and reflective properties of materials), relative perspectives, groupings and so on and so forth.

Such laws as those set down by Wertheimer (see Woodworth, 1938) are of great relevance at this point, as is the whole work of the Gestalt school, although we must be careful to distinguish the *actual* (or physical) characteristics of potential stimuli—in so far as they are knowable other than by someone's perceptions—from the effective stimuli and interpretation, which are a function of the organism's interaction (or transaction) with its environment. Thus Wertheimer's laws of perceived movement which show a perceived relationship between similar things, or things moving with similar speeds, etc. (see Boring, 1942), and more obviously, the division of the stimulus-field into figure and ground, and so on, are part of the activity of the organism; and binocular vision, flicker fusion, inferences, and so on, become part of the essential features of *perception*. Gradients, texture gradients, indeed gradients of all kinds (including, on a different level, the physiological gradients of C. M. Child) are part of the method or language of description of the organism's activity, the activity of classification, categorization and, in general, that of response.

It is as well to remember here the non-sensory figures of Hebb (1949), and the research that appears to show that there are various possible interpretations of sensorimotor activity. There may, for example, be motor activities which are not the direct result of causal stimulation;

indeed, many people have suggested that it would be incorrect to regard the sensory and motor components of the reflex arc as, in any sense, mirror-images of each other. One, for example, may arouse (or partially arouse), while the other may direct, and not merely respond, in a manner already discussed in Chapter 10 where we described Pribram's homeostatic type of control. Our models will certainly be capable of mirroring these facts, as a careful reading of Chapter 5 will already have revealed.

Psycho-physics

The essential connection between the *objective* state of affairs and the *subjective* is covered by the field of psycho-physics. It should be noted here that explicit assumptions are made that connect stimulus and sensation; for example, the Weber–Fechner Law can be stated:

$$R = K \log S/S_0$$

where S is the stimulus, R is the sensation, and S_0 is the smallest stimulus which leads to sensation. The adequacy of psycho-physics clearly depends upon the degree of precision of the fit between the parameters of stimulation and the parameters of sensation. There are examples in the psychophysical field, such as quality control, where the fit does not always seem sufficiently good for the purpose in hand. But now, the method of testing the validity of the psycho-physical methods becomes important, and this line of approach will not be continued further. The problems are clear enough (in one sense at least), and much experimental work needs to be done in this field to clarify more completely the status of psychophysics; its methodological vagueness is a direct function of the mind–body problem.

The psycho-physical methods, which are the methods of constant stimuli, single stimuli, limits, sense-ratios, reaction-times, etc., are essential to the design of experiments with respect to the sensory modalities. The general form of all psycho-physical experiments can be characterized:

$$R = f(a, b, c, \ldots n \ldots t \ldots x, y, z)$$

where a, b, c, $\ldots$ refer to specified aspects of stimuli; $\ldots x$, y, z refer to specified conditions of the organism; R means response; n is the number of presentations and t is time. The precise specifications of the variables

T B C   24

in this equation are, as Graham (1952) says, matters for further research and theoretical analysis.

Many books could be written on the diverse and widely ranging subject matter of this chapter. It is not our aim to review, as might a textbook, all the details of the variables and problems of perception. Our aim, rather, is to illustrate the cybernetic application to it by selected examples, and to seek generalities that will help us towards a general theory of perception.

To summarize this section, we may say that what is being emphasized, when questions are asked about the nature of the effective stimulus, is the fact that there is a selective process operating, and that what is effective in stimulating the organism is dependent not only on what appears in objective space at any moment, and the configuration in which it appears, but the state of the store which, in conjunction with previous stimulation, introduces states of 'set'.

What about the complex configuration which has been the subject of investigations by the Gestalt theorists? This is a matter we must consider, but here at least there seems to be a case for considering what is normally regarded as a perceptual problem (as opposed to a sensory problem) after our discussion of receptor mechanisms.

Form perception

We shall now consider the problem of form perception in terms of the models that have been suggested. Deutsch (1954) has suggested the six main facts that a theory of 'shape recognition'—as he calls it—must explain:

(1) Animals can recognize shapes independent of their location in the visual field. It is not necessary to fixate the centre of a figure in order to recognize it, nor need the eyes be moved around the contours of a figure.

(2) Recognition can be effected independently of the angle of inclination of a figure in the visual field (this means the tilt of an image in two dimensions, and not the tilt of the figure in depth such as occurs in shape constancy experiments).

(3) The size of a figure does not interfere with the identity of its shape. This, of course, does not hold at the extremes of size for reasons which seem sufficiently obvious.

(4) Mirror images appear alike. Both rats and human beings tend to confuse these. This would appear to rule out any 'template' theories of shape recognition, according to which, a contour is rotated in two dimensions until it coincides with one of the many patterns already laid down. But such a superimposition cannot take place in the case of mirror images, and no room is left, therefore, for this particular type of confusion.

(5) Visually primitive organisms such as the rat and the octopus find it hard (perhaps impossible) to distinguish between squares and circles. This does not seem to be a limitation imposed by the peripheral characteristics of the optical systems, but appears to be a more central defect as these organisms can distinguish shapes which are *far more alike geometrically*. This type of evidence tends to cast doubt on theories which base themselves on the angular properties of figures.

(6) These abilities, which appear to be mediated by the striate cortex, survive the removal of the major part of it. It is therefore reasonable to suppose that this ability to disentangle shape is common to all parts of the striate area, and that one part of the striate area is not essential in helping the next one to operate.

Deutsch feels that this would tend to rule out notions based on a scanning process. It is difficult to see how a regular scan could be maintained in the presence of extensive damage. Further, any system which requires the fixation of the centre of a figure so that it coincides with the centre of the visual field must also be ruled out. The ability is maintained even where there are extensive scotomata of central origin.

We should notice that, of this list, we might question the truth of (1), at least in the initial stages of perception (Hebb, 1949), and there may be doubts about Deutsch's inference in terms of (6). Furthermore, these six points lay no claim to completeness, but they are suggestive as a general starting point. We should note here that possibly the static approach mentioned is a special case of the more dynamic process which normally occurs in human beings.

Culbertson (1948), Rapoport (1955), Deutsch (1955) and Selfridge (1956), among others, have suggested models for systems that would be capable of carrying out the task of form recognition.

Culbertson has used logical nets for describing his own system of shape recognition; he in fact suggested some effective, although probably biologically implausible, form abstractors for the purpose.

24*

The first abstractor is a translator, which simply passes an image from one set of elements to the right, say, to an adjacent set, and on, indefinitely, across a surface, and in particular where the surface is a cylinder, around its face.

The second abstractor is a rotator which is made up of two disc-shaped arrays between which is a cylinder. This device is able to rotate any pattern indefinitely. Incidentally, both the translator and the rotator would be easy for the reader to draw, using the logical nets of Chapter 5.

Dilators and expanders can be constructed to make the image as large or as small as we please. Then we have the image centring system, and all these taken together in an appropriate combination can be shown to be sufficient to process a shape for the purposes of recognition. It is of interest, too, that the whole form abstraction system requires only 2×10^7 elements and the reaction time of the whole net is less than a quarter of a second.

The possible objection to this model of Culbertson's is, of course, Deutsch's point (4), which puts the argument against straightforward 'template' techniques.

It seems certain, to answer Deutsch's first point, that whereas image centring may not be necessary later, during *the learning of* a perception, it may be absolutely necessary.

Rapoport has constructed his perceptual model partly in terms of logical nets and partly in terms of information theory. This all implies that one must start with fairly idealized ideas about how the nervous system works. Rapoport regards the retinal photoreceptor layer as a mosaic that could be specified by, say, spherical polar co-ordinates, and uses the shortest refractory period of all the cells as his unit of time; then the effective mosaic at each instant, which is the time-unit, is uniquely specified.

Now let us assume that each instantaneous state of the retina is a potential message, which means that for n receptors there will be 2^n messages. If the photoreceptors were all independent of each other, and if in the rth instant the probability of firing the ith receptor was given by p_i, and if we said, by analogy with Laplacian probability, $q_i = 1 - p_i$, then the information content of the source would be given by

$$H = p_i \log p_i + q_i \log q_i$$

and if $p_i = \frac{1}{2}$ for all i, $H = n$ bits per message.

Now to consider what value n, the number of photoreceptors, might have. Cajal has suggested $n = 10^8$, and Fulton has suggested that 10^{-3} is about an average refractory period. If the independence of the receptors is maintained we can conclude that the production of information in the retina is at 10^{11} bits per second. This result is far too large, judging by all our other evidence of human capacities for reaction to visual stimulation.

The next step, then, is to consider—as does Rapoport—the possibility of regions sending messages, where the actual number of photoreceptors firing in each region constitutes the message. This gives us a more complicated expression for H; and then we can consider the interaction of the elements in the regions, which will make our expression for H more complicated still.

Physiologically, we have a lot of evidence that suggests that the retina is highly organized, and that there is a great deal of interdependence in the successive states of the visual field. Looking at an object under normal circumstances, we will generally see it from various slightly different angles successively. This implies a high measure of redundancy in the retina, and it is this redundancy that enables the visual system to operate at well below the level of what is suggested by the formula derived (above) by Rapoport. This is what we meant by our previous reference to a dynamic approach to perception.

The next problem is to consider the information as to the state of the visual field, as exemplified by successive states of the retina. We know that there is a bottleneck effect which operates between the retina and the representation of visual events in the cortex, possibly in area 17, in much the same way as they were originally at the retinal level. This bottleneck suggests not only lost information but, what is more important, the method by which information is selected. The extent of the bottleneck as suggested by Polyak is that 10^8 photoreceptors map on to 10^6 ganglion cells, which implies a ratio of 100 to 1 on the average. This average covers a range of 1 to 1 at the fovea, to many hundreds to one in the periphery of the retina. The reintegration of information at the end of a bottleneck is characteristic of the nervous system and depends on temporal summation.

Sir Henry Head's distinction between epicritic and protopathic vision, and the nature of these connections, suggests that detailed vision of the cones presents no serious bottleneck; the bottleneck applies only to the protopathic or generalized visual states, recording only crude character-istics of change of brightness.

Rapoport's model does not consider the distinction that is raised by the difference between epicritic and protopathic vision. He addresses himself rather to the general problem of transmission of information with minimal loss.

The system of minimizing the loss of information involves the suitable choice of a code. The reader will know that codes can be constructed for various purposes and, to take cognizance of the epicritic–protopathic distinction, two sorts of codes, at least, seem to be necessary for the visual system. One must retain detail, and this will be easiest at the region of least bottleneck. The other must try and retain as much information as possible, while maximum attention will be given to speed of signal. The mere recording of movement and so on for peripheral photorecep-tors, and great detail in the areas of great acuity.

This problem of the appropriate coding suggests the need for detailed anatomical knowledge. In the lack of this we can construct neural or logical networks as models, and consider what code should be used for systems that are nearer the known structure of the optical system.

Rapoport and Culbertson have suggested models that have a fair measure of realism and can be suitably coded to transmit information in the manner necessary to retain as much information as possible.

Selfridge's visual pattern recognition model

In the Selfridge (1956) model an original image made up of 90×90 0's and 1's is transformed into a secondary image by one of three operations. The secondary image itself may be transformed a number of times. After the image has been transformed by the operations, the 1's left in the image are counted. A typical original image is tranformed sequen-tially showing the secondary images at each step.

The final count is then compared with the numbers stored for that particular sequence under the various symbols. If, after a number of sequences have been run on an image, the counts check sufficiently well with the stored distributions of symbol 1, say, the computer may identify that image as symbol 1.

It is not supposed that the operations mentioned are an exhaustive set.

They are of three kinds, and they are all local and isotropic. The first, local averaging, replaces each datum by an average of the neighbouring data. In this way, *inter alia*, it eliminates granular noise, isolated 1's in a field of 0's, and isolated 0's in a field of 1's, emphasizing local homogeneity. The second operation, local differencing, replaces each datum by an average of the logical differences of the neighbouring data, thus emphasizing local discontinuities and tending to sharpen contrasts, edges, and corners. The third operation, 'blobbing', replaces each relatively isolated conglomeration of 1's by a single 1.

Many kinds of visual features cannot be handled by these particular operations; *for example, this model cannot distinguish a capital C from a capital U*. The latter may be merely the former rotated to an angle of 90 degrees, and all the operations are *isotropic*.

The kinds of things the model could recognize have been deliberately restricted because the digital computer was small and slow. Even though it had 65,000 bits accessible within 10 microseconds, and five times that many in slightly longer, it still took as long as 15 minutes to process an image.

It can be seen, though, that the operations are powerful enough to detect and count critical points. They are actually powerful enough to compute some measure of curvature.

Other kinds of operation will occur, as Selfridge says, 'to the curious'. One can, for example, project along any direction, which will reduce any two-dimensional set of data to a one-dimensional set, or one can 'thin', i.e. change the exterior 1's of an image to 0's so long as one does not alter the topological connectivity.

Furthermore, it is not necessary that the final data reduction be counting. The topological connectivity might be stored instead.

The instructive part of the Selfridge machine, however, is not the particular sequences of operations it uses to recognize symbols, but the way in which it hunts for good sequences. Every sequence is good or bad according as the numbers, which are obtained by applying two images, tend to differ consistently for different symbols. The essence of learning, it seems, lies in having the computer recognize the pattern of good sequences. At the beginning it selects sequences in a random fashion, but as soon as some of the sequences are 'seen' to be better than others, it fashions and tests new sequences that are like the successful ones (this is precisely the sort of thing we suggested in Chapters 5 and 7). The concept of similarity of sequences is built in, and is governed merely by a matrix of transition frequencies. All the sequences to be tested are fashioned, in the Monte Carlo manner, by this matrix of transition frequencies, which is initially flat. As soon as a successful sequence appears, its transition frequencies are used to bias that matrix, which then represents a hypothesis about (the pattern of) good sequences. This hypothesis can be tested by using it to build up new sequences, and discarding or accepting it and them according as they prove useless or useful.

It is not maintained that this method is necessarily a good way of choosing a sequence, but only that it should work better than ignoring all the knowledge of the kinds of sequences that have worked in the past.

Deutsch's visual model

Deutsch has suggested a paper-and-pencil model for shape recognition. It is made up of a two-dimensional array of elements joined to the retina, such that a contour falling on the retinal elements will fall on the equivalent elements of the array. Furthermore, as each new retinal excitation arrives, so a pulse will be sent down the 'final common cable' (f.c.c.) as well as exciting its neighbour. This system is like Culbertson's in effecting a translation of the figure so that, with a rectangle, there will be a set of pulses fired into the f.c.c., and then another set will be fired as it comes into coincidence with the opposite side. In this way the brain can receive information about the length of sides and also of shape. On the other hand, it depends upon the brain being able to make temporal distinctions, and this recoding in terms of time seems to demand a clock, which may not be too implausible.

It should be mentioned that Sutherland (1959) has suggested the possibility that the coding should be done in terms of intensity, and this notion is one that will be used in a further partial model which we shall outline at the end of this chapter.

Hebb's model for perception

There are many cases of perceptual models which are on the borderline between molar and molecular theories. Hebb's, like that of McCulloch and Pitts for pattern recognition, is primarily intended to give a plausible physiological account.

Of Deutsch's six points, the most obvious one which affects Hebb's theory, and which a theory of shape recognition must explain, is that of scanning. Deutsch argues that a careful perusal of the contour lines surrounding the figure is unnecessary, whereas Hebb, with supporting evidence from von Senden (1932) and Riesen (1947), believes that the *learning* of shape perception involves the process of counting corners, or more generally, of fixating successive points on the outline of a complex pattern. This successive fixation process is the basis of the cell assemblies. This argument is perhaps especially important at the time of learning to perceive, but is less important in adult perception, which may be the reason for the apparent disagreement here.

Let us consider Hebb's theory a little more carefully. In the first place Hebb assumes that connections from the primary visual projection area in the brain are originally random. The thresholds at synapses are supposed to vary in a random way from moment to moment as a function of recency of firing of a post-synaptic nerve cell. By repeated firing of particular sets of retinal cells the probability of the same cell assembly being fired is increased.

The possibilities of this theory are not perhaps clear, but Taylor has constructed a model which helps us to see what the implications of Hebb's theory are. This is one of many instances where it is useful actually to build a hardware system to mimic a theory.

The arguments against Hebb, mostly stated by Sutherland (1959), are that while the scanning of contour lines during the learning of the shape of a figure is all right for figures of equivalent size, this theory does not account for recognition without eye movement.

Now although Collier (1931) and others claim to show that such recognition is possible without eye movement, there are in fact two difficulties. The first is to ensure that all eye movements have really been eliminated; and the second is that eye movements may be only necessary to the learning and not to the recognition process. During learning the figure may have to be brought into standard positions by scanning, but after learning, the barest sample of the figure is usually enough for recognition purposes, even though in practice there is, of course, still the availability of eye movements for confirmation of the identity of a figure.

Certainly Sutherland's arguments against the generalized approach to perceptual models are only partly effective, and this can be seen again in his criticism of Uttley. Sutherland has argued that Uttley's system does not lend itself to generalizations other than from a subset to those sets of which it is a possible subset. Now it is obvious that this is not necessarily true, since it is easy to arrange for generalizations to depend upon the notion of similar sets, which similarity is defined in terms of so many common elements. Sets with different elements can also be identified with respect to having a common resultant, and so on. This sort of argument has really no bearing on the relative advantages of regarding specific analysing mechanisms as against general systems.

At the same time, Sutherland produces much relevant evidence to support the idea that we should not wholly overlook specific analysing mechanisms.

The fly-catching behaviour in newts seems certainly to depend on specific analysers (Sperry, 1943), and the work of Sharpless and Jasper (1956) and Hernándos-Peón, Sherrer and Jouvet (1956) supports clearly the idea of ordered sensory processing.

In the experiment of the latter group, peripheral blocking on the part of a cat was inferred when a cochlear potential to clicks was completely inhibited by the sight of a mouse. It was suggested that this might be a function of the reticular formation.

While accepting the fact that a too complete adherence to general principles in perception is probably false to fact, it would seem unwise to go as far as does Sutherland in supporting what he sees as the only alternative. In fact, of course, it is not a matter of alternatives, but rather of modifying a general approach to fit the particular experimental facts that Sutherland so ably presents.

Perceptrons

This is an example of what Rosenblatt calls a 'Genotypic model', as opposed to a 'Monotypic model'. By 'genotypic', Rosenblatt means that which is given a functional description only, whereas by 'monotypic' he means to imply a detailed structure over and above a function. It has been suggested that to some extent this distinction between anatomical detail and physiological function cuts across another distinction between general-purpose and special-purpose models (George, 1965). The Osgood and Heyer model is very much a special-purpose model dealing with visual perceptual matters alone, whereas Hebb's cell assembly system, for example, is general purpose and deals with the total organization of the brain. However, it must be added that, as usual, these distinctions generally speaking are matters of degree and not absolute distinctions. They show a tendency in the modelling rather than an absolute difference between the models.

As a result of it being classed as a genotypic model, it is no longer supposed in Rosenblatt's perceptrons that the neurons or elements and the topology of the nets underlying them are fully specified. Here we have a type of modelling that partially specifies the organization of the net and offers probabilistic constraints which generate a whole class of models. Indeed the 'perceptron' is the name for a class of models rather than a single model.

As Rosenblatt puts the whole matter himself: 'The genotypic approach is concerned with the properties of systems which conform to designated laws of organization, rather than with the logical function realised by a particular system.' Let us look at Rosenblatt's definition of a perceptron: 'A perceptron is a network composed of stimulus-unit, association-unit, and response-unit with a variable interaction matrix V which depends on the sequence of past activity states of the network.' A stimulus (S) and response (R) unit generate 'internal' and 'external' signals, respectively. 'Internal' means within the network, and 'external' means within the environment. An association (A) unit receives signals *and* emits them.

Now a *simple perceptron* is defined as satisfying the the following five conditions:

(1) There is only one R-unit with a connection from every A-unit.
(2) The perceptron is series-coupled, with connections only from S-units to A-units, and from A-units to the R-unit.
(3) The *values* of all sensory to A-unit connections are fixed.
(4) The *transmission time* of every connection is either zero or equal to a fixed constant.
(5) All signal generating functions of S-, A- and R-units are of the form $u_i(t) = f(\alpha_i(t))$, where $\alpha_i(t)$ is the algebraic sum of all input signals arriving simultaneously at the unit μ.

Now we must define 'transmission function', 'value' and 'interacting matrix'.

A *transmission function* of connections in a perceptron depends on two parameters, the transmission time of the connection τ_{ij} and the *value* of the connection U_{ij}. Variable values are called *memory functions*.

The *interacting matrix* V for a perceptron is the matrix of coupling coefficient ij for pairs of units U_i and U_j. If U_i and U_j are unconnected then $U_{ij} = 0$. An interacting matrix is what has sometimes been called a 'structure matrix'.

A perceptron can be represented as a logical net, so that any of the logical nets which have been described in this book would qualify for the name 'perceptron'. Rosenblatt has suggested other pictorial representation of perceptrons for different levels of precision. So far then, Rosenblatt has achieved only a slightly new notation. Let us look at his first 'experimental' perceptron.

An 'experimental system' can be called a simple perceptron coupled to a reinforcement control system and in an environment. This again merely restates the simplest sort of cognitive situation.

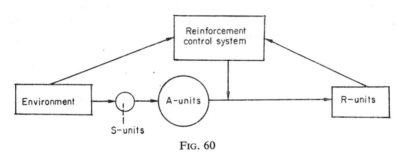

FIG. 60

From these beginnings, Rosenblatt builds up a 'Universal perceptron' which can now be thought of as generalized nets, where the detailed topology is replaced by the general constraints previously mentioned.

A retinal set of S-units can now be constructed so that 'differential' stimulation from different shapes can be achieved. If we now project two distinguishable shapes X_1 and X_2 on to the retina we have sets of A-units which simply fire or not according to whether the equivalent S-units fire.

Step by step, Rosenblatt constructs perceptrons or logical nets that can distinguish shapes, and shapes in connection with typical 'shape-names' like 'triangle', 'circle', etc.

What distinguishes Rosenblatt's work from that of Culbertson, say, is precisely what Rosenblatt describes as the difference between mono-typic and genotypic models. Culbertson specifies in logical detail the topology of his system, whereas Rosenblatt leaves open these topological considerations and replaces logically defined detail by probabilistic functions. It seems that there is scope for both approaches to the modelling of biological systems. Indeed it seems to the present writer, as already hinted, that Rosenblatt has overstated the difference between monotypic and genotypic systems and has obscured the fact that one can quite easily be made into the other.

As far as pattern recognition is concerned, Rosenblatt has been able to show that discrimination of shapes in an environment can always be carried out by the analysis of the statistical distributions of impulses arriving from suitably connected S-units. The whole picture built up is a great deal more complicated than this. The great value of Rosenblatt's work, however, stems from the fact that it supplies a means of transition from well-defined (monotypic) logical nets of the kind that can be drawn from such models as those of Uttley and Culbertson to the more statistical theories of Shimbel, Rapoport and others.

The classifying system with conditional probabilities, which is the Uttley model, differs from Rosenblatt's perceptrons, in that it is deterministic and classifies precisely as a basis for learning. Rosenblatt's system is, on the other hand, learning to classify, and does so on the basis of a statistical analysis of the input data.

This statistical analysis depends on the connectivity from S-units to A-units and the reinforcing procedure, which in the course of time can bring about the discrimination between different shapes. We shall next look briefly at Culbertson's model.

Culbertson's model

Culbertson (1950) was concerned with the way in which our visual patterns are recognized. He compiled a 'retina' from many layers of neurons—or logical nets—which, in effect, had the properties such that any figure projected on to the retina was processed by taking it through all transformations necessary to provide a comparison with a set of templates or standard set of available figures.

It is easy to see from the following logical net diagrams how a figure may undergo all sorts of transformations which allow it to be tested in all possible positions.

The first transformation is simply a linear one, and this may include dilation or expansion (see Figs. 61, 62 and 63). The next transformation is by rotation and this is shown in Fig. 64.

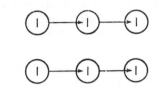

FIG. 61. SIMPLE LINEAR TRANSLATION.

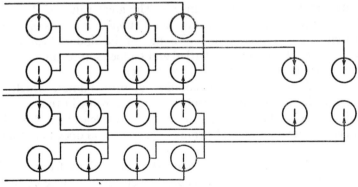

FIG. 62. DILATION FROM FOUR SETS of four elements onto one set of four elements.

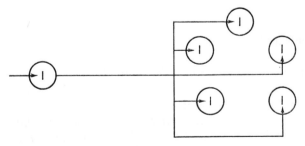

FIG. 63. EXPANSION FROM ONE TO FIVE ELEMENTS.

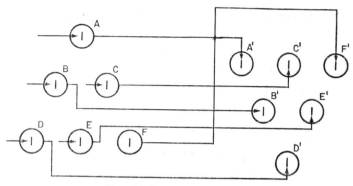

FIG. 64. SIMPLE ROTATION.

So the process continues, so that if a figure is, for example, a triangle, then sooner or later, under transformation, it will appear in a particular standard position and be recognized as such. This is the essence of a 'template' theory of perception, whereby a figure is compared with a standard kept in the memory store, and thus identified by direct comparison.

Banerji's model

Banerji (1964, 1968) has developed a language (BL) as being suitable for 'pattern recognition'. The basic idea—one we accept and wish to use—is that *concepts* are made up of the conjunction and disjunction of properties. Thus concepts may become extremely complex, and we wish to know whether concepts can be built up by logical operations on classes or properties which, of course, are publicly observable.

The basic operation of BL is that given an object named by the metalinguistic variable X is a metalanguage M, and a property A, we write $A(X)$ to mean 'the value of the property A in X'. So,

$$A(X) = B$$

means 'the value of $A(X)$ is B'. To give a concrete example we could say 'the colour of the ball is red'. We use $\cap$, $\cup$ and $\rightarrow$ from the Propositional Calculus (alternative symbols to ., V and $\supset$) to carry out the process of generating such concepts.

For two properties conjoined we can write

$$(A(X) = B) \cap (C(X) = D)$$

or, to take a particular example,

$$(\text{colour } (X) = \text{Red}) \cap (\text{Resilience } (X) = \text{Bouncy}).$$

So a ball may be regarded as a whole set of properties conjoined. BL now uses quantities such as:

$$(Ax) F(x)$$

which means, as usual, the universal quantifier: 'x is a variable whose range is a certain set, a value of x is an element of the range of x, while F is a one-place predicate, such that $(Ax) F(x)$ means that the value of x has the property F; this is asserted for the whole range of x.' So:

$$(Ax) (F(x) = C(x)).$$

We now write statements of the form

$$\text{IN } C = B$$

where C is the name for the concept C, IN is the object language equivalent to X, while $\cap$ and $=$ are the usual connectives of the propositional calculus. BL divides the language used into levels. The object language is the calculus itself, while a metalanguage describes the object language. We are using English as a meta-metalanguage to describe the metalanguage.

In BL is developed a formalism which we shall not describe here in detail. It is a convenient means of description for the making of inductive inferences and acts as a basis for naming. Let us give one of Banerji's simplest examples: Using a ternary number system, he defines a digit as follows:

$$\text{IN digit } (value \text{ (IN)} = 0) \, v$$

$$(value \text{ (IN)} = 1) \, v(value \text{ (IN)} = 2)$$

where *value* is the mapping of *terms* (such as a variable) to objects and *symbols* (a string of lower-case Latin letters and numbers).

It should be made clear that Banerji is trying to supply a formalism *for the internal representation of external states.* Let us quote him directly:

While other attempts at flexible information processing language have generally attempted facile man-machine communication in English, we have restricted ourselves to strengthening the internal representation alone: the problem of translating from English to internal representation (the semantics) has been left out as a separate problem.

Banerji also makes the point that such descriptions of concepts and languages for pattern recognition can become impossibly large.

We should say here that one of the main points of a *definition* is to reduce the enormous size of an internal description. This occurs in much the same way as in ordinary linguistic definition, so that we can refer to a man in general or to Mr. Smith in particular, and do not attempt to prescribe man in terms of his almost infinite number of defining properties. This recoding procedure, or definitions as we call them in more familiar terms, must be used in any language to make that language economic to handle. Furthermore, we do not attempt exhaustive definition, but refer to as many properties as are necessary to distinguish one class from another in a particular context, and for a particular purpose.

Banerji draws a firm distinction between the internal representation of concepts and percepts and the communication of those concepts and percepts and this is totally analogous to the use of symbolic logic for internal representation and natural language, such as English, for communication between people. Therefore one of the most important steps involved in brain-like processes must be the translation to (both ways) and from symbolic language form to natural language form.

We have in quoting Banerji's model for pattern recognition moved somewhat from the perceptual to the conceptual and in doing so are in some measure anticipating some of the thinking which will be discussed in the next chapter. We shall leave the matter at this point and merely describe what seems to be a reasonable general model of perception.

A model for perception

We will take the retinal model first. This will obviously be mirrored by an array of elements in duplicate, both mapped onto the inside of a roughly spherical shell. For practical purposes, and to clarify the argument, we can think of it initially as a single array that may be set out in any plane whatever. The particular shape and its duplication we shall at first regard as incidental to the major properties we shall be interested in mirroring, although clearly this will have the effect of temporarily eliminating matters dependent upon binocular vision.

In this single array we may label the elements as the elements of a square matrix, and we will make some tentative suggestions as to what properties such a matrix must have to carry out such functions as shape recognition, colour vision, and various other visual functions that are, at least partly, determined by the retina.

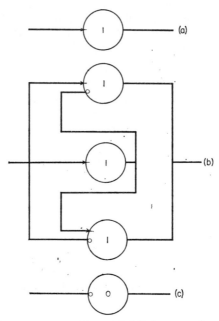

FIG. 65. VISUAL NETWORK ELEMENTS. (a) shows an element that fires when stimulated, (b) a network (three elements) that fires when the input is fired and not after and when it stops firing (on–off element), and (c) an element that does not fire when it is stimulated (off element).

Figure 65 shows a sample of some of the elements that the retina might contain. Figure 65 (a) shows an element which fires steadily all the time it is stimulated. Figure 65 (b) shows an on–off element that fires with a change of stimulation, either as firing stops or as firing starts. Figure 65 (c) represents an element that does not fire whenever it is being stimulated.

Cells which fire only at the outset or cessation of stimulation may be said to be a special case of the on–off element; they will be called 'on' and 'off' elements. The type of Fig. 65 (a) will also be called 'on' elements. Let us assume, to begin with, that these elements are randomly and densely packed all over a square array. The outputs from these elements will be assumed to run across the surface of the array and funnel through one point called the 'blind spot'. It should be borne in mind that the use of words like 'blind spot' is intended to remind us of the functional analogy with the human retina, without necessarily committing us to the statement that it is in any sense exactly the same. On–off elements and the like may be capable of being mirrored in many different ways, and we are not intending, at this stage, to be committed to biological verisimilitude.

Let us now suppose that the fibres that are led away through the blind spot are connected to a classification system, and we will also suppose for the moment that every fibre from every retinal element is connected to the storage system directly and called by its retinal name. A *retinal name* is used here merely for *our own* naming purposes, and for retinal names we shall use, as before, the letters $A, B, \ldots, N$, and combinations of these letters.

If we now place a figure, such as a solid triangle, against the retina so that its projected shape fires those cells that lie inside its boundaries and not those that lie outside, then a certain set of retinal on-elements will be fired and its complementary set will remain unfired. The off-elements will not fire (be inhibited) inside the triangle, but the on–off will, of course, have fired.

Suppose now that the set fired is recorded in a storage system that is attached to the classification system. Here, each output from the classification system has a storage set so that it is fired, and stores the information each time a set of pulses is received, as well as giving off responses. The particular set fired we shall call the 'triangle' set; if fired again it might be said to produce the identical response with the one originally elicited; but by the nature of the connections in the storage system it will be seen that the whole of the triangle set will not subsequently need to fire on every occasion for the same response to be elicited as was originally elicited.

At this point we will temporarily change our description of the operation to a simple set-theoretic description, since this is what is implicit in our classification and storage system. This means that any subset of the total triangle may be able to elicit the triangle response. What will in fact decide this matter will be the extent to which subsets in the past, assumed to be samples of the triangle subset, have been responded to 'without mishap'.

This last point requires some elucidation. If our recognition is to be *effective* it must be able to tell us whether a particular subset is a sample of a certain larger set or not. If, according to a probability measure, it is 'said to be' a sample of some particular set, then confirmation of this can be achieved through the prolonged sampling of the sets in the visual field, or by acting on the assumption of correct identification, and then observing the subsequent outcome of the whole context of some piece of behaviour to discover whether or not there is any discrepancy. Naturally, such a probabilistic system will be liable to error. But more of this later.

We must now look again at the retina itself and discover its limitations. The first and most obvious is that if we project on to the retina another triangle which is slightly larger or smaller than the one already 'learned', it may fire no element in common with the first set; we may therefore ask why there should be any similarity between the first set and the second.

To answer this objection we can introduce the notion of *scanning*. To make the new triangle elicit many of the same responses at the level of the subsets, we must arrange that the contours of the figure which is presented to the retina are scanned, and to do this we must effect a gradient across the face of the retina such that the retinal centre (or central area) will move along the contour lines. This means, of course, that already we have destroyed the random nature of our retina.

Before discussing how this might be achieved we should mention that, to conform with the facts of eye movements, there must be a certain oscillation of the eye around whatever line is being fixated. This is in keeping with the results of experiments on the fixated eye, and has the effect of keeping the on–off elements on the contour lines firing steadily, and so transferring a total outline of the figure to the classification system. But this, of course, is insufficient to elicit the same subset of responses from the classification system, and it is here that we must add the condition of scanning; indeed we might guess that the fact of eye movements is a direct result of the scanning operation of the eyes. Even in the fixated eye it is supposed that scanning cannot be wholly suppressed, and it appears to show slow 'damping' properties.

At any instant that the retina is stimulated by the presentation of a figure, there will be a localized centring response that moves the figure towards the point of maximum excitation. Should it happen at any instant that there are a number of equi-excited points at equi-distance from the centre of the retina, then those eye movements which occur even in the resting state, partly through slow 'damping', will immediately bring one point into the maximum place and so cause movements along the contour lines to this local maximum. As the maximum is reached, so the feed-back effect is diminished to a minimum, thus causing the next point to become a maximum. This is simply because the feedback causing the movement increases with distance from the retinal centre, as well as with intensity of stimulation. This means that the scanning of a figure will proceed indefinitely unless or until the tendency to scan can be removed by the storage which suppresses the scanning operation, although the suppression is never so complete that no incipient scanning movements in the form of eye movements are observable. The question of this storage control must be left for the time being.

Figure 66 illustrates the point of the feedback which leads to scanning. The effect of centring and scanning need not be achieved exactly as we have described it, since there are many ways in which such a mechanism could effect a scan of a field with differing potentials, and such that a

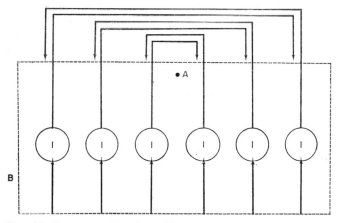

Fig. 66. CORRECTOR. The figure illustrates the very simple principle involved in making correcting movements with respect to a stimulated point.

point of maximum becomes diminished as it travels across a graded scanner, setting up new maxima and thus producing further movement. What is important at this level of cybernetic analysis is that we can see how to construct a system in electronic form that would have this sort of ability.

Two important points should be noted in passing; firstly the gradient across the retina may divide into two parts, the part that brings the figure on to the central area of the retina, where in fact the sense of movement gives way to sense of detail, and the movement that still remains on that retinal area sensitive to detail but which now is necessary to the actual scanning operation. It is not being suggested here that two separate mechanisms are necessary for this, though there is some biological evidence that this is so. The evidence is, crudely, that peripheral photoreceptors have more many–one connections (perhaps a measure of feedback strength for centring) with their bipolar cells than do the more central photoreceptors; yet eye movements will still occur when the whole figure is within the virtually rod-free area. This is clearly a matter that can only be decided by further experiment.

Our second point is that classification and storage are not necessarily effected in a single stage. It seems indeed likely that classification proceeds by stages in a hierarchical fashion, with the first stages being retinal and the final stages being cortical.

This last point is closely concerned with another important fact. It is being suggested that the visual (and other sensory) systems are primarily set-theoretic in their mode of operation. This implies that a particular *concept*, such as a *corner* or *line*, or a figure like a *triangle*, must involve the sequential firing of closely related subsets of elements. If this is so, then the nature of the classification system—in however many stages it may occur—will use an astronomical number of elements, since it must take account of every possible figure as well as every actual figure. This suggests that we should also be able to show a method for self-classification.

A system that has the necessary properties of self-classification has in fact been designed (Chapman, 1959). It is simply a system that constructs its connections as those connections are needed, or, more properly, as a function of the times that they have fired together, the actual firing of the subsets increasing their probability of firing in the future. Chapman's system will become relatively stable when the majority of the environ-

ment has become familiar, and his model should be regarded as representing the growth of the classification process with learning.

While Chapman's system in no way precludes the possibility of some
fixed connections being built in—genetically, or through a process of
maturation—it does not require that the classification system be fully
connected. From a logical point of view, Chapman's model is illustrated
by Fig. 26 (Chapter 5) where it is necessary to have some storage registers available to increase and decrease the sensitivity of connections
as a result of their frequency of use. In the logical net system, however,
it is necessary to have all the connections initially made before the sensitivity can be changed, and this may be neurophysiologically undesirable.

This whole question of appropriateness of description is bound up
with the concept of *growth*. Chapman's 'growth nets' have advantages
which suggest that their potentialities should be given detailed investigation. This is itself bound up with the present trend in cybernetics,
which is towards the manufacture of models using chemical and chemical-colloidal fabrics. A chemical self-classifying system is one that is
envisaged, and it is hoped to build such a system in the near future.

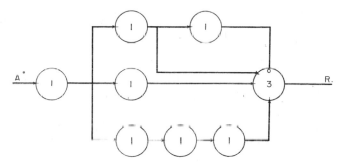

FIG. 67. CODED INPUT. A logical net which fires if and only if it receives
an input of the form 101, where 101 is an ordered event of length three
involving firing, non-firing and firing of *A* in that essential order.

Figure 67 shows a logical net that will clearly fire a specific pulse code
down the optic nerve where, we shall be tempted to say, the code represents a specific characteristic, such as colour. This, of course, sheds
very little light on the biochemical states of the retina which produce the
different codes, but something of value may come of such an analysis
even here, since we can construct two, three, or more basic sets such

that their mixture, coming from two or three different types of 'colour' element spread throughout the retina will produce a coded input at area 17 that represents the various spectral colours. It is easy to see how the process might be carried through, and this immediately suggests a certain range of experiments (see a similar method outlined in Landahl, 1952).

What is the distribution of the colour elements on the retina such as to be able to reproduce the Bezolde–Brucke phenomenon, or the Purkinje phenomenon, both of which are changes in the hue of spectral colours with a change in the level of illumination? The Purkinje phenomenon in particular shows that, as light increases from zero, the blues appear first and the reds last. These various effects have been observed with colours on the human eye (Granit, 1947, 1955; Wilmer, 1946). Here, if anywhere, our analytical device shows through clearly, since we shall certainly want to substitute a more analog, ultimately chemical, model for the logical net model of the retina.

There are obviously a vast number of questions that we should now start to ask of our model, especially on the lines of: can it do this, or that? We should expect it to be able to produce effects already observed, or now capable of being observed, in the human eye, but it is necessary now to bear in mind the nature of the storage and the nature of motivation. We must also just mention the matter of dimensions.

Suppose the optic nerve contains about one million fibres (Stewart, 1959), and they act in the binary fashion we have assumed, then a complete classification system of the form shown in Fig. 26 (Chapter 5) would call for $2^{1,000,000}$ elements, which is clearly ridiculous. Actual estimates have suggested 10^{12} as something like an upper bound for the whole of the central nervous system, so we can immediately see the need for incomplete classification, whether or not that classification is self-selecting.

Jacobsen (1951) has estimated that the optic nerve would have to be fifteen times larger for the nerve fibres to be used as inefficiently as they are in the ear. This is again an economy in the nervous system, achieved by incomplete classification. This whole problem of redundancy and economy in nervous organization is one that will repay the most careful study in the future (Barlow, 1959); it is of course essential in bringing our conceptual models into line with the biological facts.

Our present problem about the nature of the storage system is simply as to whether we should postulate many different types of store, or not.

Certainly it is tempting to suggest that the storage arrangement of Fig. 26 (Chapter 5) refers to the learning process, and that the information so learned is then moved on to some more permanent store; but while this can be shown to be possible with a logical net system, it offends our need for economy in the brain model. At the same time we do envisage the classifying and storage system occurring in stages, so that visual classification may itself occur at various levels and, at the highest level, information will be stored and associated from the visual, auditory, and indeed all the special senses, as well as from the internal organs.

The above storage system has of necessity the property of working on the basis of weighted frequencies, so that where the number of occurrences are less than the number of available storage elements, the response is a function of a Laplacian probability. If the alternative state holds, then the probability is weighted for recency. When we add the motivational system to the storage, we immediately add the differentiation factor of 'value' into the building up of the storage. If we wish to separate 'value' from the probability of occurrences, we can do so by keeping a duplicate set of storage elements; but this, in general, and in the interests of neuro-economy, will hardly be plausible.

Since it is not our primary interest here to discuss storage systems in logical net models, we shall cut short this particular discussion. They have been mentioned only in so far as they are clearly bound up with vision.

Before we leave the matter altogether we must mention again the problem of language. This is only just beginning to be studied, and it will obviously prove extremely complicated since it should go some way to focus on the overlapping interests of logicians, semanticist, philosophers and psychologists, as well as biologists.

All that can be said here is that a system of labelling can be associated with objects perceived, actions made by the automaton itself, and relations between the two. This association can be achieved by an automaton in exactly the same way as we have already described for learning shapes. The problem is largely bound up with the gradual reconstruction of human language with respect to human environment, such that a whole syntax can eventually be reconstructed. For our purpose here it is important to note two very crucial facts. Language, while apparently involving an astronomically high number of elements, will also have the effect of allowing the automaton to use linguistic generalizations as a succinct store of information. This implies that in the human brain there must be the possibility of operating by an overriding control of ordinary associations as a result of language. This could be taken as an argument for a separate store for linguistic generalizations, as distinct from the storage system so far discussed, and to some extent this must be so. It seems likely, indeed, that this extra storage works with information from the storage elements already referred to, so that conceptual operations can be performed. These operations will include deductive and inductive inferences, and will also include what we call 'imagination', since it will be possible to initiate firing of the storage elements from inside the store, and not just by sensory control alone.

This matter of language is almost certainly directly connected with vision in the human being, since the words (concepts) such as 'line', 'corner', 'curvature' and so on, will all arise as a result of associating words with particular sensory experiences. It can be seen from this that certain familiar figures will immediately produce the response of naming, and certain words such as 'corner', 'line', etc., will be aroused in the storage, and a small sample may be enough for the response 'triangle', or 'square', on an almost instantaneous sample of the environment. This is in accordance with suggestions about the perception and recognition of shapes, and the learning of this perceptual process, which goes back to the work of Hebb (1949).

We shall now return to some of those problems of the visual system that might be regarded as relatively independent of the central organization, bearing in mind that we have already had occasion to realize that many of the visual acts we perform are so completely bound up with the brain-as-a-whole that they cannot be studied adequately in isolation.

Let us then briefly consider some of the functional details of our model of the visual system so far suggested in outline. It must be emphasized that the purpose here is not to try to give great detail—since our main purpose is methodological—but merely to say enough to allow the reader to see how the process might be continued.

We will first consider what is known as the 'figural after-effect', which we described at the beginning of this chapter. This has been explained by Osgood and Heyer (1952), using the model of the visual system suggested by Marshall and Talbot (1942), by reference to an excitation that was set up along a double contour line that brought about a wedge of excitation in area 17. The wedge of excitation was an approximate integration of separate excitations whose maximum was assumed to represent the line 'actually seen' by the individual. The superposition of a second line, after 2 minutes' fixation of a point near to the first line, caused the second line to be displaced to a position further away from the fixation point. This was thought to be the result of the relative 'fatiguing' of the cells, caused by continued firing in the period of fixation, leaving the second line falling on an area which is below the resting state of excitation of the rest of the retina. The two curves of excitation are superimposed, and the maximum is simply moved away from the position it would otherwise have taken up.

In our own retinal model of the last section, exactly this state of affairs pertains, although not designed for. After the initial excitation there is a decrement in the excitation curve due to the falling off of the on-element's firing, except at the edges of the line. This conforms with the assumption we made in discussing scanning, when we said that the points of maxima died away on being reached, leaving another maximum for the eye to move on to. The eye, being fixated by central control alone, still shows limited movement, and the excitation for the equivalent part of the visual cortex must fall below that of the surrounding retinal elements; cortical representation and the figural after-effects could be accounted for exactly as in the Osgood and Heyer model. The reason for the fall of excitation with fixation could most easily be accounted for by saying that at the central retinal point the off-elements are in excess of the on-elements, and when the on–off fall below a critical level, the state of excitation becomes less at this *focal* point than in the surrounding areas. This could also be accounted for in a variety of other ways, one of which is mentioned below.

It need hardly be said that this is by no means the only way in which the scanning operation can be made effective, and the biological plausibility of the explanation should now be seriously considered. The off-effect has been regarded by Granit (1947) as a release from inhibition, which suggests that the off-elements are elements that fire in the resting state and therefore, with an area that is stimulated, the off-fibres might be regarded as being inhibited.

This problem of the diminution of excitation with a fixated eye accounts, on the Marshall–Talbot hypothesis, for figural after-effects, and requires further consideration. It is something that seems to be quite necessary to an explanation of the functioning of the eye, and perhaps represents the same physiological fact that is called 'fatigue'. This could, of course, be accounted for by considering a decrement in the on-elements, where more and more of the cells cease to fire with increasing stimulation. A logical net can easily be drawn to represent this state of affairs.

The points so far mentioned also link up with evidence on the formation of contours in the visual system. The Werner effect is shown in a simple experiment where a black disc is presented on a white background, quickly followed by a black ring whose inner radius is exactly the same as the radius of the disc. This causes loss of ability to see the disc if the ring is presented sufficiently quickly after the disc. The Werner effect is thought to obtain because the contour of the disc is not formed before the same contour is used in the ring, and so the black disc is suppressed altogether. This fact is certainly one that would occur in our model, provided it is arranged that the horizontal cells of the retina are functionally interdependent in their connections with the on–off elements on the periphery of a figure, and this again can easily be arranged.

The degree of stimulation, of course, can be achieved by frequency of firing, as well as by the number of elements that fire, and both will be expected to occur in our model.

In this same connection one might seek to explain the α-rhythm by appeal to the synchronous firing of the off-elements, or at least some of them. We should here seek to relate the characteristic waves with the observed frequency and amplitude of the cells themselves. In much the same way we would try to replace the coded elements suggested in Fig. 67 for colour vision by codings that represent a direct function of the frequency and amplitude of the primary colour waves.

In a similar way we may expect to find an explanation of contrast effect. With two adjacent black and white patches there will be a maximum difference in excitation, since in any case all the on-elements will fire, and immediately next to this will be an area with a minimum number (zero) of on-elements firing. The change here from a maximum to a minimum will thus be maximal. This effect could clearly operate in the same way for complementary colours, and it should be possible to work out a code that shows precisely the necessary relations between neighbouring areas to achieve this end. The contrast effect will be further emphasized by the horizontal cells which fire elements in the surrounding black areas, and not all in the white areas, as we have already suggested above.

So much for the present outline of Cybernetics and perception; some more general suggestions will be made about these matters in the next chapter.

Summary

This chapter has tried to give a brief integrated account of perception, taking into account the physiological and philosophical evidence, as well as the experimental psychological evidence.

There is some repetition of our earlier discussion, in Chapter 5, of the methods of classification and of the perceptual models based on classification.

Uttley, Deutsch, Selfridge, Culbertson, Rapoport, McCulloch, Pitts, and others have formulated models for perception which we have briefly considered, and a new model is suggested that incorporates some of the characteristics of these other models, as well as the model of the visual system due to Osgood and Heyer.

A little general discussion has also taken place with respect to the well-known psychological evidence on perception. The evidence we take to be well known includes constancy, after-effects and after-images, perception of space and, of course, the perception of forms which is so essential to recognition. It is to be remembered that, while it is truly necessary to show how recognition can occur under conditions of minimal cues, it can also, and does normally, occur under conditions permitting of a vast redundancy of information from many different sensory sources.

This chapter is directly continued in the next one, which continues to deal with the perceptual problem.

CHAPTER 12

PATTERN RECOGNITION

THIS may be an appropriate moment to summarize some of the advantages and benefits that cybernetics has to offer in the analysis of perceptual and cognitive problems.

In the first place we are, of course, to understand 'cybernetics' as implying effective methods, and not merely as the construction of hardware models or the programming of computers. This means that much of experimental psychology can already be thought to be included in the field of cybernetics. In a narrower view, however, we may expect to find value coming from the simulation of all aspects of the nervous system and human behaviour.

In particular, we need more computer programs to illustrate learning, which is directly connected with the organization of the storage system, and this eventually includes recognition, recall, and every aspect of cognition including perception, and, above all, pattern recognition.

The primary problem for the future of cognition, and one which has been much neglected so far, is that of language; and language is also capable of analysis by computer methods, and also involves pattern recognition.

At the same time as we need to simulate by digital and analog computers, we also need to build models of different parts of the nervous system. These models may be at various levels of generality; some need to simulate its electrical activity, some its chemical activity, some the relations between neurons, and so on. While we can hope to simulate much of the structure and organization of human behaviour, we also need to do the same thing for other organisms. We also need to build models that modify their own structure, or grow and change, as well as the models that are prewired and only change functionally.

Finally, we need to build our models of every kind of fabric, from electronic and other physical systems to chemical and chemical-colloidal ones.

This is the search, and it carries a promise of which experimental psychologists have only recently become aware.

We shall now return to a reconsideration of some of the problems of perception and cognition, with an eye to making the conceptual models, so far discussed, more nearly meet the experimental facts of human behaviour.

We have called this chapter pattern recognition, as a reminder that this is a central theme running throughout cybernetics. In a sense it is unfair to sort out one particular chapter and call it pattern recognition and thereby run the risk of implying that the rest has been concerned with something other than pattern recognition, because this is not so. The words 'pattern recognition' have often been understood in two different senses. One is sensory pattern recognition and this particularly has been applied to the visual sense, and conceptual pattern recognition which applies to all learning, problem solving and thinking as well as even language. This particular chapter is primarily concerned with models of a visual system although the principles involved refer to other sensory systems in some measure and to some extent refer to central cognitive activity. The earlier chapter on problem solving (Chapter 7) was also concerned with pattern recognition but quite specifically of a central kind, and Chapter 8, since it also dealt with learning and adaptive behaviour even though in the form of computer programs, was also concerned with pattern recognition. The earlier chapters on automata theory and games theory was necessarily concerned with pattern recognition in the sense that what we were trying to construct were pattern recognizers and only the chapters on the nervous system (Chapters 9 and 10) were not primarily addressed at the problem of pattern recognition but again were addressed at the type of systems which are capable of achieving this end. It is important to be absolutely clear that this is the central theme of the whole of cybernetics and must be the central theme of the whole of cognition, and in this chapter we are taking a slightly limited view of it and although we are paying some attention to the central issues much of the discussion will be about what are sometimes called perceptual models.

Perceptual models

The particular outline of perceptual models and the eventual set of suggestions made in the last chapter, suffer from many doubts and possible defects. Two of the most prominent ones surround the question of eye movements, and the necessity for a scanning operation as a preliminary to recognition.

Let us first consider the problem of eye movements. Work by Riggs *et al.* (1953) lends credence to the claim that figural after-effects of various kinds do not depend upon eye movements and this was suggested as a result of using contact lenses, which allowed the figures perceived to move with the movements of the eyes.

While it is not certain that by such means all relative eye movement is eliminated, it is certainly minimized. Bearing in mind Deutsch's (1956) objection to the Osgood–Heyer model for figural after-effects, we might feel that the attempts to model either these or other related perceptual phenomena are on the wrong track.

Deutsch's argument is simply that eye movements are not essential to the figural after-effect, and that the Osgood–Heyer model depends on an interaction of the normally distributed excitations in the visual cortex. But, he argues, if such excitations can summate over such a wide visual angle, how are two lines normally discriminated, as they are known to be, in terms of a much narrower retinal angle?

The problems so posed can be 'solved' or 'resolved' in a number of ways, none of which is immediately and *completely* testable. In the first place, if eye movements are *not necessary* to these after-effects, then the distribution of excitation of a single stimulus line (double contour line) will tend to be very narrow indeed, and thus, apparently, greatly reducing this possibility of summatory effects. Indeed, we know that no effect will occur *unless* a further condition is introduced, namely, that the inspection figure must be mapped on to the retina for some period of not less than 1 minute, and preferably 2 minutes. The implication is that the spread of excitation which is necessary to the summatory effect is derived only under conditions of steady stimulation. George (1962) has carried out an experiment which is aimed at settling this point, and the results are, to say the least, encouraging. By taking two vertical lines at varying distances apart, and at varying distances from a fixation point, it was found that, after steady fixation for one minute, the ability to discriminate between the two lines had entirely vanished; at least, many subjects—significantly many subjects— claimed that this was so. This appears to justify the argument that, with spread of excitation under 'fatiguing' conditions, summation will occur and discrimination will be lost.

There are other theoretical suggestions that could be made to overcome the Deutsch objection, but in view of the apparent success of the first tentative suggestion, the matter need be pursued no further. The only weak link in the logical chain is that, under the ordinary conditions of figural after-effect, eye movements certainly do occur, and the spread of excitation that seems to occur with fatigue has not been shown to occur independently of eye movement. This will not greatly concern us now, though, since the occurrence of a summatory spread of effect certainly seems to take place normally, and it is rather too much to ask us to believe that it will not also occur in the eye when all movement is eliminated *if* figural after-effects still occur. The doubt is as to whether all eye movements are really eliminated, or whether the spread of effect occurs anyway. The two points are by no means mutually exclusive, but the second seems to be true in any case.

Now let us look for a moment at the scanning operation of the eye. This is one way in which similar figures in different retinal locations could be brought into positions of comparison. If this is to be ruled out by the elimination of eye movements or scanning movements, even *during* learning, then we will have to use some other indicator of retinal position, such as one conveyed by temporal coding (Deutsch, 1955; Dodwell, 1957). There are some difficulties with this idea as we have already remarked, and the Culbertson model achieves its coding by having the equivalent of retinal scanning more centrally placed. It seems that either method could be effective, and further evidence casts some doubt on the idea of scanning that we have suggested, and that was previously suggested by Hebb (1949).

This might be said to be one major point which can only be settled by further experiment, since there is plenty of evidence that, from the purely conceptual point of view, any of these models might suffice. An alternative that, as far as the writer is aware, has not been taken very far, is that the retina, as a classifying system, might simply represent the relations between sets of points, so that the stores may indeed receive subsets that have no element in common, and yet use the same word—such as 'triangle' or 'circle'—to describe them, because they bear certain characteristic and similar relations to each other.

The principle suggested is exactly that by which we represent different families of curves in Cartesian coordinates, so that anything of the form $ax+by+c = 0$ represents a straight line, three such lines represent a triangle, a form such as $x^2+y^2 = a^2$ would represent a circle, and so on.

It is not being suggested that the nervous system converts geometrical patterns into sequential patterns exactly in the Cartesian, or even the projective manner; but some such a principle would overcome the need for postulating scanning eye movements as necessary to recognition during the learning period.

It is not intended that this matter should be pursued further here, for this would need exploratory construction of new models, combined with new research on the physiology of the visual system, while this book is endeavouring only to summarize what has been done to date.

As far as this particular problem is concerned, we cannot rule out the more central theories which might account for the effects to which we refer as 'movement after-effects' and 'figural after-effects'. As an instance, there is something to be said for regarding the *set* to move the eyes—which indeed might not actually need the eye movement itself, although generally it would be accompanied by it—as setting up a central storage state such that, when the movement is stopped, the actual physical stimuli will make relative movements in the opposite direction. To put the matter crudely, this means that if the movement was to the left, the lines will be discovered persistently to the right of the anticipated position. Wohlgemuth (1911) has demonstrated many of the properties of the movement after-effects, but little has been suggested by way of explanation. One approach may be to try to develop the Osgood–Heyer theory, and we shall do this shortly. Another way is to assume that the Osgood–Heyer effects are negligible, and that the matter should be centrally explained.

This last question naturally suggests that we should look at figural after-effects from the same point of view. Could figural after-effects be explained more plausibly in a central manner? Although we cannot discuss the matter in detail here, it is essential that we look again at the basic process by which contours are formed in the visual cortex. The results of Werner (1940) and Fry and Bartley (1935) make it clear that there is an intimate relation between contour formation and perception of brightness of surfaces. It is also known from the work of the Transactionalists that brightness and size are interdependent, and there is the possibility that the figural after-effects represent the work of central interpretation, where a figure becomes distorted as a result of the subject seeing the test and inspection figures together as a meaningful whole, even though they do not overlap.

One piece of evidence that bears on this last suggestion seems to imply the opposite (George, 1953c), for when the test and inspection figures were actually superimposed for a particular case, the result was the opposite to what our suggestions above would lead one to expect. However, this case is not really a parallel, since we are not suggesting that they should appear as one pattern, but rather that the effect of the inspection figure is to present a certain space, and that when the test figure is presented, the test figure is distorted accordingly.

A real possibility is that when an inspection figure of two unequal squares, say, on either side of a fixation point is seen, they are seen as three-dimensional, and therefore the one which is smaller distorts the

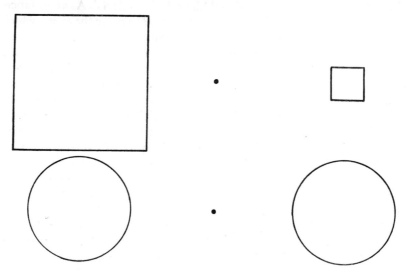

FIG. 68. FIGURAL AFTER-EFFECT. If the eye fixates the dot half way between the two squares at a distance of about eighteen inches and then after about 30 seconds is transferred to the dot immediately below, the left-hand circle can be seen to be smaller than the right-hand one.

spatial framework (as centrally interpreted) and this would naturally result in the equal circles, say, of the test-figure being seen as unequal. The difficulty, here, is that this same figural after-effect can be derived with other figures that do not readily lend themselves to interpretation in three-dimensional terms.

A more sinister thought of course is that it is both the Osgood–Heyer effect and the interpretative effect occurring together that causes the many after-effects. But we shall not pursue that possibility any further.

Perception of movement, as we know from work on actual and apparent movement, depends upon sequential contour formation, but the fact that apparent movement occurs reminds us that the actual discrimination between contours is a function of successive stimulation.

When we have solved the problem of visual perception to the extent of providing a model of discrimination of brightness, constancy, etc., we can tackle the problems presented by clinical psychologists (Zangwill *et al.*). In the meantime their findings—such as that destruction of parts of the optic radiations seem to destroy constancy, perhaps by way of brightness discrimination, which was also destroyed—are valuable as contributing to our present model, and a reminder that all these things are closely interdependent.

Movement after-effects

Let us now explicitly address ourselves to the problem of movement after-effects. The problem is as to whether the Osgood–Heyer model is sufficient to account for these effects as well as for the figural after-effects. It should be noticed that Osgood himself (1953) has applied the model to the case of apparent movement. He suggested that two contour lines interact when their peaks are mutually shifted. Indeed, the same sort of explanation could be used to explain movement itself, although presumably it would only be necessary to do so in the case of the fixated eye. Either way, the idea is that the two excitation distributions interact in such a way as to produce a single moving peak in apparent movement, while in actual movement the peak is already an integrated one from a single source, or if a series of lines, from a series of sources.

In the case of apparent movement, the problem of the Osgood–Heyer model is again simply to explain how summation takes place here, and not when two lines are discriminated. The answer in the fixed case of the figural after-effect seems to be, as we have already said, that during the fatiguing operation, which is taking place while the inspection figure is exposed, a broad distribution of reduced excitation occurs and the question now arises as to whether this changes our interpretation of the moving line case.

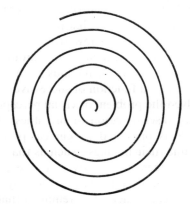

FIG. 69. THE PLATEAU SPIRAL. This figure has been used to produce movement after-effects in the eye (see text).

We can put the matter to a similar test. We know that if a series of lines moves sufficiently quickly across the retina, or rotates quickly enough as, for example, the blades of a fan, then the lines or blades are not separately seen, but an impression of continuity is created. This could be interpreted as the failure to achieve any separate distributions at all, and confirmation that summation is taking place.

But if the lines are moved slowly enough they can be seen individually, which shows, on the theory, that summation is not taking place. So far, so good, but we must now try to account for the after-effect. The lines stop, and an impression of movement in the opposite direction occurs. Fatiguing must certainly occur in the retina, since the movement after-effects only occur after a period of inspection, and prior to stopping the movement to derive the effect. If, then, our supposition about the broad spread of fatiguing is correct, we should expect that when the lines are stationary after the inspection period, they set up an excitation that interacts with the fatiguing excitation and creates, at the least, a shift in the opposite direction. This shift in the opposite direction will be maintained in the same way as the figural after-effect, and thus create an apparent movement of much the same kind as Osgood suggests for ordinary apparent movement.

It must be mentioned here that there is a difficulty over such effects as the Plateau spiral, which creates movement after-effects in roughly radial directions away from the centre of the spiral. If, as Osgood and Heyer assume, the excitation distribution depends on eye movements, one is faced with the somewhat perplexing thought that the eye must move in all directions at once. The answer to this can take one of two obvious forms: either eye movements are unnecessary, and a spread of excitation with peaking does not depend upon eye movement, or the spiral effect is derived by sampling the visual environment and generalizing from this sample. This last explanation might be worked into something plausible, but it seems much more likely that eye movements, although they may contribute to the effect, are in practice unnecessary to it, and that the movement after-effect needs only the interacting spreads of excitation. The theory proposed requires that the discrimination between two adjacent lines is greatly reduced again as fatigue sets in during the inspection period, and this seems very likely to be true.

One problem that now arises is an effect that occurs when a wheel with, say, four spokes is rotated fairly rapidly. The effect is that the number of spokes is greatly increased phenomenally. The explanation of this problem probably lies in the fact that in such circumstances there is no way of identifying the individual spokes, which are forming contours at a rate below the level of summation, and at a rate that makes it impossible for the eye to do any sort of count. The effect should be reduced with fatiguing of the eye after lengthy fixation of the centre of the rotating wheel. The method, on the theory here proposed, is to start with a slow rate at which each spoke is visible, and increase the speed through the successive stages of multiplying (and perhaps finally decreasing again) and the integrating.

No more will be said here about these models of the visual system. It is hoped that when further experiments have been carried out it will be possible to give a more integrated account of the perceptual activities. The model in hardware mentioned in the previous chapter will be used to try to build up every aspect of perceptual theory: contrast, movement (apparent and real) and so on; but of course there will be some difficulties in showing that the method used in the hardware model will give the same result as that used in the human eye. It will be noticed, again, that our technique has marked behaviouristic implications.

Other perceptual models

We have so far discussed only general models based on classification, and some specific analysing mechanisms such as that of Osgood and Heyer. There are, of course, many more of both of these types of model that we shall meet and have to examine, and here we must at least make mention of the Perceptron (Rosenblatt, 1958, 1959), the Pandemonium (Selfridge, 1959), and some of the models that have been constructed to deal with problems such as speech perception (Fry and Denes, 1959; Ladefoged, 1959). These are all efforts, mostly similar to those we have analysed, to meet the problem of modelling perceptual systems, and therefore of the greatest interest from the cybernetic viewpoint.

Pattern recognition and central cognition

We have said quite a lot about cognitive problems, with rather particular attention to perception and learning, but so far we have scarcely considered the problem of thinking as such, and the nature of cognitive terms such as 'thinking', 'problem solving', and so on. Cybernetics apart, the last few years have seen a great deal of progress in the process of trying to construct models of cognitive processes, and it might be said that cybernetics has merely lent further emphasis to this particular development.

Most people have tended to accept the Reichenbach (1938) dictum that the context of discovery and the context of justification are quite different from each other. We have taken this to imply a very pronounced difference between the manner in which humans actually think—by taking big jumps, making guesses, etc.—and the manner in which they subsequently justify their intuitions.

We should notice that while learning theorists have themselves paid scant attention to thinking, most experiments on thinking have been built up around human subjects. But from the behaviouristic point of view, thinking is something that we infer from performance, in the same way as we infer learning from performance, and we should perhaps ask about the differences between learning and thinking and even, for that matter, problem solving, which often seems to merit a separate chapter in books on psychology. Again from the behaviouristic point of view, we shall want to say that thinking must apply not only to what we are conscious of doing, it must also include processes of which we are unaware. This means that a solution to a problem, whether arrived at during waking or sleeping, could be said to be the result of thinking; and since we would also want to say that learning, almost always—if not always—involves solving a problem, it can be seen that all these apparently different questions could be collapsed into one.

The Reichenbach distinction, namely (as already mentioned) that the context of *discovery* is wholly distinct from the context of justification, is only obviously true when we refer to thinking as a process of which we are consciously aware, and we cannot say that actual internal changes which proceed towards a solution are anything like so haphazard as the scraps of information we have about our own thinking processes. Bartlett (1958) has pointed out that, in the series of experiments he conducted on human beings, there were fairly systematic changes going on, usually moving towards a solution. Of course the problem may not be solved, but we should not want to say on that account that thinking had not taken place. Just as solutions to situations may not be learned, so thinking, or some internal changes, will go on whether or not they lead to learning, or solve particular problems. This is perhaps the nucleus of a distinction between the various terms.

There have been many studies of thinking (Humphrey, 1951; Bartlett, 1958; Bruner, Goodnow and Austin, 1956) and they have all dwelt on the human being, and on the layout of input information and its importance for the results of problem solving; this, of course, was well known to be a source of Gestalt theory (Kohler, 1925).

It is a question as to whether we should think of thinking as being unified or not, and it is a semantic question, typical of the kind we feel cybernetics can help us to solve. In the first place, as with perception and learning, it was impossible to establish exactly where thinking started and where it finished; indeed, it has seemed to be a matter of convention. Certainly it is clear that there are many different facets to the internal organization of any system that solves problems, since there are different sorts of problems to solve. Some demand a relationship between inputs alone, others between inputs and outputs; some occur in a closed situation, and are mathematical or deductive in part of their form, others require what Bartlett calls 'adventurous thinking' and are more obviously inductive in form, although the differences in the examples he gives are more in terms of the type of problem than in the differences of suggested solutions. The way information has to be put together to form a solution is at least different on the surface in various problem situations, though the differences may be more apparent than real.

Bartlett's definition of thinking is, 'the extension of evidence in accord with that evidence, so as to fill up gaps in the evidence; and this is done by moving through a succession of interconnected steps, which may be stated at the time or left until later to be stated'.

This seems curious at first sight, and Bartlett himself recognizes that it may be a special case; in fact it is a statement which brings out fairly clearly the inductive nature of thinking. His suggestion that thinking is a high-level form of skilled behaviour is most acceptable from the cybernetic viewpoint.

Humphrey (1951) defines thinking, as 'what occurs in experience when an organism, human or animal, meets, recognizes, and solves a problem'. He also points out that the term 'reasoning' may be preferred, and he further admits that there is no hard and fast distinction between learning and thinking. All this is in agreement with our argument.

Bruner *et al.* (1956) impinge upon another aspect of thinking when they talk of categorizing activity and its relation to the making of inferences and to the general field of cognition. Concept formation, or 'concept attainment' as they call it, is discussed at some length, and they are also interested in 'selective strategy', which is concerned with the order in which hypotheses (or beliefs) are tested.

George (1960a) has suggested a simple model for an inference making system in terms of logical nets. It is based precisely on the discussion of finite automata, and therefore involves classification of temporal sequences of events, and the association of such events (or event names) whereby new consequences may be derived by 'conceptual' activity alone. Since then the author has made a number of suggestions for models appropriate to thinking. They are all pattern recognition models and in the main in the form of computer programs (George, 1970).

At this stage the subject of language obviously needs some further discussion. Language is certainly used by human beings in their problem solving activities, but whether it should be said that all thinking either depended directly on language, or was carried out entirely in language, it would be more difficult to decide. Judging from our computer work in Chapter 7, it looks as if the natural and easy way to solve problems is by making, and applying, generalizations derived from some previous circumstances. The learning, of course, goes deeper than this, because the use of signs and symbols has itself to be learned, and after that, further learning may take place within the language so learned. It is conceivable that organisms could think in other than symbols, since the word 'thinking' could be used simply for a type of awareness and association, accompanied perhaps by images, without the occurrence of language, but whether this is so is quite a different problem.

We should perhaps mention that attempts to understand consciousness from a behaviouristic point of view—and therefore from a cybernetic point of view—are not likely to provide more than a rough, heuristic idea of what constitutes consciousness, because this throws us right into the problem called by philosophers 'Other Minds'. We cannot know what it is to be another person, and still less what it is to be a machine. Naturally we experience great difficulty in imagining a machine having consciousness in the human sense, and perhaps the only kind of constructed system that could be thought to have the same sort of consciousness as ourselves is one that is constructed from the same chemical colloidal materials as is the human being. This has really little to do with cybernetics as such, but it is perhaps worth saying here if only to remind us of our behaviouristic commitment.

By the same token, thinking can really only be meaningful in the cybernetic situation when considered as the method by which the automaton proceeds to try and solve problems, learn about the environment, or perhaps freely associate with respect to some stimulus. This point is of some importance. A human being will often say, 'Let me think'; and if he thinks aloud he may say something like, 'I had it on Tuesday... Tuesday I was in London... then I came back on the train...I had it on the train, so I must have lost it when I got back... Now what did I do?... I went to the garage...'. This sort of operation, which seems very common in human beings, appears to be a restimulation of the memory store. It might be described as a chain of stimuli and responses that are elicited by the organism, although they are to some extent tied to the environment. Work on sensory deprivation (Bexton, Heron and Scott, 1954, and others) has shown fairly clearly that this sort of organized self-stimulation cannot be carried on indefinitely when the subject is deprived of sensory stimulation. In any case, it could be said to be an act of memorizing rather than of thinking, which only helps to remind us of the semantic confusion that is liable to cloud the whole subject.

In the case of a finite automaton, we could easily arrange for it to run through its store, taking item after item in some definite order according to its method of storage, and then draw logical inferences as they are needed to some specific end, i.e. to solve some specific problem, for example 'to discover the place where I lost my fountain pen'. We should expect to find the memory store organized on the basis of recency, frequency and value, at the very least, and thus some information would be available and some not.

It is tempting to say that a finite automaton which could perform deduction and induction (by induction we shall mean: able to make generalizations of an empirical kind on the basis of probabilities) can easily assess the credibility of statements as a function of their objective probabilities, coupled with the weighting that certainly seems to occur because of the emotional and motivational systems. Indeed, these systems do seem to have the effect of weighting events in terms of desires and prejudices and so on, which could be characteristics of the counting and other mechanisms that vary with different individual systems, no doubt as a result of their experience, and of whatever built-in characteristics they have. Here we see the relevance of the decision procedures of the theory of games; games will be learned by different people, perhaps often through accidental factors, and certainly as a result of environmental considerations.

The task of constructing a program on a computer which will show the variety demanded in mimicking a human being is certainly a colossal one, and the sheer magnitude of the system might well be considered somewhat daunting. In the meantime, a manner of approach has been adopted which involves showing particular functions, building greatly extended memory storage systems, and making use of autocoding devices, especially of the compiler kind (Minsky, 1959; Backus, 1959).

In the language developed in Chapter 5 as a preliminary to applying program techniques and building finite automata, it would be suitable to describe thinking simply as the utilization of beliefs in any situation whatever. Especially would this apply to the manipulation of existing beliefs to make deductions and inductions—which means to form new beliefs—and the processes involving regurgitation of beliefs when suitably stimulated. This is all part of the activity of what we have called the C-system. We have postulated that this must itself depend on the motivational system, or M-system; but this is really a statement that is analytic rather than one capable of being tested.

It is not for a moment felt that this brief section on thinking does justice in any way to the vast ramifications of human thought; what it might do is to shed some light on the relatively unified nature that thinking takes.

Another cognitive word in frequent use is 'imagination'. The basis of this might be sought in the recombination of previously existing items in the storage system. It is well known that it is impossible to give any knowledge by way of explanation to another person by any means other than by appeals to concepts already familiar to that other person, which suggests that thinking is very much tied to previous experience. Whether the imagination takes the form of referring to events that have happened but have not actually been witnessed, or whether to events that have never happened, the function of the automaton will be the same. It must selectively recreate an event name of some length which is taken to represent the event itself.

This statement is, again, quite inadequate to account for all the ramifications that occur under the names of 'imagination', 'creative thinking', etc., indeed it makes no such attempt, but it says enough perhaps to show how such problems may be quite easily fitted into the scheme of the finite automaton.

The fact of being able to stimulate the sensory storage systems directly, i.e. other than by actual external stimulation, offers an obvious approach to the problem of imagery, since by this means some shadowy picture of the original scene is given to the automaton. The idea is, of course, obvious enough, and it is mentioned only for the sake of some attempt at completeness.

It seems to the writer that the big problem that cybernetics has to solve in the future is that of language. It ought to be possible to teach an automaton a complex language—this can quite easily be done for a computer with a simple language—and the automaton could then be shown, under a variety of different conditions, to recreate the development of, say, the English language, in a manner to which we have already drawn attention. This is a huge undertaking, but it is one in which it should be possible to show that it would be natural to separate events in the environment (nouns) and their properties (adjectives) and the computer's own outputs (verbs).

Eventually a linguistic system could be reconstructed which would be extremely helpful in confirming the correctness or otherwise of our conceptual systems, since quite a lot is known of the quantitative side of linguistics (Osgood, 1953), and this must certainly link up with the other cognitive knowledge we have, as well as with our philosophical knowledge.

One of the principal features that we have to acknowledge is that the names we have come to give to cognitive operations by no means lie in a one–one correspondence with different structures or mechanisms. As a result, one may construct a model and then interpret the model from different points of view with respect to our cognitive terms.

'Perceptual learning' (Drever, 1960) is a term increasingly used in the literature of cognition, and this, like 'discrimination learning', really lays emphasis on the fact that some learning is much more immediately tied to perceptual activities than other learning. This should not in any way make us think of such perceptual learning as a new process; rather it is a familiar process which is to some extent distinctive, because it tends to one end of a continuum of learning (and perceptual activities), for we knew from the start that learning and perception were not wholly separable.

Summary

This chapter has directly continued the discussion of perception started in the previous chapter, although it has concentrated attention mainly upon the Osgood and Heyer model for the visual system, and thought explicitly in terms of pattern recognition. It seems likely that this sort of model, with modifications to be expected as it becomes more frequently tested under new conditions, would be appropriate for the visual system, and that it should be directly attached to a classification system which may be expected to operate in stages, eventually integrating sensory information with information from the other sensory sources.

This summary of perception is followed by a very brief description of some of the other principal features of cognition. Language is necessarily mentioned, as are the obvious cognitive terms such as 'thinking', 'problem-solving', 'imagination', and so on.

It is suggested that, with the integration of perception with learning, the main cognitive problems are solved; but as far as human behaviour is concerned it is language that has failed to receive, so far, sufficient attention from experimental psychologists.

It might even be claimed in a general way that we now understand the type of physiological processes that are necessary to cognition; but even if this were true—and it might be thought to be just plausible—the amount of detail that we still have to work out is tremendous.

CHAPTER 13

ARTIFICIAL INTELLIGENCE

ONE of the central themes of cybernetics is artificial intelligence; it is, in a sense, indeed the fundamental problem of cybernetics, and this is so regardless of whether the aim is *simulation* of human behaviour and the human brain, as much of our book has assumed, or *synthesis*, where it is intelligent activity that is the goal, regardless of whether the methods are humanlike or not.

We shall in this chapter outline some of the basic characteristics of an artificially intelligent system. There is now a considerable body of literature surrounding this subject and this chapter can only serve as a summary of some of its most important features.

There are many possible approaches to artificial intelligence, but in this chapter the emphasis will be on the synthesis and simulation of cognitive processes. It will indeed by especially concerned with the synthesis of cognitive processes, although synthesis and simulation inevitably overlap.

If we were able to manufacture any set of models of cognitive activity which purport to show anything like the 'richness' observed in human behaviour, then we need *at least* to be able to model the following features:

(1) Concepts
(2) Structures
(3) Hypotheses
(4) Language
(5) Logic

(6) Pattern recognition
(7) The representation of problems
(8) Date retrieval
(9) Evidence

Let us briefly consider each in turn.

Concepts

By concept we mean either a *class* or a *property* (this is, itself, a distinction which can be confounded, although here we shall keep the concepts separate). *Green*, *red* or *blue* or *Armenian gentlemen* are all concepts. Such entities are the basic building bricks on which the human intelligence operates, but concepts are not equally basic. A concept such as *Armenian gentlemen* is a multiple concept whereas the concept of *blue* is a singular concept, that is, we can make further discriminations if we want to; concepts can either be simple or complex.

In principle it is possible to manufacture concepts, either *ab initio* or from old concepts. Concepts come from old concepts by the operations of conjunction and disjunction or operations such as replacement and substitution. New concepts may emerge if our domain of observation is increased, although even here our understanding of whatever is conceptually new must relate to something which is already conceptually familiar. There is a clear and obvious relationship between concepts and the labels (words or symbols) which are used to represent those concepts in a field of discourse.

We are not arguing, of course, that the above list represents a *sufficient* set of characteristics to exemplify artificial intelligence, only that they are certainly *necessary*. In fact, the concept is almost the atom of the artificially intelligent system, since upon it we construct all the other features such as hypothesis making, evidence and the like, and generate more complex theoretical structures and languages based on the notion of a concept and a label for that concept which means the word.

We can treat concept learning as a type of discrimination learning, or as do Bruner, Goodnow and Austin (1956) we can think of it in terms of information processing routines. We come somewhere near this view as do Newell, Shaw and Simon (1963) but we prefer to think explicitly of concepts as basic units in the 'meaning' situation where given red (x) and round (y) the statement that an object (s) is both red and round is given by

$$s = x.y \tag{1}$$

and objects which are either blue (z) or red and still round are given by

$$s' = (x \ v \ z).y \tag{2}$$

and so on, where s' is another object and where concepts involve naming and the derivation of inductive hypotheses, such as 'all red or blue long objects are heavy (q)', i.e.

$$h' = (As')(s' \rightarrow q)$$

or

$$h' = (As')\big(((x \; v \; z).y) \rightarrow q\big) \tag{3}$$

where $\rightarrow$ means 'implies' in the ordinary sense of 'if it has property x then it necessarily has property q', not therefore in the sense of ordinary material implication.

The main problem is as to whether concepts can ever be other than a reordering or recombining of existing concepts, or whether by enlarging our sensory experience we can derive new concepts. Even then though they are not apparently explicable, except in terms which are already familiar. This in turn raises the question as to whether or not we can think of certain concepts as basic and others as derived, so that in the above example x and y are basic, but s and s' are derived. If so, then this must refer to our own capacities and the building up of historically given experience and not necessarily something inevitable and typical of all nature. It should be noticed that we are here coming close to the reductionist argument which, for example, 'reduces' all statements of a biological kind to physico-chemical statements. If the forms are sufficiently similar then the question is as to whether (1) could be rewritten with x as the independent variable, in some form such as

$$x = f(s, y)$$

for some function f. The answer to the question though appears to be in the negative and that there is a one-way process involved as far as part-to-whole is concerned.

We shall also take into account Banerji's (1960) work on a language for conceptual analysis which he regards as being quite distinct from a natural language for external communication. Since Banerji's languages are set-theoretic and in symbolic logic form, this is wholly consistent with our view that ordinary language needs to be translated into symbolic logic for internal processing.

Structure

By structure we mean the 'essence of knowledge', and by this we mean the relationships, including the orderings, that exist (1) between concepts and themselves and (2) between concepts and the linguistic structures which represent those concepts. We have already drawn attention to the fact that concepts and words are similar, but they are certainly not the same. To identify an object with the word which denotes it or a statement with what the statement represents is simply to encourage confusion (Korzybski, 1933).

There are a certain number of basic operations which occur in all knowledge and they include structure, which is the anatomy of the system, order, which is the way in which the structure occurs in terms of order if order is involved as it usually is, where one distinguishes *function* from structure. Bearing in mind that the physiology of a system and the anatomy of the system are structured and ordered and these two particular types of description make up the whole of any system whatever.

The concepts of structure and order (Oliver, 1951) are basic and on them depend the concepts of time, organization and the like. Much of this basic framework we are subsuming under the flag clearly marked Realism and hope it is a 'Critical Realism'.

Hypotheses

The formation of hypotheses from concepts takes us firmly into the linguistic field. Hypothesis formation is basic to knowledge and essential to problem solving; it is one of our central interests in artificial intelligence. Hypothesis formation is a linguistic activity which is very similar to induction. We need to carefully distinguish between the counting operation which is most frequently necessary to the formulation of a hypothesis which is subsequently formulated. This is rather like distinguishing the method by which we sum a series from the actual sum itself, or the method by which we arrive at an induction from the induction itself.

We should recognize that stochastic processes, especially Markov nets, are important for generating hypotheses but they are not, of course, the hypotheses themselves. One of the basic problems here will be to translate numerical data into linguistic data.

What we need to do is to supply a method such as that of using Markov nets, although *any* method might be used, to generate hypotheses from concepts. We have already illustrated this with (3), i.e.

$$h' = (As')(s' \to q).$$

We can add any number of examples, but what is so important is that in the computer model, or in any cybernetic model of the process, the activity should be goal-directed. Logic is permissive and we are not told by logic what arguments to develop. What tells us in practice is what goals we are, at any moment, trying to achieve. The development of hypotheses can therefore be likened to the development of strategies in the theory of games.

What is so interesting here is that hypothesis formation is precisely strategy development in the context of empirical games; the method used is the method of induction.

Language

We have already introduced language into our discussion but we now have to make this introduction more explicit and we have to recognize that there are many different levels of language even if we take the word 'language' in its broadest possible sense. In other words, there are languages of the nervous system (some might say codes rather than languages); there are languages like mathematics whether involving a metric or not; there are languages with a syntax like English, and also other natural languages with very different syntaxes.

Some of these languages are particularly useful for internal representation of data and others are more convenient for external communication. It does not follow that they are both equally suitable for the same purpose. Banerji (1960) has already made the point that his own language of concept formation is designed for internal representation and for internal logical processing and data processing, but it is not necessarily convenient for external communication *between* people or between computers. Nevertheless, we should be interested in both types of language. This is so since natural language programs such as are exemplified by NAMER, SIR, SINTHEX, LIP, ORACLE (Simons, 1965) and many others besides, are extremely relevant to our attempt to build up a total picture of artificial intelligence.

Simons (1965) has made a survey of natural language programs written for the computer and has divided them up into a series of subsets. He refers to them as:

(1) List structure data based systems.
(2) Graphic data based systems.
(3) Text data based systems.
(4) Logical inference systems.

To take each of these in turn and briefly describe them we should say that the list structure data based systems are well illustrated by SAD SAM. This is essentially a question answering system where SAD SAM itself stands for Sentence Appraiser and Diagrammer and Semantic Analysing Machine (Lindsay, 1963). The programs for SAD SAM written by Lindsay are all written in IPLV hence the list processing subset.

There were basically two sections to his program, one the parsing section dealing with the syntax. In this parsing section he breaks a sentence down into parts which he calls nouns, verbs, noun phrases and the other usual grammatical components of sentences. Then a treelike structure is generated showing the grammatical relationships existing between the parts. This output to the parsing section, which is a separate part of the program, becomes the input to the semantic section. The semantic section of the program searches for a subject complement combination especially those associated with the verb 'to be'. For example, 'John's father, Bill, is Mary's father', 'John's father' is the 'father of Mary and is called Bill' and 'Mary and John are brothers'.

So we can break this down into attribute value statements where we have the attribute husband has value Bill, the attribute wife has unknown value; attribute offspring equals John and Mary values; husband's parents, attribute, equals unknown value; wife's parents, attribute, equals unknown value and so on. If we now know that John and Mary are brother and sister we then learn Bill's wife is called Carol and we can also know the name of the mother of John and Mary and so we can gradually by the simplest sort of inference making build up the relations from the semantics.

The simplest graphic data based system is NAMER where the only problem presented to the program is that of recognizing and discriminating between different shapes such as circles, elipses, squares, etc., and attributing an appropriate name to each, thus the word 'circle' applies to the circular shape, the word 'square' to a square shape and so on. It would be easy to generalize on this system and attribute any number of properties to any of the discriminable shapes and this pattern recognition system linked to language could be complementary to the list structure data based system exhibited by SAD SAM.

We now turn to text based systems and the example here we give is that of PROTOSYNTHEX (Simons, Klein and McConlogue, 1963) or SYNTHEX as it is sometimes more briefly called. PROTOSYNTHEX answers questions posed in English and answers them from an encyclopaedia. The language itself indexes the text, using a synonym dictionary and an intersection logic and a simple information scoring function to extract from the text those sentences that most resemble the questions being processed, to question the text which has been retrieved or parsed and then compared. The sentences which are most similar to the question are the ones given in the answer subject to one final semantic analysis.

SYNTHEX, as we shall call it, deals in VAPS words, they earmark the Volume, the Article, the Paragraph and the Sentence for the whole of the text and the index word in the original question, key terms, as we sometimes call them in the LIP language, are then looked up and their frequency of occurrence borne in mind so that if words like 'foot' and 'hand' occur then they are clearly related words and they may go with head, with muscle, with fingers and we look for the greatest number of intersections of these related terms derived from the synonym dictionary, and then by taking the maximum score the appropriate bits of text are capable of being reproduced.

The parsing in SYNTHEX depends on a dependency logic (Hayes, 1962) where questions of the form 'Where do flies go in the wintertime?' get an answer of the form 'Flies go ... in the wintertime', and the thing to be looked for, of course, is the words to fill in the blank. The structure of the sentence is put into the usual treelike form and the look-up operation depending on intersection, and then the scoring operation lead to a final look to see if the answer as a whole makes sense in terms of attribute value and semantic rules; finally the answer is printed out. Clearly this is heuristic in essence since there is a chance of giving incorrect information and therefore one must think of it, as one should most natural language programming, as being a many-pathed effort. The final category of inference-based languages we shall illustrate by LIP (George and Sarkar, 1970; George, 1970). LIP in fact can occur in any of the different categories we have mentioned so far since there are simple LIP languages which are mere data retrieval languages and there are more complex ones which give full parsing as opposed to fixed linguistic and syntactic forms and you can get full parsing and full inference making besides.

The inference making is somewhat similar to the way it occurs in SIR (Raphael, 1964) and also somewhat similar in the simplest instances to the very simple inference making of SAD SAM.

With the more complex LIP programs a question is asked and data retrieval takes place to see, in somewhat the same way as the parsing operation in SYNTHEX, if there is a possibility of getting the information directly from the data base. If this is not possible, then we go through again to pick up statements in the data base which have some variables in common. Thus to take a simple instance, we may have a form such as *Bab* which means '*a* is the brother to *b*' and another *Bac* meaning '*a* is the brother to *c*' and if the question is 'Is *b* brother to *c*?', that is '*Bbc*?' then by picking up the other two instances and using the entailment rule for B... — it is possible to draw the inference that in fact *b* and *c* are brothers. More complicated logical inferences can be made when the statement is translated into logical form, primarily using the calculus of relations, and subsequently comparing the relational statements and their entailment and deriving the necessary inferences.

In fact, it is possible to build a full axiomatic system with full sets of semantic rules so that everything referred to in the system refers to something in 'reality'. Logical inferences, both of a deductive and an inductive kind, can be made because the game can be thought of in real time and therefore the sort of goal-directed game can be played according to certain strategies and scored in terms of degree of success.

The issue of language is especially important because many of the inductive inferences we learn as human beings are derived from other people telling us the details and procedures, rather than we ourselves deriving them directly from our experience. We learn from both *description* and direct *acquaintance* with the environment, and almost certainly human beings learn a higher proportion of what they know from description than they do from acquaintance; useful artificial intelligences will have to do so as well. This alone is sufficient to indicate the importance of language, and a reminder that knowledge is only cumulative as a *result of language*.

Logic

Deductive logical methods can be used in more than one way as rules and parts of artificially intelligent systems. For example, Hao Wang has used a method of pattern recognition which is more nearly algorithmic than the heuristic methods used by Shaw, Simon and Newell. In one sense Hao Wang's (1963) formulation is more 'satisfactory' than a heuristic approach. But for an artificially intelligent system that is required to learn rather than being an entity that has learned, then Newell, Shaw and Simon's methods are basic.

In particular if the learning of a processing language is already more or less complete (it never is completely so) then Hao Wang's methods are more economical and useful. If we are concentrating on the use of logic we should use every possible algorithm, truth-tables and the like. On the other hand, if language learning is still going on we are, by definition, concerned with the derivation of logic itself, and thus we need to consider the heuristic methods by which logic is acquired.

A great deal of work has already been done on theorem proving on computers (Wang, 1960a, 1960b; Newell, Shaw and Simon, 1963; Gelerntner, 1963; Gelerntner, Hanson and Loveland, 1963), especially in geometry and logic and this is directly relevant to the process of decision-making on computers. In saying this we are, of course, presupposing that decision-making will sometimes at least entail inference-making.

We have already made the point in discussing language that many natural language programs, certainly in the case of LIP programs, require the translating of natural language statements into logical form. The logical form needed is most often the calculus of relations where the terms used are all terms with denotation and therefore have semantic rules which include the entailments of the operators, where the operators refer to either connectives or verbs in ordinary English.

We have already mentioned also that axiomatic systems of an applied kind can be constructed and in so far as they are playing in real time in a goal-directed manner, strategies or heuristics can be worked out which lead the user of the strategy to the goals and he has to evaluate the routes. This can be done either by deductive inference from the axioms in the light of the goal-directed nature of the activity or it can be done by going through the activity and then finding out whether it was done well, either by literally carrying it out or simply formulating a strategy and seeing what would have happened if you had done it, i.e. by simulating the actual game itself.

We should add that it is not only inference-making that allows us to draw inferences if one can state the matter somewhat paradoxically, you also have causal change of relationships where A causes B and B causes C, etc., and knowing that A causes B and B causes C allows you to know that A causes C. This is not so much a logical relationship as a causal relationship, although the relationship between causal and logical relationships is a complicated one and underlines the well-known argument in the world of philosophy between 'formal' and 'factual'.

With that we shall leave our brief discussion of inference-making, again reminding the reader of the tremendous importance that logic, both inductive and deductive, plays in the problem of artificial intelli·· gence.

Pattern recognition

Pattern recognition is implicit throughout the above arguments since search for similarities among differences and differences among similarities is basic to the sort of data processing exemplified by artificial intelligence. There are particular models of sensory pattern recognition such as those of Rapoport, Culbertson, Uttley and others, but there are also questions of conceptual pattern recognition which are implicit in the work of Selfridge, Minsky and other similar approaches to the above problems.

We shall say no more about pattern recognition here since it is the subject of the preceding chapter.

This is a central issue in artificial intelligence in much the same way as language and logic and overlaps them in so far as, for example, Hao Wang (1963) as we have mentioned, used pattern recognition as a means of formulating theorem-proving systems for the computer, so in perceptual models and conceptual models depend on the concepts of pattern recognition which is a universal type of activity of the utmost importance. Again, we see that pattern recognition is a central issue for artificial intelligence.

Representation of problems

It has become increasingly clear in recent years, particularly as a result of the work of Amarel (although others have been involved), that the way a problem is presented is important for the manner in which a solution is proposed, and sometimes found. In other words, to use Michie's terms, a problem may be trivialized by transformation to a suitable form of representation; this is certainly the case.

One of the things a problem-solver may be expected to have to do is to continue to provide a number of transformations until the problem takes on an easy aspect. This easy aspect may well appear by translating the problem into a form which is easily recognizable as a special case of an existing standard problem.

There is another sense, of course, in which representation is important and that is in the semantic context. We have already drawn attention to the distinction between language and the things represented by language, and we also must be aware that language represents a degree of abstraction from the 'reality' described. Here again the representation is vital; how precise and how explicit is it at any particular level of abstraction? Are all the concepts involved in the discussion at the same level of abstraction? This leads to a discussion of definitions and introduces the attendant difficulty of finding a basis for knowledge. That question in turn can bring up all the epistemological disputes between phenomenalists and realists—both naive and critical—which are relevant to our own artificially intelligent system; it was Mackay (1956) who was among the first to draw attention to the epistemological problem of artefacts.

One interesting facet of the problem is as follows. There are stages in empirical inference making which involve knowledge of facts. Such stages certainly play a vital role in most human intelligent activities. Thus, for example, if you know the left-hand side of a chemical equation, it is an empirical matter whether you know the right-hand side of the equation. This may merely be a matter of logical inference, since if enough properties of the context in which the chemical formula is embedded are known to the owners of the left-hand side of the formula, then without knowledge of the right-hand side that knowledge can be deduced from the empirical facts; by a form of 'empirical logic'.

Data collection

It is clear that no intelligent system, whether real or artificial, could conceivably behave intelligently in its environment, let alone survive and evolve, without the ability to collect data. Concepts, the structure of the environment or the knowledge we have of the environment, and the hypotheses derived from our concepts with respect to such structures all demand data. Language which refers directly to the notion of concepts, structures and hypotheses is intended to relate data, and even though in the form of logic we can study the forms that we use to relate the data as such, still whole description of the data would be vacuous were it not for the empirical information, which relates what is essentially a set of numbers and units to the 'real world'. We have discussed the problem of pattern recognition and its closely related problem of perception so here we shall simply say that any intelligent system must be able to interact with its environment in some manner and be able to collect and utilize information, by storing it, so that when some new circumstance arises memory of experience in what seems like sufficiently similar situations allows it to behave in an intelligent way.

Clearly the whole classical problem, as it now is, of data retrieval suggests not only that it is necessary to be able to collect and retain data, but also that it should be organized in the memory store, perhaps the human brain primarily, in such a way that it is easily accessible particularly under conditions of urgency and risk.

There are many aspects to this very complicated problem. On the one hand there is the question of how the nervous system is actually constructed so that information is stored there, as it is, and how it can be retrieved. There is also the question of what form the information should take and how much storage space is available for the collecting and retaining of such information. And whether it is because of the relatively small finite nature of the storage space available in the human brain relative to the amount of information available in the environment, that processes of generalizations and simplification tend to replace the sheer loss of information.

In fact the whole question of whether information is ever lost is in itself a relevant one, since we have some reason to suppose that under certain circumstances, such as hypnosis in the case of human beings, that information apparently lost can be rediscovered. It is well known, of course, that information which is stored is not always immediately available hence one is often in the situation where one knows that one knows but one cannot remember exactly what it is that one knows. There is though some evidence that certain information is lost altogether in spite of the fact that much more is retained than might seem possible at first glance.

The relationship between the collecting and storing and retrieving of data and problems of natural languages is obviously very close. Since one way of regarding the human problem-solver is to think of him as recording all his information in terms of events all of which are in some measure named. The very processes of language which involve the naming, and involve therefore the fractionation of the environment, themselves present a considerable number of problems. We shall not attempt to discuss this in any detail here, merely to note that they are of extreme importance to the overall understanding of an intelligent system.

Evidence

Being able to reason and being able to collect and utilize information and, perhaps even more relevant to our immediate interests, being able to formulate hypotheses from which we can make decisions about the environment, are not enough unless we have some way of trying to decide whether what it is that we think we know is in some sense valid.

There are many fields here which are extremely relevant to that of decision-taking which is our primary interest. If we have information, we have to ask whether it confirms or refutes some particular belief or hypothesis. We have to push it further and then ask to what extent it confirms or refutes some particular hypothesis, and this automatically raises the question of the consistency of the hypotheses that have been formulated in different circumstances. Or to put it in other words, the internal consistencies of the beliefs we as individuals may hold about the world around us.

The notion of confirmation cannot be taken entirely in isolation since we also have to appeal to personal credibility. Personal credibility, that is, the extent to which one finds oneself able to believe a statement to be true, is in some ways reflective of the totality of the things one believes. It also represents the fact that the things we believe are beliefs with different degrees of strength and it may well be that the strength with which certain beliefs are held are not necessarily reflective of the actual weight of evidence, the factual support or the degree of confirmation that has been obtained objectively.

When we are trying to objectively justify things which we 'objectively' believe, we have to go through certain processes which are intended to provide evidence for our beliefs. The difficulty is primarily that we cannot be sure whether certain further sets of statements is really even relevant to the belief that they are supposed to be supporting and even if they are, we cannot be very clear as to what weight they supply. In certain simple cases, such as trying to justify some particular fact of history, we may simply appeal to the record book and say that was the result of that particular football match and all the football manuals agree about the result, there cannot be any reason to doubt it.

We are, in general, thinking of very much more complicated situations which are not mere records of relatively simple events, but hypotheses which have been confirmed to a greater or lesser extent or with the nature of science or knowledge. To some extent (Hempel and Oppenheim, 1950) weight of evidence can be separated from confirmation as can factual support. To some extent there are certain facts which are more or less indubitable or unlikely to be doubted because of their high probability and a certain weight of evidence which related these facts where relevant to certain hypotheses and confirmation is something which should take both of these factors into account as well as to some extent incorporating credibility and the consistency of the total belief structure of any particular individual.

We may wish to support a Peircean view that the totality of human beliefs tend to converge and converge towards the truth, but this in itself is a hypothesis which needs some sort of confirmation. It is like so many other principles of testability and the simplicity criterion of Occram's razor, something which we tend to believe and certainly has credibility for us but in themselves are principles difficult to prove and can only be exemplified by the extent to which they are pragmatically useful.

Concluding remarks

A consideration of all these matters is needed in order to build up an 'artificially intelligent system'. It goes without saying that the artificially intelligent system must have models of the external world at varying degrees of abstraction—this is implied by all that has been said so far— and also must have models with evaluations of each individual human source in the environment, otherwise it cannot assess and evaluate data from verbal 'descriptions'. No doubt other specific methods need to be used such as minimax regret and Bayes rule, strategies which allow the system to arrive at particular decisions in particular contexts.

The real problem of artificial intelligence is to integrate these methods into one complete model.

CHAPTER 14

SUMMARY

IN THIS chapter we shall attempt to summarize briefly all that has been considered and discussed in the book as a whole.

Cybernetics is the science of control and communication, and cybernetics can be used as a method to analyse the facts of human behaviour; but it is only one such method of analysis, and it must take its place alongside animal work, ethological and comparative, as well as experimental work on humans, and physiological studies of animals and humans.

Cybernetics represents the application of an old idea, the idea that human beings and animals are essentially very complicated machines. It asserts that they are deterministic systems which could be constructed (or reconstructed) in the laboratory, but whether or not this is actually true is not of the first importance, since the statement is only making explicit what is implicit in the behaviouristic approach to psychology and the mechanistic approach to biology in general. To take this assertion beyond the level of the trivial would necessitate an examination of what is meant by 'behaviouristic' and 'mechanistic'.

Cybernetics as a science of behaviour emerges mainly from three considerations:

(1) The development of servosystems and computers that are far more like human beings than any machines made previously.
(2) The need for developing a degree of precision in the models and theories used in any science, particularly the biological sciences of which an essential part is experimental psychology.
(3) This may be regarded as a corollary of (2), in that it lays emphasis on the need for mathematical descriptions. It may be confidently argued that any science develops quickly if it can be made mathe-

matical, and we should therefore try to introduce mathematics
into biology.

The usefulness of computers and servosystems is very great indeed,
particularly because it allows us to build models with them, and like them,
by other methods such as paper-and-pencil methods.

Computers, as we have seen, can be programmed to learn and also to
perceive, and it seems reasonable to say that they can also be programmed
to think, since thinking and learning are not, in the last analysis, of great
difference.

The problem, as seen from the point of view of computer programming,
was how to organize the storage system and how to program for the
process of generalization which is so essential to learning in computers,
as of course it is in human beings. This is by no means easy to do with a
computer, for the simple reason that most contemporary computers have
small storage systems. It is difficult for the computer to learn the first
processes when starting from no information at all, but the subsequent
stages become progressively easier because the computer is applying
established generalizations from one situation to another, rather than
working in terms of the one situation alone.

The computer programming technique allows us to check theories of
learning and their effectiveness, as well as offering a means of studying
new learning techniques, and appreciation of this brings to life the sort of
methodological experiment called the 'mathematico-deductive theory of
rote learning', which was undertaken by Hull and his associates (1940).
This might well turn out to be a prototype of many such experiments in
the future, since a computer can be programmed to handle with great
celerity a situation which for the human being would involve an intoler-
ably lengthy and tiresome process, and one which might possibly result
in a value by no means commensurate with the effort made to attain it.

Computer programming is likely to be followed up systematically in
the future, and for this method to become a standard part of psychology,
it is essential that a computer language should be developed—like
FORTRAN or P.L.1, the special compiler *languages* constructed by IBM
for automatic programming, for example—which will allow us to state
our program in simple everyday terms, and let the computer itself put it
into computer form and test its efficacy.

Such work as has been done on computer programming and learning might be taken to suggest that existing theories of learning, such as those of Guthrie, Hull, Tolman, Olds and others, do not differ as much from each other as was once supposed, and that in many cases differences between them are more at the level of interpretation than in the precise process depicted. But there are also some actual differences, and these suggest that different theories have emphasized some and neglected other important features in the learning process. This indicates the need for some measure of integration of existing theories of learning, and indeed much the same argument is true for perception and the other features of cognition; but this book has not been primarily concerned with carrying out that integration.

The vital part played by language in human learning is a matter that has not received very detailed attention by psychologists, and this is perhaps strange in view of the amount of work that has been done by philosophers and logicians in this domain. We have at any rate tried to indicate the trend in linguistic matters, especially in the context of computer programming, where its importance is revealed fairly clearly.

Learning, thinking, perceiving and so on, are obviously influenced by language. Language may be learned, words perceived, and linguistic information stored, just like any other associative process of the kind we have discussed; but the important feature of language is that, once it has been learned sufficiently, concepts and generalizations if indeed they are different—can be conveyed linguistically rather than through direct experience.

This suggests that an analysis of language should be possible in behaviouristic terms, with the aid of programming and other cybernetic techniques, to show how language has evolved and how big a part it has played in human learning. Quite obviously, without language the accumulation of human learning would have been an impossibility, and it seems likely that the high-speed change of strategies—high-speed learning—of which humans are capable, is due primarily to language.

This is not to say generalizations and other concept-forming principles would be impossible without language, but it seems certain that they are more effective with language, for—and what is more important—a species which has symbolic skill will inevitably use it, and it thus plays a vital part in human behaviour.

In the computer itself it is important to distinguish the binary code language of the internal representation of events, from the development

28*

of language—which may also be in binary code in the computer—wherein one computer word signifies other, or a collection of other, computer words.

There are various other ways by which we could go about constructing precise models, and *of course finite automata are the ones favoured in this book*. Information theoretic models are also of great interest, and have been emphasized by Broadbent. The great advantage of either conceptual system lies in its precision and relative ease of analysis, so that logical mistakes and vagueness can be easily detected.

No attempt has been made in this book to follow up work on information theoretic models, but they can quite obviously be conveniently fitted together with automata theory. The work of Hick (1952), Crossman (1953, 1955) and Broadbent (1958) should be consulted for developments along these lines.

The models so far referred to are all pre-wired in a sense, and certainly this is true of computers and logical nets, but it is important to realize that they are not fixed in their behaviour on that account, since the programming and the input tape create variation in behaviour of much the same kind as we might expect from human beings.

Hardware models of finite automata are also generally pre-wired, and we may expect that models will also be made in abundance in the future which will have the properties of growth, not only because we want to study development in the human being as well as the developed human, but also because the growth process must itself partly determine the nature of the grown product, a product which is indeed never quite fixed. Although growth models of the kind suggested by Pask, Beer, Chapman and others, will certainly be carefully examined in the near future, as will the chemical forms of finite automata, for the present the logical net or tape type of finite automaton is perfectly adequate for the analysis of existing models and theories, and can in fact be shown to be capable of representing the same set of events as could a growth system.

There is little doubt, either, that these same methods will soon be extensively employed in the field of applied psychology. Already much work has been done in social and in abnormal psychology to prepare the way for it, and no doubt the same is true for all the relevant fields.

Apart from their practical utility, there is a deeper principle involved in this sort of model making activity; it is that the mere collection of empirical data does not make a science. Empirical data, taken from observation of the world, are most certainly the vital food on which the whole edifice of science is built, but is not built by collection and restatement alone; they must be interpreted and integrated into a form, usually linguistic, from which certain logical consequences can be derived. This means that methods by which scientific theories are constructed are of the first importance, and this is increasingly the case as our precision in theory construction advances.

It has sometimes been said that theorizing in psychology is premature, but in fact there are very few cases in which this is true. After all it is not a matter of *either* theorizing *or* experimenting; both go together.

Comprehension of this last fact has been slow, largely because so much of the early theorizing seemed to be no more than empty speculation; and indeed some theorizing has gone on in a manner that is too remote from the facts. Many of us feel that philosophers might help themselves to solve at least some of their own problems if they would add empirical evidence derived from experiment to their own armchair speculations. The great benefit philosophers have to offer to scientists is their sophisticated analysis of language and logic, for this is something that the scientist needs and will increasingly need with the progress of the behavioural sciences.

It is often denied that scientists make verbal mistakes of the kind philosophers of science tend to attribute to them, but there is more than an element of truth in the allegation. Certainly it is true that a part of a science may be fairly clear-cut, and its problems not primarily verbal; but for other parts it is also true that a verbal tangle may ensue, and the more the scientist is persuaded that he doesn't get into verbal tangles, the more likely he is not to recognize them when he meets them. The words 'reinforcement', 'learning', 'motivation', 'perception' are words that are hardly clear-cut in their meaning, and a further complication is the fundamental fact that a description at the everyday level may use terms whose significance disappears at other levels of analysis.

This last point is clearly illustrated if we can imagine the difference in the descriptions of the performance of a car by, on the one hand, a casual observer, and on the other hand by the same observer after he has driven the car himself. A description by an expert mechanic would be different again, for he would have developed a different vocabulary. For example, while the casual observer might attribute separate causes to different manifestations such as skidding, bad cornering and erratic steering, the expert's description would be in terms fundamental to all three: the car's centre of gravity, length of wheel base, condition of tyres, etc., and the driver's lack of skill. Any number of other examples will readily come to mind to show that at a given level of description variables may be seen to be related, and at other levels they may seem unrelated.

It is on this account that the writer believes that any model-theory for behaviour must be at many levels, and that these levels must be closely integrated with each other. Hence, of course, the need for neurophysiological and, ultimately, biochemical descriptions of behaviour.

As to the use of particular methods in science, it must be recognized that there are various ways of making progress. The method suggested by Broadbent, which involved local theorizing, keeping close to experimental facts, is one, and one that is essential; but to follow this alone would involve a narrowness of outlook which would make for lack of integration with neighbouring scientific disciplines.

The hypothetico-deductive method has been much maligned of late, and mostly for the wrong reasons. It is true that the method as such is not well defined, and the name covers lots of different forms of theory construction; Hull's use of the method with his quantification is sometimes uneconomical and unwieldly, but a great deal can be said on behalf of using hypothetico-deductive methods, since they have the property of effective testability which we look for in a cybernetic system. Indeed, axiomatic systems are closely connected with cybernetic systems, and we should therefore encourage their use.

This is not meant in the sense of excluding the use of the *ad hoc* explanation, but rather to draw attention to the fact that, in general, we need to fit these *ad hoc* explanations together into a complete model if we are to have an effective science.

Turning now to the actual problems of cognition, it must be said again that these problems have not been explicitly dealt with in detail.

Hull, Tolman and Guthrie as individual learning theorists have become somewhat submerged in the general discussion of problems, and no doubt this placing of the emphasis on the problem rather than on the person and his theory represents healthy progress in the subject. There are, of course, many new theorists emerging in the field: Olds, Glanzer, Deutsch, Uttley, Broadbent and others have written extensively, and most illuminatingly, on the current problems of learning theory.

Nevertheless, our present emphasis is on method. Recent years have seen the development of mathematical models for learning theory, and those of Estes, Bush and Mosteller, Gulliksen and London, are among the first to come to mind. The methods are either the application of the differential calculus or the use of statistical analysis, which is of course essentially stochastic in its nature.

These mathematical models bear some relation to the conditional probability theory of learning suggested by Uttley; indeed his system is capable of being restated in stochastic form.

Conditioning of the classical and instrumental kind is naturally a subject to demand explanation, and the major problem is still the matter of reinforcement. Can learning take place without reinforcement? The answer is that without some selective process it would be difficult to see why learning should not be totally indiscriminate. Now discrimination can take place through a selective filter, but what is it that makes the filter selective? Whatever it is could, of course, represent the reinforcer.

But apart from the selective factor that may occur at the perceptual end, the field of latent learning suggests that learning may take place without reinforcement, and we are now faced with untestable statements to the effect that either learning always depends on reinforcement, or it doesn't. Either statement is untestable while we judge the presence of reinforcement by the fact of learning *having taken place*.

The alternative is to show in each case what the reinforcer is, and this quite obviously will not generally be possible.

Uttley's model, which has been a major influence on the writer's own views, suggests the basic nature of classification, conditional probability and reinforcement. But it should be noted that reinforcement might not be adequately represented by drive reduction, since we know from a number of experiments that sham feeding will often reduce food searching activity, and that reinforcement is not merely need-reduction in the crude sense.

Contiguity may itself supply learning, just as concepts may supply needs. Such a development of the idea of needs from physiological states, such as hunger and thirst, becoming associated with concepts which allow a person simply to think of something and, as a result, to want it, could easily occur in a finite automaton, and can be shown to occur in an appropriately programmed computer.

The problem is perhaps ultimately a neurophysiological one, or one that will be settled only by neurophysiological experiment. In the meantime, we can at least say that a reinforcement principle seems essential, and this principal should be generalized beyond its form in Hull's writings to deal with the more sophisticated types of reinforcement met in conceptual activity.

A great deal has been said recently about perceptual learning and discrimination learning, and this serves to remind us of the healthy fact that learning and perception are being increasingly seen as a unified process, and that learning perceptually is not something different from ordinary learning. The emphasis is now on the fact that some learning is more immediately tied to perception than other learning.

We may now summarize the cybernetic models described in this book.

(1) Models of the visual system. These include especially the models of Culbertson, Pitts and McCulloch, Selfridge, Rapoport, Osgood and Heyer, Uttley, Deutsch and George.

(2) General classification systems that may apply to any or all of the special senses; these include especially the models of Uttley, Chapman, George and Pask.

(3) The central process of conditional probability, counting and association. In the simpler associative cases this especially includes the hardware models of Shannon, Grey Walter, Deutsch, and in more complex form, the conditional probability computers of Uttley and the models of Stewart.

(4) Broadbent's auditory theories must also be mentioned here.

(5) Memory stores, including delay line and magnetic core storage, one form of which has been described by Oldfield.

(6) Motivational systems, especially in Uttley's models, in logical net form, and as exemplified by Ashby's Homeostat.

(7) Natural language programming. This includes the methods of such programs as SIR, NAMER, LIP, and many others. These are in the process of being developed now.

(8) Inference-making programs. There are a whole series of logic theorem proving methods which have been developed in various different forms by such people as Wang, Newell, Shaw and Simon and others and all these are also in the process of being developed.

(9) Heuristic methods. Heuristic methods, which are the equivalent of creative capacity or *ad hoc* rules, rules of thumb, etc., probably supply the most important type of modelling so far to enter into the cybernetic field.

The list could be greatly extended to include in particular the learning theorists such as Hull and Tolman, neurophysiologists such as Pribram, and neurophysiological theorists such as Hebb and Milner. We would also remind the reader of the many other models, both in hardware and paper-and-pencil, due to Turing, Church, Bridgman, and many others, that have a direct bearing on our problem.

Information theorists have undertaken to model many of the same systems from slightly different points of view. Usually the emphasis is more operationally inclined, and is more directly concerned with performance.

It seems fairly clear that, from the models we have, we can supply sensory and motor systems, a central control with temporary storage, probability counters, and a permanent storage system, in a variety of different ways. Many of the models would certainly be workable, and could be made in more than one fabric. However, we still have a very long way to go before we can fit all the empirical facts together, especially at the molecular level, to supply anything like *the* working model we need. We are well aware, also, that all this says little or nothing about modelling the social situation.

The trouble is that we have reached a point where many of these problems can be understood in a general way, and yet the very size of the model-making undertaking is so large as to defy conceptual clarity.

At the moment there are two strikingly pressing problems in cybernetics, the first one being the need for a notation that allows an easy, detailed description of a vast iterated system. Obvious places to look for help are in algebra, set theory, statistics and logic, and the best that can be done involves all these means; but to develop a suitably integrated language or notation in which we could construct conceptual or paper-and-pencil models will be a major task indeed. Of course an answer may lie in computer programming, and especially in auto-codes, but those particular auto-codes called generating routines which are so vital to learning are not as yet sufficiently developed.

The second big problem for cybernetics is to find an inexpensive unit, or set of units, so that very large-scale special-purpose computers may be constructed. This problem is partly answered by general-purpose digital computers and partly by transistors, and in the future it is likely to be greatly helped by new storage techniques, and by the micro-module method of computer construction.

There are, of course, many other problems to be solved before we have effective theories which will allow us to predict the behaviour of individuals and groups of people, but from the cybernetician's point of view the two mentioned above are the most urgent.

We shall now outline very briefly what we consider to be the most likely principles applying in the construction of the human organism. This could have been the subject of the whole book, and it has been to some extent interwoven with a discussion that has been more concerned with the development of conceptual models and the methodological implications of these models. In the main the model will be concerned with only one sensory input, vision, and the reactions that are involved with this, though of course the system could be extended to include all the other senses. The main points are:

(1) In the first place we have to decide between different models of the visual system. The Osgood–Heyer model still seems the most promising in describing the actual transmission of patterns to the visual cortex. The method by which colour vision may be fitted into this particular model is not yet entirely clear, but it should not prove a major problem to simply associate colour properties with the various configurations transmitted from retina to cortex. Conceptually, there are many possible methods by which this might be done, but the question has not been discussed in this book.

(2) Information in the visual cortex is assumed to be classified, and may proceed by stages where each sensory modality starts its partial classification independently. Ultimately the information from the various special senses is integrated.

(3) It seems likely that information from all the senses could be described in terms of a filter, and the partial classification process is itself a temporary storage system—it certainly could be—such that information is processed in terms of its urgency, the urgency factor operating at some level of classificatory recognition.

(4) The process of visual recognition depends upon classification, either with or without eye movements. Eye movements are certainly normally involved, but whether it is possible to learn to perceive without eye movements remains an open question.

(5) Learning is dependent upon the principle of selective association. The storage system at the earlier levels is assumed to store spatial and

temporal associations, and these associations are kept in the first storage while conditional probabilities about their associations are being established. The most frequent, the most recent and the most valuable are the ones for which the conditional probabilities are first sought, and in terms of which, at some critical value, they are transferred to some other store as having been learned.

(6) The second store, for information actually learned, is primarily a verbal storage system where what is remembered is a linguistic form of description in particular or general terms. Words, and languages, are learned like all other associations, and transferred into the second storage in the same way. This means that the logical operations that can be enacted on information in the secondary storage are, in fact, a set of operations on words.

(7) Thinking is in no essential way different from learning—although the emphasis is here on language—and consists in the formation of linguistic hypotheses from the conditional probabilities in storage that are themselves derived logically from storage, or directly transferred from the first storage system.

(8) Memory is ordered storage of information and, when needed, its reconstruction is effected by stimulation, either through an internal association process or through an external sensory process.

(9) Recall involves the internal partial firing of centres that are normally sensorially elicited.

(10) Motivation is presumed to operate in a reinforcing manner on the associations dealt with at all levels of the system, where secondary motivation occurs to transfer positive or negative values to associations that did not originally have those positive or negative values. This allows the thinking operation to produce a need since, when an association with a value—particularly a strong value—occurs, it may itself change the direction of behaviour towards satisfying a new need.

(11) From the last comment it is clear that needs are to be thought of as being organic, representing states of hunger, thirst, etc., and also conceptual in that 'thinking about something' may lead to a need. The satisfaction of a need may be either organic or conceptual, and here curiosity will be regarded as a basic, although rather general, drive.

(12) Emotions are thought to be closely associated with states of need, so that with satisfaction of need pleasant feelings occur, and conversely, with the frustration of needs, unpleasant feelings occur. The built-in

principle of the organism that must survive is that the pleasant feelings should be maximized and the unpleasant minimized. Here, the words pleasant and unpleasant are being stretched somewhat beyond their everyday meanings, since they must also include activities that are not inherently pleasure-giving or otherwise, but whose operations may be vitally important for survival.

(13) The apparatus for 11 and 12 is built in, as is the basic principle of association. From these beginnings the principle of generalization (concept formation) is acquired by experience.

(14) Learning may sometimes be closely integrated in a sequence with innate components, and it may be centred around primarily perceptual material, in which case we call it perceptual learning. When we learn in terms of relations rather than properties, we call it discrimination learning; and when we learn in terms of concept formation we simply call it learning, or conceptual learning. When it involves the use of logic and language we call it thinking.

(15) 'Thinking', when used behaviouristically, means just what we said in (14) although, as far as one can tell, when the word is used in the everyday sense it may mean only those logical and linguistic operations of which we are *conscious*.

(16) Thinking may ramify in curious ways which represent the operations of extrapolation (induction) and the drawing of consequences (deduction). These are by no means only linguistic processes, for they involve the associations of the store system where the association is simply between event-names, and not the names for event-names. This is a rather clumsy distinction made necessary by the fact that there is a sense in which *everything* inside the nervous system is at least in coded form.

(17) Consciousness is not a property of a system that can be examined cybernetically, and in the shadow of the problem of 'other minds' we should simply say that it probably represents a certain neural activity whereby we are given a private glimpse of our own cerebral activity, through images and sensations.

(18) The basic associations on which the system is founded have a large compass of complexity, ranging from simple habits, through commonplace 'beliefs' or 'expectancies', to highly complex pieces of problem solving, which we might call hypothesis formation.

(19) Perception is assumed to be essentially the same as the process of recognition, which is simply the classification of objects, events, etc.

(20) Problem solving is assumed to be essentially the same as the process of learning or thinking, as opposed to the subsequent stage of 'having learned'.

(21) Receptor systems are assumed to be available so that they may be switched into the system where they may actively change the central state, in a homeostatic manner. They may also be classified as a particular case, and respond only to internal elicitation. The ideas of Deutsch are relevant here, and his type of homeostatic responding system seems the most likely type of output.

(22) The main key to the development of creative thinking, problem solving, planning and decision taking lies almost certainly in the use of heuristic methods and the inclusion of specific models, such as Bayes model, in the heuristic methods. It is here that we see one of the major developments in cybernetic thinking.

This list has grown long, and we must now summarize the more molecular level of description.

Neurologically speaking, we have already seen how much current neurophysiological thought is running parallel to the type of closed loop homeostatic processes we have been assuming. The work of Pribram, mentioned in Chapter 10, paints a picture with which we are in essential agreement.

(1) The cortex is a storage and analysing system. It has input systems connected directly to it, and their cortical representation makes up the bulk of the storage system. These input representations are relatively well established in terms of localization.

(2) The cortex also has the two stages of storage system to which we have already referred. The first stage is ramified, and starts even in the sensory endings, such as the retina, and continues to classify throughout the visual cortex. Similarly, the process may be supposed to operate through the rest of the sensory cortex and the areas of cortical elaboration.

(3) The second storage system is presumably in the temporal-parietal regions of the cortex and in the frontal regions as well.

(4) The cortex is presumed to be partially localized in that the density of particular functional connections tend to occur together in particular areas. Nevertheless, there is a considerable amount of cortical

overlap, due to the different functions being represented by neurons, or collections of neurons, with widely ramified connections.

(5) It is assumed that the sub-cortical areas are concerned with the channelling and timing of information flow from the lower and to the lower centres. The hypothalamus is representative of the emotional centres, and is connected with the activating reticular system in mediating feelings and sensations from internal states of the organisms, the limbic system then representing sorts of pleasure and pain centres.

(6) The cerebellum is concerned with the integration of motor activating information.

(7) The reflex arc unit of nervous activity is a special case of a homeostatic unit whereby there exist graded neural responses which modify the homeostatic control associated with cortical and subcortical centres.

(8) It is assumed that there is a feedback of information from effectors that modify the central state.

(9) It is assumed that sets of neurons fire together circuitously in something like the manner suggested by Milner-cell assemblies with differential inhibition.

(10) The logical net analysis, which has been used prominently in clarifying principles expressed in this book, while not appropriate for a description of the details of the neurophysiological picture as they stand, comes sufficiently near for a direct comparison to be made between a model couched in neurophysiological terms, such as Milner's, and the logical net equivalent.

A brain model in outline

In this book it is being explicitly assumed that the brain is a data-processing system, with a very large store, or set of stores (such as fast and slower stores), which is working on coded information which travels along the pathways of the nervous system, as a function of certain complicated conditions. These conditions being supplied both by the environment and the internal state of the system.

We are not, of course, assuming a ready-made resemblance between computers and brains. But we are assuming that the computer can be appropriately programmed to simulate a brain, and that the computer can carry a model of the brain. It is also the case, of course, that the brain can carry a model of the computer (Apter, 1970).

We assume that the sensory pathways are primarily concerned with input, and this input activity is integrated into the complex selectivity reinforced processing of the brain. It seems clear that sensory inputs are independent classification systems, and are partial and adaptive in their function. They act, in hierarchical fashion, as filters to a higher integrated partial classification system which is the central store. They are also possibly processors in their own right.

All the information which is stored in the brain occurs at various levels of generality in the hierarchy, and it is reasonable to expect to be able to distinguish short-term from long-term memories: this is indeed connected with core as opposed to backing types of store. This indeed is not the only possible distinction, as the human brain may store in a whole variety of stages.

Much evidence derived from observations and experiments upon lower organisms is misleading when applied to the human brain, which is far more complex and has far greater storage capacity, allowing the human being to be seen no longer as a passive receptor of, and reactor to, stimuli. What is called 'free' (as opposed to 'tied') thinking is a reminder that activity is often intiated by the human brain as a result of its conceptual activities. This makes the brain a dynamic selector system, as much influenced by its internal states as by external stimuli.

Another problem we have to deal with is that of the frontal lobes and their role. More evidence is now available which suggests that cortical locations are the seat of the higher level memory stores where the conceptual processes of handling data, performing logical inferences, and the like occur; this particularly applies to the frontal lobes. The whole question of the role of cortical localization is renewed, but viewed as a dynamic rather than a static one. It seems certain that the cortical areas overlap and play very many different roles, according to whether an organism is learning, utilizing information already learned, hypothesizing or whatever. Information is stored in an overlapping manner and detailed information, like data placed in computer registers, may vary from person to person and from time to time in the same person. The comparison with list-processing is an obvious one and suggests that the human brain has, in fact, compromised on localization in the interests of flexibility.

The reticular formation (another important part of the brain) seems to be associated with motivation and drive. These features themselves though are complicated and concerned with selection, activation, priorities, emergencies, etc., all within the compass of a homeostatic principle which serves the organic needs of the body for survival: they are though obviously interconnected with the higher cortical (conceptual) activities in the hierarchy. The limbic system is almost certainly connected with motivational activity and is, as Pribram suggested, probably the regulator of the dispositions of organisms, this function being performed by the use of graded neural homeostats.

There are still $S-R$ activities of a reflex kind occurring (Spinelli and Pribram, 1970) in the brain, but they become something of an artefact as far as the human brain is concerned, if they are thought of as the basis of the total neural activity. Dotey (1965) has shown, while still using conditioning terminology, the greater detail of the workings of associations and classifications in store, which also suggests the very close association between equivalent areas in different hemispheres. It also suggests though that the growth of store has changed the reflex notion from a dominant to a recessive one. The whole question of reflexes, whether conditioned or otherwise, is a central one in the study of the brain, but the consensus tends now to think of them as limited special cases of a more general process, rather than the other way round.

Visual information is initially processed in the occipital areas of the cortex, auditory information in the temporo-parietal areas, and so on. The regions which process language are probably the so-called 'speech areas'. Here, however, there is a problem since speech for the brain is complex. Human beings 'vocalize' as a motor activity of a relatively simple kind, while they symbolize as a very high-level conceptual activity. Sounds can be formalized as words and sentences and their utterance leads to an auditory response, which leads to translation into symbols.

This leads us to the question of language. Language is both motivated and itself motivates. Words may remind us of, or initiate, needs and drives. Language is also closely associated with imagery, so that when humans 'image' or 'imagine' something, somehow some subset of the total set of sensory inputs which are involved in the actual sensory experience is stimulated. Humans, it seems, learn to associate noises, such as those that represent words, with objects, relations and other conceptual factors, so that it must be assumed that the human brain stores language and data separately. Although separately stored, they are intimately associated by something like a list-process or a complex cross-referencing association system. Human beings can 'image' an event from the past and can make statements about that event, such as giving a verbal description of it. In fact, humans tend to speak about events as they 'image' them, and can hardly speak about something without 'imaging' it. Alternatively they usually either write about or talk about what they are imaging. This reminds us that to some extent thinking is similar to a process of talking to oneself.

The whole process of conceptualizing is a process which is intimately bound up with language, and is thought to be a function closely associated with the frontal areas of the brain; there is some considerable behavioural and neurophysiological evidence for this belief. The hierarchical nature of the brain suggests that the generation of new principles, recursion formulae, meta-rules, etc., which allow the solution of new problems is primarily a frontal-lobe activity.

Research in cybernetics, particularly from the domains of computer synthesis and simulation, suggests that the brain is, as has been said, a complex and flexible hierarchical store with the ability to make inferences, both deductive and inductive, and perform computations, where the computational activity of mathematics has to be previously learned and conceptualized. Such formal mathematical models and methods are readily available already in a digital computer, because of the programmer, who makes them available. Although we should note that no one programmer will appreciate the significance of all the models and methods he makes available.

One question of importance is why is there not a higher correlation between cortical damage and impairment of function? Search for memory traces of a dynamic character, suggested by Lashley and others, have been largely abandoned, so that it would seem to be necessary to accept instead the fact that the detailed information contained in any one cortical area varies according to the order in which it has occurred in the history of the owner, or at least partly by this and partly by his cross-referencing system. In other words, information is contained in the detailed structures of the nervous system in a way which allows complicated overlapping of both functions and detail; this still retains the notion of a sort of statistical localization.

One way of fitting and testing the essential rightness of the views expressed is for a large team of scientists to build a large and detailed simulation of the brain on a computer, filling in all the detail that is known with some measure of confidence and adding on 'plausible' detail until the model is fully connected and effective: this is a sort of empirical axiomatic system. The main test then is that of seeing whether it, as a brain, can successfully program its environment, and to see if it can do so in the same way that human brains do. In this discussion of the general organization of the human brain we have intentionally skirted around the neurological detail. Thus, it would be desirable to be able to assert exactly what function the amygdaloid bodies or the Brodman area 27 performs, but this is not possible. It is a picture rather like that of the organization of a 'fourth-generation' multi-processing computer and it has dynamic properties.

We now think of the brain as a hierarchically organized, highly adaptive partial and partitioned classification system, which has a high degree of specialization which merges with a high degree of integrated function which is both anatomically and physiologically overlapping. The basic units are Pribram's 'graded function' homeostats, and it is possible to locate principal areas, statistically speaking, of importance in the cortex—for example, for integrated conceptual behaviour involving memory or the interpretation of the special senses. The 'vertical' system, including the thalamus and limbic systems, are primarily emotional representations in store which are concerned with drive and reinforcement and are closely integrated with the other activities of the cortex. The cerebellum and the associated tracts and closely connected areas are part of the motor control system which is so necessary to organized overt body movements, and also has overlap with other higher (cortical) areas of the brain.

There can be little or no doubt that the cortex is the primary representational centre for all the cognitive activities of its owner, and must contain 'models' of the 'world outside' and the people in it as well as a 'model' of the person himself. This last function is essential to consciousness and seems to be connected also with the function of the reticular formation. We could guess reasonably at this point that the modelling processes, especially that of internal modelling, leads through consciousness to self-consciousness and the general awareness which people have of themselves. But here the world of existing evidence (especially neurological evidence) is left and the world of speculation entered. It is accordingly at this point at which to stop.

Before we complete this text we should note that many people have regarded the computer as quite unsuitable as a brain model, and some have even thought it unsuitable as a method of simulating the intelligent behaviour, but we strongly take the view that the computer can enormously add to our knowledge and understanding both of the brain and of human behaviour. The reason for this is partly an economic one. It is that the computer is the only large-scale universal machine available which is only made specific when a suitable program has been inserted and that program as we have seen, especially in the context of heuristic and adaptive methods, can be made as flexible as the ingenuity of the programmer allows.

Von Neumann himself regarded the computer as being unsuitable as a brain model because of the logical constraints on its organization and we accept that this is true, that there are such constraints, but we would emphasize the opposite side of the coin and that is that many of the features of any system, however complex, can be suitably simulated and the only sensible economic way of carrying out such a simulation is through the digital computer.

We should also emphasize that a number of other aspects of cybernetics, apart from those which have been explicitly discussed in this book, have been developed in the last few years and one thinks immediately, here of Findler, who studied the laboratory decision-making problem in which subjects set their own control variables. There is another program called ALDUS constructed by Loehlin who in it tried to simulate a face-to-face interaction with records of attraction, anger and fear and attempts to reproduce more realistic aspects of human interaction. ALDUS responded to new objects by setting indices representing approach, attack and avoidance and the like and must go some way to fill the gap left by our lack of complete and explicit understanding of emotional behaviour. Clarkson (1963) and others have developed heuristic methods in problems such as investment analysis and appraisal and these same methods have been applied in some measure (George, 1970) to decision taking, diversification, expansion and acquisition, all features of problem solving in the business context. So with the 'open-ended' thought that there is a lot more involved in cybernetics than we have attempted to describe, even briefly, in this particular text, we shall leave the matter at that.

On finishing a book such as this, even at the second attempt, one is very conscious that fresh information is coming in with each succeeding journal and each new book, and for that and for other reasons, much has inevitably been left unsaid. This book has been written in the hope that it will encourage more people to realize that cybernetics has a serious contribution to make to our understanding of behaviour, and that most readers will find the arguments sufficiently clear and cogent to convince them that there is a perfectly good sense in which we should want to say that the 'brain is a computer'.

SOME RECENT BRAIN MODELS

A WHOLE variety of brain models have been suggested over the years and we have dealt with a number of them in this book. We have particularly concentrated attention on mathematical models of a logical kind (Woodger, McCulloch–Pitts nets, von Neumann nets, etc.) of a stochastic kind (e.g. Bush and Mosteller), and we have mentioned the relevance of theory of games. We have also discussed Cybernetics and brain models in the more informal terms of natural language. In recent years particularly, a whole host of new models have been developed and we should, in this appendix to the second edition, mention some of the more recent models that have been suggested, and which have not been mentioned in the main text.

Before looking at particular examples, let us say that the difficulty implicit in applying mathematical models to brains or behaviour—or indeed to anything at all—is to recognize the appropriateness of the mathematics to be used. If you can, as did Heisenberg in the case of quantum mechanics, appreciate that matrix algebra is particularly suitable, or as Dirac did, also in the field of quantum mechanics, appreciate that vector analysis is extremely appropriate, so much the better. The very fact that Heisenberg and Dirac could have found two different but equally appropriate descriptions serves as a reminder that we can interchange (and translate between) different descriptions of the same system. It therefore comes about that many different brain models have been couched in many different terms and one of our problems in the future will be to translate from one descriptive language to another.

We shall in this appendix mention first the recent models of a Servo-system type (Grodings, 1963; Deutsch, 1967). Such models are greatly influenced by engineering considerations such as engineering mathematics. This inevitably means that we quickly become involved in differential equations, transfer functions and the like. Such methods have been highly successful in engineering science and control theory, but have been thought by many to be too detailed for our present (more statistical) understanding of the structure and function of brains.

Deutsch, in talking of memory-storage theories (1967, chapter 11) refers to conditioning theory, and distinguishes short- from long-term memory. He also mentions the important developments in holograms (Willshaw and Longuett-Higgins, 1969). He then develops models of audition and vision and lends neurophysiological plausibility to the theory by reference to experimental work (e.g. Hubel and Wiesel, 1959, 1963) and finally discusses the thought processes, although by now any attempt to provide detailed mathematical descriptions have been dropped.

More neurological in orientation is the work of Marr (1970) and Olds (1969). The essence of Marr's model is that the basic operations of the cerebral neocortex involves the use of past experience to form so-called 'classificatory units' which are used to interpret subsequent experience. Frequency of stimulation of the brain and a high rate of redundancy are two of the essential conditions for the formation of such classificatory units.

Marr's subsequent description of his brain model is in information theoretic terms and he prescribes neural models to perform the role of *diagnosis* and *interpretation* and he points out that the model's ability to perform diagnosis automatically enables it to interpret. The rest of the discussion is concerned with the correspondence between the model and the human brain.

Olds thinks of the neuroanatomy of the hippocampus as a focal point for learning and reinforcement. He compares his ideas with respect to the hippocampus to computer storage systems and points out both the differences and the similarities. He suggests that what he calls 'emotional integrators' of the subcortex and lateral hypothalamus might project into computer-like grids in the cerebellum, tectum, hippocampus and neocortex. These grids are then closely associated with what the author calls a Hullian type of reinforcement.

Next we come to the very much more mathematically orientated work of J. S. Griffith (1967, 1971). As far as his own theory is concerned, Griffith assumes (in a manner somewhat reminiscent of Hebb) a growth process between two cells and he feels there may be many different chemicals involved, since there are many different brain structures.

Griffith asserts that a structure matrix showing possible stimulus–response relationships defines the structure of the brain and he assumes that what he calls the *mode* is the main flexible neural link in the nervous system, and that with the positive reinforcement of a situation there is an increase in the synaptic connections in the appropriate areas of the nervous system. Conversely, with negative reinforcement, there is a decrease in such synaptic connections.

Griffith's view of the brain as a sort of stochastic automaton has two great virtues. One is that he has developed with it the appropriately precise mathematical descriptions and the other is that his model directly suggests certain experiments, some of which he himself outlines in his book.

Griffith, in his later work (1971), goes on to generalize on his own theory and points to the general development of mathematical neurobiology, which includes the study of Pitts–McCulloch nets, random nets (Rapoport, 1952), information theory and non-linear equations. It may be that Griffith's work is the most promising of all the models mentioned in this appendix. It is also perhaps closest in thinking and attitude to that of this book.

REFERENCES

ADAMS, D. K. (1929) Experimental studies of adaptive behaviour in cats. *Comp. Psychol. Monog.* **6**, 1.

ADEY, W. R. (1961) *Brain Mechanisms and Learning*, F. DELAFRESNAYE (Editor), Oxford, Blackwells.

ALBE-FESSARD, D. and FESSARD, A. (1963) *Progress in Brain Research* **1**, 115.

ALBINO, R. C. (1960) A lecture given at Bristol University on 'The Organization of the Cerebral Cortex.'

AMAREL, S. (1960) An approach to automatic theory formation. *Proceedings of Illinois Symposium on Principles of Self-Organization*, Urbana, Univ. of Illinois Press.

AMAREL, S. (1962) An approach to automatic theory formation. In: H. VON FOERSTER and G. W. ZOPF, Jr. (Editors), *Principles of Self-Organization*, Oxford, Pergamon Press.

AMAREL, S. (1965) Problem solving procedures for efficient syntactic analysis. *A.C.M. 20th National Conference.*

AMAREL, S. (1967) An approach to heuristic problem solving and theorem proving in propositional calculus, *Computer Science and Systems*, University of Toronto Press.

AMAREL, S. (1968) On representations of problems of reasoning about actions. In: D. MICHIE (Editor), *Machine Intelligence-3*, University of Edinburgh Press.

APTER, M. J. (1966) *Cybernetics and Development*, Oxford, Pergamon Press.

APTER, M. J. (1970) *The Computer Simulation of Behaviour*, London, Hutchinson.

ARBIB, M. A. (1965) *Brains, Machines and Mathematics*, McGraw-Hill.

ARNOT, R. E. (1949) Clinical indications for pre-frontal lobotomy. *J. nerv. ment. Dis.* **109**, 267–9.

ASHBY, W. R. (1947) Dynamics of the cerebral cortex. XIII. Interrelation between stabilities of parts within a whole dynamic system. *J. comp. Psychol.* **40**, 1–8.

ASHBY, W. R. (1948) The homeostat. *Electron. Eng.* **20**, 380.

ASHBY, W. R. (1950) The cerebral mechanisms of intelligent action. In: D. RICHTER (Editor), *Perspectives in Neuropsychiatry*, H. K. Lewis, London.

ASHBY, W. R. (1952) *Design for a Brain*, Chapman & Hall, London.

ASHBY, W. R. (1956a) Design for an intelligence amplifier. In: C. E. SHANNON and J. MCCARTHY (Editors), *Automata Studies*, Princeton University Press.

ASHBY, W. R. (1956b) *An Introduction to Cybernetics*, Chapman & Hall, London

BACKUS, J. (1959) Automatic programming: properties and performance of FORTRAN systems I and II. In: *Mechanisation of Thought Processes*, Natural Physical Laboratory Symposium, H.M. Stationery Office.

BANERJI, R. B. (1960) An information processing program for object recognition. *General Systems* **5**, 117.

BANERJI, R. B. (1964) A language for the description of concepts. *General Systems* **9**, 135.

BANERJI, R. B. (1968) *Some Results in a Theory of Problem Solving*, Case Research Center Monograph, Parts I and II.

BARD, P. (1934) On emotional expression after decortication with some remarks on certain theoretical views. *Psychol. Rev.* **41**, 309–29.

BARLOW, H. B. (1959) Sensory mechanisms, the reduction of redundancy and intelligence. In: *Mechanisation of Thought Processes*, N.P.L. Symposium, H.M. Stationery Office.

BARONDES, S. H. and COHEN, H. D. (1966) Puromycin effect on successive phases of memory storage. *Science* **151**, 594–95.

BARTLETT, F. C. (1932) *Remembering*, Cambridge University Press.

BARTLETT, F. C. (1958) *Thinking*, Allen & Unwin, London.

BEACH, F. A. (1958) Neural and chemical regulation of behaviour. In: H. F. HARLOW and C. N. WOOLSEY (Editors), *Biological and Biochemical Bases of Behaviour*, University of Wisconsin Press.

BEER, S. (1959) *Cybernetics and Management*, English Universities Press.

BEER, S. (1960) Towards the cybernetic factory. Paper delivered in symposium on *Principles of Self-Organization*, University of Illinois.

BEKHTEREV, V. M. (1932) *General Principles of Human Reflexology*, International, New York.

BELLMAN, R.E. (1957) *Dynamic Programming*, Princeton University Press.

BELLMAN, R. E. and DREYFUS, S. E. (1962) *Applied Dynamic Programming*, Princeton University Press.

BERITOFF, S. (1932) *Individually Acquired Activity of the Central Nervous System*, GIZ Tiflis.

BERLYNE, D. E. (1960) Novelty and curiosity as determinants of exploratory behaviour. *Brit. J. Psychol.* **41**, 68–80.

BEURLE, R. L. (1954a) Activity in a block of cells capable of regenerating pulses. RRE Memorandum 1042.

BEURLE, R. L. (1954b) Properties of a block of cells capable of regenerating pulses, RRE Memorandum 1043.

BEURLE, R. L. (1962) Functional organization in random networks. In: H. VON FOERSTER and G. W. ZOPF, Jr. (Editors), *Principles of Self-Organization*, Oxford, Pergamon Press.

BEXTON, W. H., HERON, W. and SCOTT, T. H. (1954) Effects of decreased variation in the sensory environment. *Canad. J. Psychol.* **8**, 70–6.

BISHOP, G. H. and CLARE, M. H. (1952) Sites of origin of electrical potentials in striate cortex. *J. Neurophysiol.* **15**, 201–20.

BLODGETT, H. C. (1929) The effect of the introduction of rewards upon the maze performance of rats. *Univ. Calif. Publ. Psychol.* **4**, 113–34.

BLUM, J. S., CHOW, K. L. and BLUM, R. A. (1951) Delayed response performance of monkeys with frontal removals after excitant and sedative drugs. *J. Neurophysiol.* **14,** 197–202.

BLUM, M. (1962) Properties of a neuron with many inputs. In: H. VON FOERSTER and G. W. ZOPF, Jr. (Editors), *Principles of Self-Organization,* Oxford, Pergamon Press.

BORING, E. G. (1942) *Sensation and Perception in The History of Experimental Psychology,* Appleton-Century-Crofts, New York.

BORING, E. G. (1952) Visual perception as invariance. *Psychol. Rev.* **59,** 141–8.

BOWDEN, B. V. (Editor) (1953) *Faster than Thought,* Pitman, London.

BRAITENBERG, V. (1967a) Is the cerebellar cortex a biological clock in the millisecond range? In: C. A. Fox and R. S. SNIDER (Editors) *The Cerebellum. Progress in Brain Research,* Vol. 25, Amsterdam, Elsevier.

BRAITENBERG, V. (1967b) On the use of theories, models and Cybernetical toys in brain research. *Brain Research,* **6,** 2, 201–15.

BRAITHWAITE, R. B. (1953) *Scientific Explanation,* Cambridge University Press.

BRIDGMAN, P. W. (1927) *The Logic of Modern Physics,* Macmillan, New York.

BROADBENT, D. E. (1954) The role of auditory localization in attention and memory span. *J. exp. Psychol.* **47,** 191 6.

BROADBENT, D. E. (1958) *Perception and Communication,* Pergamon Press, London and New York.

BRODMANN, K. (1909) *Vergleichende Lokalisationslehre der Grosshirnrinde in ihren Prinzipen dargestellt auf Grund der Zellenbaue,* Leipzig.

BROGDEN, W. J. (1939) The effect of frequency of reinforcement upon the level of conditioning. *J. exp. Psychol.* **24,** 419 31.

BROOKS, C. McC. and ECCLES, J. C. (1947) Electrical investigation of the monosynaptic pathway through the spinal cord. *J. Neurophysiol.* **10,** 251 75.

BROUWER, L. E. J. (1924) *Beweis, dass jede volle Funktion gleichmässig stetig ist.* Proceedings of the Koninklijke Nederlandse Akademie van Wetenschappen, Amsterdam. **27.**

BRUNER, J. S., GOODNOW, J. J. and AUSTIN, G. A. (1956) *A Study of Thinking,* John Wiley, New York.

BRUNSWICK, E. (1939) Probability as a determiner of rat behaviour. *J. exp. Psychol.* **25,** 195–7.

BRUNSWICK, E. (1943) Organismic achievement and environmental probability. *Psychol. Rev.* **50,** 255–72.

BUCHWALD, N. A. and HULL, C. D. (1967) Some problems associated with interpretation of physiological and behavioural responses to stimulation of caudate and thalamic nuclei. *Brain Research,* **6,** 1, 1–11.

BUCY, P. C. (1944) *The Pre-Central Motor Cortex,* University of Illinois Press.

BULLOCK, T. H. (1959) Neuron doctrine and electrophysiology. *Science* **129,** 997–1002.

BURNS, B. D. (1950) Some properties of the cat's isolated cerebral cortex. *J. Physiol.* **111,** 50–68.

BURNS, B. D. (1951) Some properties of isolated cerebral cortex in the unanaesthetised cat. *J. Physiol.* **112,** 156–75.

BURNS, B. D. (1958) *The Mammalian Cerebral Cortex,* Edward Arnold, London.

BURSTEN, B. and DELGADO, J. M. R. (1958) Positive reinforcement induced by the cerebral stimulation in the monkey. *J. comp. physiol. Psychol.* **51**, 6–10.

BUSH, R. R. and MOSTELLER, F. (1951a) A mathematical model for simple learning. *Psychol. Rev.* **58**, 313–23.

BUSH, R. R. and MOSTELLER, F. (1951b) A model for stimulus generalization and discrimination. *Psychol. Rev.* **58**, 413–23.

BUSH, R. R. and MOSTELLER, F. (1955) *Stochastic Models for Learning*, John Wiley, New York.

CAJAL, R. Y (1952) *Histologie du système nerveux de l'homme et des vertébrés*, Institute Ramon y Cajal.

CAMPBELL, A. W. (1905) *Histological Studies on the Localisation of Cerebral Function*, Cambridge University Press.

CAMPBELL, R. J. and HARLOW, H. F. (1945) Problem solution by monkeys following bilateral removal of the prefrontal areas. V. Spatial delayed reactions. *J. exp. Psychol.* **35**, 110–26.

CANNON, W. B. (1929) *Bodily Changes in Pain, Hunger, Fear and Rage*, Appleton-Century, New York.

CANTRIL, H., AMES, A., HASTORF, A. H. and ITTELSON, W. H. (1949a) Psychology and scientific research. I. The nature of scientific inquiry. *Science* **110**, 461–4.

CANTRIL, H., AMES, A., HASTORF, A. H. and ITTELSON, W. H. (1949b) Psychology and scientific research. II. Scientific inquiry and scientific method. *Science* **110**, 491–7.

CANTRIL, H., AMES, A., HASTORF, A. H. and ITTELSON, W. H. (1949c) Psychology and scientific research. III. Transactional view in psychological research. *Science* **110**, 517–22.

CARNAP, R. (1937) Testability and meaning. *Phil. Sci.* **3**, 419–71; **4**, 1–40.

CARNAP, R. (1952) Empiricism, semantics and ontology. In: LEONARD LINSKY (Editor), *Semantics and the Philosophy of language*, University of Illinois Press.

CARNAP, R. (1958) *An Introduction to Symbolic Logic and Its Applications*, Dover Publications, New York.

CATE, J. TEN (1923) Essai d'étude des fonctions de l'écorce cérébrale des pigeons par la méthode des reflexes conditionnels. *Arch. Néerl. Physiol.* **8**, 234–73.

CHANCE, W. A. (1969) *Statistical Methods for Decision Making*, Irwin.

CHAPMAN, B. L. M. (1959) A self organizing classifying system. *Cybernetica* **2**, 3, 152–61.

CHOW, K. L. (1952) Further studies of selective ablation of associative cortex in relation to visually mediated behaviour. *J. comp. physiol. Psychol.* **45**, 109-18.

CHOW, K. L. (1954) Effects of temporal neocortical ablation on visual discrimination learning sets in monkeys. *J. comp. physiol. Psychol.* **47**, 194–8.

CHOW, K. L., BLUM, J. S. and BLUM, R. A. (1951) Effects of combined destruction of frontal and posterior 'association areas' in monkeys. *J. Neurophysiol.* XIV, **1**, 59–72.

CHURCH, A. (1936) An unsolvable problem of elementary number theory. *Amer. J. Math.* **58**, 345–63.

CHURCH, A. (1944) *Introduction to Mathematical Logic*, Princeton University Press.

CLARK, G. and LASHLEY, K. S. (1947) Visual disturbances following frontal ablations in the monkey. *Anat. Rec.* **97**, 326.

CLARKSON, G. P. E. (1963) Model of the trust investment process. In: E. A. FEIGEN-BAUM and J. FELDMAN (Editors), *Computers and Thought*, McGraw-Hill.

COBURN, H. E. (1951) The brain analogy. *Psychol. Rev.* **58**, 155-78.

COBURN, H. E. (1952) The brain analogy; a discussion. *Psychol. Rev.* **59**, 453-60.

COGHILL, G. E. (1929) *Anatomy and the Problem of Behaviour*, Cambridge University Press.

COLLIER, R. M. (1931) An experimental study of form perception in indirect vision. *J. comp. Psychol.* **11**, 281.

COWAN, J. (1962) Many valued logics and reliable automata. In: H. VON FOERSTER and G. W. ZOPF Jr. (Editors), *Principles of Self-Organization*, Oxford, Pergamon Press.

CRAWSHAY-WILLIAMS, R. (1946) *The Comforts of Unreason*, Routledge & Kegan Paul, London.

CRAWSHAY-WILLIAMS, R. (1957) *Methods and Criteria of Reasoning*, Routledge & Kegan Paul.

CREED, R. S., DENNY-BROWN, D., ECCLES, J. C., LIDDELL, E. G. T. and SHERRINGTON, C. S. (1932) *Reflex Activity of the Spinal Cord*, Oxford University Press.

CROSSMAN, E. R. F. W. (1953) Entropy and choice time: the effect of frequency un-balance on choice response. *Quart. J. exp. Psychol.* **5**, 41-51.

CROSSMAN, E. R. F. W. (1955) The measurement of discriminability. *Quart. J. exp. Psychol.* **7**, 176-95.

CULBERTSON, J. T. (1948) A mechanism for optic nerve conduction and form percep tion. *Bull. Math. Biophysiol.* **10**, 31-40.

CULBERTSON, J. T. (1950) *Consciousness and Behavior—a Neural Analysis of Behavior and Consciousness*, Brown, Dubuque, Iowa.

CULBERTSON, J. T. (1952) Hypothetical robots. Rand. Project P-296.

CULBERTSON, J. T. (1956) Some uneconomical robots. In: C. E. SHANNON and J. MCCARTHY (Editors), *Automata Studies*, Princeton University Press.

CULLER, E. and METTLER, F. A. (1934) Conditioned behaviour in a decorticate dog. *J. comp. Psychol.* **18**, 219-303.

DA FONSECA, J. S. (1966) *Neuronal Models*, Lisbon University.

DARROW, C. W. (1947) Psychological and psycho-physiological significance of the electroencephalogram. *Psychol. Rev.* **54**, 157-68.

DAVIS, D. M. (1958) *Computability and unsolvability*. McGraw-Hill, New York.

DELAFRESNAYE, J. F. (Editor) (1954) *Brain Mechanisms and Consciousness*, Blackwelly Oxford.

DE LEEUW, K., MOORE, E. F., SHANNON, C. E. and SHAPIRO, N. (1956) Computabilit, of probabilistic machines. In: C. E. SHANNON and J. MCCARTHY (Editors), *Automata Studies*, Princeton University Press.

DEUTSCH, J. A. (1953) A new type of behaviour theory. *Brit. J. Psychol.* **44**, 304-17.

DEUTSCH, J. A. (1954) A machine with insight. *Quart. J. exp. Psychol.* **6**, 6-11.

DEUTSCH, J. A. (1955) A theory of shape recognition. *Brit. J. Psychol.* **46**, 30-7.

DEUTSCH, J. A. (1956) The statistical theory of the figural after-effects and acuity. *Brit. J. Psychol.* **47**, 208-15.

DEUTSCH, S. (1967) *Models of the Nervous System*, Wiley.

DEWEY, J. and BENTLEY, A. (1949) *Knowing and the Known*, Beacon Press.

DODWELL, P. C. (1957) Shape recognition in rats. *Brit. J. Psychol.* **43**, 221.

DOTEY, R. W. (1965) Conditioned reflexes elicited by electrical stimulation of the brain in macaques. *J. Neurophysiol.* **28**, 623–40.

DREVER, J. (1960) Perceptual learning. *Ann. Rev. Psychol.* **11**, 131–60.

DUSSER DE BARENNE, J. G. and McCULLOCH, W. S. (1937) Local stimulatory inactivation within the cerebral cortex, the factor for extinction. *Amer. J. Physiol.* **118**, 510–28.

DUSSER DE BARENNE, J. G. and McCULLOCH, W. S. (1938) Functional organization in the sensory cortex of the monkey *(Macaca mulatta)*. *J. Neurophysiol.* **1**, 69–85.

DUSSER DE BARENNE, J. G. and McCULLOCH, W. S. (1939) Factors for facilitation and extinction in the central nervous system. *J. Neurophysiol.* **2**, 319–55.

DUSSER DE BARENNE, J. G., GAROL, H. W. and McCULLOCH, W. S. (1941) Functional organization of sensory and adjacent cortex in the monkey. *J. Neurophysiol.* **4**, 324–30.

ECCLES, J. C. (1946) Synaptic potentials of motoneurones. *J. Neurophysiol.* **9**, 87–120.

ECCLES, J. C. (1953) *The Neurophysiological Basis of Mind*, Oxford University Press.

ELWORTHY, P. H. (1956) The physical chemistry of the lecithins. *J. Pharm. Pharmacol.* **8**, 1001–18.

ELWORTHY, P. H. and SAUNDERS, L. (1955) Surface forces of lecithin sols in the presence of some inorganic salts. *J. Chem. Soc.* 1166–9.

ERLANGER, J. and GASSER, H. S. (1937) *Electrical Signs of Nervous Activity*, University of Pennsylvania Press, Philadelphia.

ESTES, W. K. (1950) Towards a statistical theory of learning. *Psychol. Rev.* **57**, 94–107.

FARLEY, B. A. and CLARK, W. A. (1961) In: E. C. CHEARY (Editor), *Information Theory*, London, Butterworth.

FEIGE, H. (1950) Existential hypotheses. *Phil. Sci.* **17**, 2, 35–62.

FITCH, F. B. and BARRY, G. (1950) Towards a formalization of Hull's behaviour theory. *Phil. Sci.* **17**, 260–5.

FRANKENHAUSER, B. (1951) Limitations of method of strychnine neuronography. *J. Neurophysiol.* XIV, **1**, 73–9.

FREGE (1893, 1903) *Grundgesetze der Arithmetik*, Vols. I and II.

FRY, D. B. and DENES, P. (1959) An analogue of the speech recognition process. In: *Mechanisation of Thought Processes*, N.P.L. Symposium.

FRY, G. A. and BARTLEY, S. H. (1935) The relation of stry light in the eye to the retinal action potential. *Amer. J. Physiol.*

FULTON, J. F. (1943) *Physiology of the Nervous System*, Oxford University Press.

FULTON, J. F. (1949) *Functional Localisation in the Frontal Lobes and Cerebellum*, Oxford University Press.

FULTON, J. F., LIVINGSTON, R. B. and DAVIS, G. D. (1947) Ablation of area 13 in primates. *Fed. Proc. Amer. Soc. exp. Biol.* **6**, 108.

GALAMBOS, R. (1956) Suppression of auditory nerve activity by stimulation of efferent fibres to cochlea. *J. Neurophysiol.* **19**, 424–37.

GALE, D. and STEWART, F. M. (1953) Infinite games with perfect information. *Ann. Math.* Study No. 28 (Princeton, 1953), 245–66.

GELERNTNER, H. (1963) Realization of a geometry theorem-proving machine. In: E. A. FEIGENBAUM and J. FELDMAN (Editors), *Computers and Thought*, McGraw-Hill.

GELERNTNER, H., HANSON, J. R. and LOVELAND, D. W. (1963) Empirical explorations of the geometry theorem machine. *Proc. Western Joint Computer Conference.*

GELLHORN, E. and JOHNSON, D. A. (1951) Further studies on the role of proprioception in cortically induced movements of the foreleg of the monkey. *Brain* **LXXIII,** 513–31.

GEORGE, F. H. (1953a) Logical constructs and psychological theory. *Psychol. Rev.* **60,** 1–6.

GEORGE, F. H. (1953b) Formalization of language systems for behaviour theory. *Psychol. Rev.* **60,** 232–40.

GEORGE, F. H. (1953c) On the figural after-effect. *Quart. J. exp. Psychol.*

GEORGE, F. H. (1953d) On the theory of the figural after-effect. *Canad. J. Psychol.* **7,** 167–71.

GEORGE, F. H. (1956a) Pragmatics. *J. Phil. Phen. Res.* 226–35.

GEORGE, F. H. (1956b) Logical networks and behaviour. *Bull. Math. Biophys.* **18,** 337–48.

GEORGE, F. H. (1957a) Behaviour network systems for finite automata. *Methodos* **9,** 279–91.

GEORGE, F. H. (1957b) Epistemology and the problem of perception. *Mind* **65,** 491–506.

GEORGE, F. H. (1957c) Programming a computer to learn. *Times Review of Science.*

GEORGE, F. H. (1957d) Logical networks and probability. *Bull. Math. Biophys.* **19,** 187–99.

GEORGE, F. H. (1958) Probabilistic machines. *Automation Prog* **3,** 19–21.

GEORGE, F. H. (1959a) Models and theories in social psychology. In: LLEWELLYN GROSS (Editor), *Symposium on Sociological Theory,* Row, Peterson & Co., Evanston, Illinois.

GEORGE, F. H. (1959b) Inductive machines and the problem of learning. *Cybernetica* **2,** 109–26.

GEORGE, F. H. (1960a) Modèles de la pensée. *Cahiers de L'Institut de science économique appliquée,* No. 98, series 3.

GEORGE, F. H. (1960b) Models in Cybernetics. In Symposium of Soc. Exp. Biol. on *Models and Analogues in Biology,* vol. 14, pp. 169–91, Cambridge University Press.

GEORGE, F. H. (1962) Acuity and the theory of figural after-effects. *J. Exp. Psychol.*

GEORGE, F. H. (1962) Simple adaptive programs for computers. Paper read at Conference on Cybernetics, U.C.L.A.

GEORGE, F. H. (1965) *Cybernetics and Biology,* Oliver & Boyd.

GEORGE, F. H. (1966) Hypothesis confirmation on a digital computer. Paper read at Conference of Bionics, Dayton, Ohio.

GEORGE, F. H. (1970) *Models of Thinking,* George Allen & Unwin.

GEORGE, F. H. and HANDLON, J. H. (1955) Towards a general theory of behaviour. *Methodos* **7,** 25–44.

GEORGE, F. H. and HANDLON, J. H. (1957) A language for perceptual analysis. *Psychol. Rev.* **64,** 14–25.

GEORGE, F. H. and SARKAR, P. A. (1970) An introduction to LIP programming. *J. Inst. Comp. Sci.* **1,** 2.

GEORGE, F. H. and STEWART, D. J. (1967) On programming digital computers to learn In: *Learning and Automaton Theory,* Academic Press.

GIBSON, J. J. (1950) *The Perception of the Visual World,* Houghton Miflin, New York.

GIBSON, J. J. (1952) The visual field and the visual world: a reply to Professor Boring· *Psychol. Rev.* **59**, 149–51.

GINSBERG, S. (1962) *An Introduction to Mathematical Machine Theory*, Reading, Mass. Addison-Wesley.

GLUSHKOV, V. M. (1962) *Synthesis of Digital Automata*, Moscow.

GODEL, K. (1931) Über formal unentscheidbare Sätze der Principia Mathematica und verwandter System 1. *Mh. Math. Phys.* **38**, 173–98.

GOLDMAN, S. (1953) *Information Theory*, Constable, London.

GOLDSTEIN, K. (1939) *The Organism*, American Book Co.

GOODE, H. H. and MACHOL, R. E. (1957) *System Engineering*, McGraw-Hill, New York.

GRAHAM, C. H. (1952) Behavior and the psychophysical methods: an analysis of some recent experiments. *Psychol. Rev.* **59**, 62–70.

GRANIT, R. (1947) *Sensory Mechanisms of the Retina*, Oxford University Press.

GRANIT, R. (1955) *Receptors and Sensory Perception*, Yale University Press.

GREGORY, R. L. (1960) A paper read at meeting of Experimental Psychology Society.

GRIFFITH, J. S. (1967) *A View of the Brain*, Oxford University Press.

GRIFFITH, J. S. (1971) *Mathematical Neurobiology*, Academic Press.

GRODINS, F. G. (1963) *Control Theory and Biological Systems*, Columbia University Press.

GUTHRIE, E. R. (1935) *The Psychology of Learning*, Harper, New York.

GUTHRIE, E. R. (1942) Conditioning: a theory of learning in terms of stimulus, response and association. Chapter 1 in *The Psychology of Learning*. Natl. Soc. Stud. Educ. 41st Yearbook, part II, 17–60.

GUTHRIE, E. R. and HORTON, G. P. (1946) *Cats in a Puzzle Box*, Rinehart, London.

HALL, K. R. L., EARLE, A. E. and CROOKES, T. G. (1952) A pendulum phenomenon in the visual perception of apparent movement. *Quart. J. exp. Psychol.* **4**, 109–20.

HANEY, G. W. (1931) The effect of familiarity on maze performance of albino rats. *Univ. Calif. Publ. Psychol.* **4**, 319–33.

HARLOW, H. F. (1949) The formation of learning sets. *Psychol. Rev.* **56**, 51–65.

HARLOW, H. F. (1959) Behavioral contributions to interdisciplinary research. In: H. F. HARLOW and C. N. WOOLSEY (Editors), *Biological and Biochemical Bases of Behavior*, University of Wisconsin Press.

HARLOW, H. F., MEYER, D. and SETTLAGE, P. H. (1951) The effects of large cortical lesions on the solution of oddity problems by monkeys. *J. comp. physiol. Psychol.* **44**, 320–6.

HAYEK, S. A. (1952) *The Sensory Order*, University of Chicago.

HAYES, R. M. (1963) Mathematical models in information retrieval. *In Natural Language and the Computer*, McGraw-Hill.

HEBB, D. O. (1945) Man's frontal lobes: a critical review. *Arch. Neurol. Psychiat.* **54**, 10–24.

HEBB, D. O. (1949) *The Organization of Behavior*, John Wiley, New York.

HEBB, D. O. (1955) Drives and the CNS (conceptual nervous system). *Psychol. Rev.* **62**, 243–54.

HEMPEL, C. G. and OPPENHEIM, P. (1948) The logic of explanation. *Philos. Sci.* **15**,

HEMPEL, C. G. and OPPENHEIM, P. (1953) The logic of explanation. In: H. FEIGL and M. BRODBEK (Editors), *Readings in the Philosophy of Science*, Appleton-Century-Crofts, New York.

HENRY, C. E. and SCOVILLE, W. B. (1952) Suppression-burst activity from isolated cerebral cortex in man. *Electroenceph. clin. Neurophysiol.* **4**, 1–22.

HERNÁNDEZ-PÉON, R., SCHERRER, H. and JOUVET, M. (1956) Modification of electric activity in the cochlear nucleus during 'attention' in unanaesthetized cats. *Science* **123**, 331.

HEYTING, A. (1934) Mathematische Grundlagenforschung. Intuitionismus. Beweistheorie. *Ergebnisse der Mathematik und ihrer Grenzgebiete*, Vol. 4, Springer, Berlin.

HICK, W. E. (1952) On the rate of gain of information. *Quart. J. exp. Psychol.* **4**, 11–26.

HILBERT, D. (1922) *Die logischen Grundlagen der Mathematik. Math. Ann.* **88**, 151–65.

HILGARD, E. R. *Theories of Learning*, Appleton-Century-Crofts, New York.

HILGARD, E. R. and MARQUIS, D. G. (1940) *Conditioning and Learning*, Appleton-Century-Crofts, New York.

HILL, D. (1950) Electroencephalography as an instrument of research in psychiatry. In: D. RICHTER (Editor), *Perspective in Neuro-psychiatry*, Lewis, London.

HINES, M. (1936) The anterior border of the monkey's cortex and the production of spasticity. *Amer. J. Physiol.* **116**, 76.

HODGKIN, A. L. (1951) The tonic basis of electrical activity in nerve and muscle. *Biol. Rev.* **26**, 339–409.

HODGKIN, A. L. (1957) Croonian lecture. *Proc. Roy. Soc.*

HOLT, E. B. (1931) *Animal Drive and the Learning Process*, Holt, New York.

HOLWAY, A. H. and BORING, E. G. (1941) Determinants of apparent visual size with distant variant. *Amer. J. Psychol.* **54**, 21–37.

HOUSEHOLDER, A. S. and LANDAHL, H. D. (1945) *Mathematical Biophysics of the Central Nervous System*, Principia Press, Bloomington, Indiana.

HUBEL, D. H. (1967) Effects of distortion of sensory input on the visual system of kittens. *Physiologist*, **10**, 17 ff.

HUBEL, D. H. and WIESEL, T. N. (1959) Receptive fields of single neurons in the cat's striate cortex. *J. Physiol.* **148**, 574–91.

HUBEL, D. H. and WIESEL, T. N. (1962) Receptive fields, binocular interaction, and functional architecture in the cat's visual cortex. *J. Physiol.* **160**, 106–23.

HUBEL, D. H. and WIESEL, T. N. (1963) Receptive fields and functional architecture in two nonstriate visual areas. *J. Neurophysiol.* **28**, 229–89.

HULL, C. L. (1943) *Principles of Behaviour*, Appleton-Century-Crofts, New York.

HULL, C. L. (1950) Behavior postulates and corollaries—1949. *Psychol. Rev.* **57**, 173–80.

HULL, C. L. (1952) *A Behavior System: An Introduction to Behavior Theory Concerning the Individual Organism*, Yale University Press.

HULL, C. L., HOVLAND, C. I., ROSS, R. T., HALL, M., PERKINS, D. T. and FITCH, F. B. (1940) *Mathematico-deductive Theory of Rote Learning: A Study in Scientific Methodology*, Yale University Press.

HUMPHREY, G. (1933) *The Nature of Learning in Its Relation to the Living System*, Kegan Paul, New York.

HUMPHREY, G. (1951) *Thinking*, Methuen, London.

HUMPHREYS, L. G. (1939a) The effect of random alternation of reinforcement on the acquisition and extinction of conditioned eyelid reactions. *J. exp. Psychol.* **25**, 141–58.

HUMPHREYS, L. G. (1939b) Acquisition and extinction of verbal expectations in a situation analogous to conditioning. *J. exp. Psychol.* **25**, 294–301.

HUNT, E. B. (1962) *Concept Learning: An Information Processing Problem*, John Wiley.

ITTELSON, W. H. and CANTRIL, H. (1954) *Perception: A Transactionalist Approach*, Doubleday, New York.

JACKSON, J. H. (1931) *Selected Writings of John Hughlings Jackson*, 2 vols., Hodder & Stoughton, London.

JACOBSEN, H. (1951) The informational capacity of the human eye. *Science* **113**, 292.

JACOBSON, C. F. (1931) A study of cerebral function in learning. The frontal lobes. *J. comp. Neurol.* **52**, 271–340.

JACOBSON, C. F. (1935) Functions of frontal association areas in primates. *Arch. Neurol. Psychiat.* **33**, 558–69.

JACOBSON, C. F. (1936) Studies of cerebral functions in primates. I. The functions of the frontal association areas in monkeys. *Comp. Psychol. Monogr.* **13**, 63, 3–60.

JACOBSON, C. F. and ELDER, J. H. (1936) Studies of cerebral functions in primates. II. The effect of temporal lobe lesions on delayed response in monkeys. *Comp. Psychol. Monogr.* **13**, 63, 61-5.

JACOBSON, C. F. and HASLERAND, G. M. (1936) Studies of cerebral functions in primates. III. A note on the effect of motor and premotor area lesions on delayed response in monkeys. *Comp. Psychol. Monogr.* **13**, 66–8.

JACOBSON, C. F., WOLFE, J. B. and JACKSON, T. A. (1935) An experimental analysis of the functions of the frontal association areas in primates. *J. nerv. ment. Dis.* **82**, 1–14.

JAMES, P. H. R. (1957) Learning sets. A talk given at Bristol University, England.

JAMES, W. (1890) *The Principles of Psychology*, Holt, New York.

JASPER, H. H. (1958) Reticular-cortical systems and theories of the integrative action of the brain. In: H. F. HARLOW and C. N. WOOLSEY (Editors), *Biological and Biochemical Cases of Behavior*, University of Wisconsin Press.

JEFFERY, R. C. (1965) *The Logic of Decision*, McGraw-Hill.

JENKINS, W. O. and STAKLEY, J. C. (1950) Partial reinforcement: a review and a critique. *Psychol. Bull.* **47**, 193–234.

KAPLAN, A. and SCHOTT (1951) A calculus for empirical classes. *Methodos* **3**, 165–90.

KAPPERS, C. U. A., HUBER, G. C. and CROSBY, E. C. (1936) *The Comparative Anatomy of the Nervous System of Vertebrates, including Man*, Macmillan, New York.

KELLER, F. S. (1940) The effect of sequence of continuous and periodic reinforcement upon the reflex reserve. *J. exp. Psychol.* **27**, 559–65.

KENDLER, H. H. (1947) An investigation of latent learning in a T-maze. *J. comp. physiol. Psychol.* **40**, 256–70.

KENDLER, H. H. (1952) Some comments on Thistlethwaite's perception of latent learning. *Psychol. Bull.* **49**, 47–51.

KENNARD, M. A., SPENCER, S. and FOUNTAIN, G. (1941) Hyperactivity in monkeys following lesions of the frontal lobes. *J. Neurophysiol.* **4**, 512–24.

KENNEDY, A. (1960) A possible artifact in electroencephalography. *Psychol. Rev.* **66**, 347–52.

KILPATRICK, F. P. (Editor) (1953) *Human Behavior from the Transactional Point of View*, Institute for Associated Research, Hanover, New Hampshire.

KLEENE, S. C. (1951) Representation of events in nerve nets and finite automata. Rand Research Memorandum, RM 704.

KLUVER, H. (1933) *Behavior Mechanisms in Monkeys*, Chicago University Press.

KÖHLER, W. (1925) *The Mentality of Apes*, Kegan Paul, London.

KÖHLER, W. (1940) *Dynamics in Psychology*, Liveright, New York.

KÖHLER, W. and WALLACH, H. (1944) Figural after effects: an investigation of visual processes. *Proc. Amer. Phil. Soc.* **88**, 269–357.

KONORSKI, J. (1948) *Conditioned Reflexes and Neuron Organization*, Cambridge University Press.

KÖRNER, S. (1951) Ostensive predicates. *Mind* **9**, 60, 80–9.

KÖRNER, S. (1959) *Conceptual Thinking*, Dover Publications, New York.

KORZYBSKI, A. (1933) *Science and Sanity*, Science Press.

KRECHEVSKY, I. (1932a) The genesis of 'hypotheses' in rats. *Univ. Calif. Publ. Psychol.* **6**, 45–64.

KRECHEVSKY, I. (1932b) 'Hypotheses' in rats. *Psychol. Rev.* **39**, 516–32.

KRECHEVSKY, I. (1933a) Hereditary nature of 'hypotheses'. *J. comp. Psychol.* **15**, 429–43.

KRECHEVSKY, I. (1933b) The docile nature of 'hypotheses'. *J. comp. Psychol.* **15**, 429–43.

KRECHEVSKY, I. (1935) Brain mechanisms and 'hypotheses'. *J. comp. Psychol.* **19**, 425–68.

KRUGER, L. (1965) Morphological alterations of the cerebral cortex and their possible role in the loss and acquisition of information. In: D. P. KIMBLE (Editor), *Anatomy of Memory*, pp. 88–139, Science and Behavior Books, Palo Alto.

KULPE, O. (1893) *Grundriss der Psychologie*, Berlin.

LADEFOGED, P. (1959) The perception of speech. In: *Mechanisation of Thought Processes*, N.P.L. Symposium.

LANDAHL, H. D. (1952) Mathematical biophysics of colour vision. *Bull. Math. Biophys.* **14**, 317–25.

LANDAHL, H. D. and RUNGE, R. (1946) Outline of a matrix calculus for neural nets. *Bull. Math. Biophys.* **8**, 75–81.

LASHLEY, K. S. (1929a) Learning. I. Nervous mechanism in learning. In: C. MURCHISON (Editor), *The Foundations of Experimental Psychology*, Clark University Press.

LASHLEY, K. S. (1929b) *Brain Mechanisms and Intelligence*, University of Chicago Press.

LASHLEY, K. S. (1942) The problem of cerebral organization in vision. *Biol. Symposium* **7**, 301–22.

LASHLEY, K. S. (1947) Structural variations in the nervous system in relation to behavior. *Psychol. Rev.* **54**, 6.

LASHLEY, K. S. (1949) The problem of serial order in behavior. In: L. A. JEFRESS (Editor), *Hixon Symposium on Cerebral Mechanisms in Behavior*.

LASHLEY, K. S. (1950) In search of the engram. In: Symposium of Soc. Exp. Biol. on *Physiological Mechanisms in Animal Behaviour*, Vol. 4, Cambridge University Press.

LAWRENCE, M. (1949a) *Studies in Human Behaviour*, Princeton University Press.

LAWRENCE, M. (1949b) *An Inquiry into the Nature of Perception*, Princeton Institute for Associated Research.

LE GROS CLARK, W. E. (1950) The structure of the brain and the process of thinking· In: PETER LASLETT (Editor), *The Physical Basis of Mind*, Blackwell, Oxford.

LEWIS, C. I. (1946) *Analysis of Knowledge and Valuation*, Open Court Publishing Co., La Salle, Illinois.

LEWIS, C. I. and LANGFORD, C. H. (1932) *Symbolic Logic*, The Century Co., New York.

LI, C. L., CULLER, C. and JASPER, H. H. (1956) Laminar microelectrode analysis of cortical unspecific recruiting responses and spontaneous rhythms. *J. Neurophysiol.* **19**, 131–43.

LIDDELL, E. G. T. and PHILLIPS, C. G. (1951) Thresholds for cortical representation. *Brain* **73**, 125–40.

LILLY, J. C. (1958) Correlations between neurophysiological activity in the cortex and short-term behavior in the monkey. In: H. F. HARLOW and C. N. WOOLSEY (Editors), *Biological and Biochemical Bases of Behavior*, University of Wisconsin Press.

LINDSAY, R. K. (1963) Inferential memory as the basis of machines which understand natural language. In: A. FEIGENBAUM and J. FELDMAN (Editors), *Computers and Thought*, McGraw-Hill.

LINDSLEY, D. B. (1951) Emotion. In: S. S. STEVENS (Editor), *Handbook of Experimental Psychology*, John Wiley, New York.

LITMAN, R. A. and ROSEN, E. (1950) Molar and molecular. *Psychol. Rev.* **57**, 58–65.

LOFGREN, L. (1962a) Limits for automatic error correction. In: H. VON FOERSTER and G. W. ZOPF, Jr. (Editors), *Principles of Self-Organization*, Oxford, Pergamon Press.

LOFGREN, L. (1962b) Kinematic and tessellation models of self-repair. In: E. E. BERNARD and M. R. CANE (Editors), *Biological Prototypes and Synthetic Systems*, Plenum Press.

LONDON, I. D. (1950) An ideal equation derived for a class of forgetting curves. *Psychol. Rev.* **57**, 295–302.

LONDON, I. D. (1951) An ideal equation of forgetting derived for overlearning. *Psychol. Rev.* **58**, 45–9.

LORENTE DE NÓ, R. (1938a) Synaptic stimulation of motoneurons as a local process. *J. Neurophysiol.* **1**, 195–206.

LORENTE DE NÓ, R. (1938b) Analysis of the activity of the chains of internuncial neurons. *J. Neurophysiol.* **1**, 207–44.

LORENTE DE NÓ, R. (1947) *A Study of Nerve Physiology*, Vols. 1 and 2. In studies from the Rockefeller Institute for Medical Research, Vols. 131 and 132.

LORENZ, K. (1950) The comparative method of studying innate behaviour patterns. Symposium Vol. 4 of Soc. Exp. Biol. on *Physiological Mechanisms in Animal Behaviour*, Cambridge University Press.

LUCE, R. D. and RAIFFA, H. (1957) *Games and Decisions*, Wiley.

MCCARTHY, J. (1961) A basis for a mathematical theory of computation. *Proc. Western Joint Computer Conference*.

MACCORQUODALE, K. and MEEHL, P. E. (1954) Edvard C. Tolman. In: ESTES *et al.*, *Modern Learning Theory*, A. T. POFFENBERGER (Editor), Appleton-Century Crofts, New York.

MacFarlane, D. A. (1930) The role of kinesthesis in maze learning. *Univ. Calif. Publ. Psychol.* **4,** 277–305.

Mackay, D. M. (1951) Mindlike behaviour in artefacts. *Brit. J. Phil. Sci.* **2,** 105–21.

Mackay, D. M. (1956) The epistemological problem for automata. In: C. E. Shannon and J. McCarthy (Editors), *Automata Studies,* Princeton University Press.

Magoun, H. W. (1958) Non-specific brain mechanisms. In: H. F. Harlow and C. N. Woolsey (Editors), *Biological and Biochemical Bases of Behavior,* University of Wisconsin Press.

Maltzman, I. (1952) The Blodgett and Haney types of latent learning experiment: Reply to Thistlethwaite. *Psychol. Bull.* **49,** 52–60.

Marsan, C. A. and Stoll, J. (1951) Subcortical connections of the temporal pole in relation to temporal lobe seizures. *Arch. Neurol. Psych.* **66,** 669–86.

Marshall, W. H. and Talbot, S. A. (1942) Recent evidence for neural mechanisms in vision leading to a general theory of sensory acuity. In: H. Kluver (Editor,) *Visual Mechanisms. Biol. Symposium.* **7,** 117–64.

Masserman, J. H. (1943) *Behavior and Neurosis: An Experimental Psycho-analytic Approach to Psycho-biological Principles,* Chicago University Press.

McCulloch, W. S. (1959) Agatha tyche: of nervous nets—the lucky reckoners. In: *Mechanisation of Thought Processes,* N.P.L. Symposium, pp. 611–26.

McCulloch, W. S. and Pitts, W. (1943) A logical calcula of the ideas immanent in nervous activity. *Bull. Math. Biophys.* **5,** 115–33.

McDougall, W. (1923) *Outline of Psychology,* Scribners, New York.

McGaugh, J. L. (1966) Time-dependent processes in memory storage. *Ann. Rev. Physiol.* **28,** 107–36.

McNaughton, R. (1961) The theory of automata, a survey. In: F. L. Alt (Editor), *Advances in Computers,* Vol. II, Academic Press.

Meehl, P. E. (1950) On the circularity of the law of effect. *Psychol. Bull.* **47,** 52–75.

Meehl, P. E. and MacCorquodale, K. (1951) Some methodological comments concerning expectancy theory. *Psychol. Rev.* **58,** 230–3.

Mettler, F. A. (1944) Physiologic effects of bilateral simultaneous frontal lesions in the primate. *J. comp. Neurol.* **81,** 105–36.

Meyer, D. R. (1951) Food deprivation and discrimination reversal learning by monkeys. *J. exp. Psychol.* **41,** 10–16.

Meyer, D. R. (1958) Some psychological determinants of sparing and loss following damage to the brain. In: H. F. Harlow and C. N. Woolsey (Editors), *Biological and Biochemical Bases of Behavior,* University of Wisconsin Press.

Miller, G. A., Galanter, E. H. and Pribram, K. H. (1960) *Plans and the Structure of Behavior.* Henry Holt.

Miller, N. E. and Dilara, L. (1967) Instrumental learning of heart rate changes in curarized rats; shaping and specificity to discriminative stimulus. *J. comp. physiol. Psychol.* **63** (1), 12–19.

Miller, N. E. and Dollard, J. C. (1941) *Social Learning and Limitation,* Yale University Press.

Miller, N. E. and Kessen, M. L. (1952) Reward effects of food via stomach fistula compared with those of food via mouth. *J. comp. physiol. Psychol.* **45,** 555–64.

Milner, B. (1958) Psychological defects produced by temporal lobe excision. *The*

Brain and Human Behavior, Research Publ. Assoc. Nervous Mental Disease, pp. 244–57.

MILNER, B. and PENFIELD, W. (1955) The effect of hippocampal lesions on recent memory. *Trans. Amer. Neurol. Assoc.* **80,** 42–8.

MILNER, P. M. (1957) The cell assembly: Mark II. *Psychol. Rev.* **64,** 242–52.

MINSKY, M. L. (1954) *Neural-analog Networks and the Brain-model Problem*, Princeton University. Microfilmed.

MINSKY, M. L. (1959) Some methods of artificial intelligence and heuristic programming. In: *Mechanisation of Thought Processes*, N.P.L. Symposium.

MOORE, E. F. (1964) *Sequential Machines: Selected Papers*, Addison-Wesley.

MOORE, E. F. and SHANNON, C. E. (1956) Reliable circuitry using less reliable relays. *J. Franklin Inst.* **262,** 191–208; 281–98.

MORRELL, F. and JASPER, H. H. (1955) Conditioning of cortical electrical activity in the monkey. *Proc. Amer. EEG Soc.* **9.**

MORRELL, F., ROBERTS, L. and JASPER, H. H. (1956) Effect of focal epileptogenic lesions and their ablation upon conditioned electrical responses of the brain in the monkey. *Electroenceph. clin. Neurophysiol.* **8,** 217–36.

MORRIS, C. W. (1946) *Signs, Language and Behavior*, Prentice Hall, New York.

MORUZZI, G. and MAGOUN, H. W. (1949) Brain stem reticular formation and activation of the EEG. *Electroenceph. clin. Neurophysiol.* **1,** 455–73.

MOWRER, O. H. and JONES, H. W. (1943) Extinction and behavior variability as functions of effortlessness of task. *J. exp. Psychol.* **33,** 369–89.

MUELLER, C. G. JR. and SCHOENFELD, W. N. (1954) Edwin R. Guthrie. In: W. K. ESTES and OTHERS, *Modern Learning Theory*, Appleton-Century-Crofts, New York, pp. 345–79.

NEWELL, A. (1961) *Information Processing Language. V. Manuel*, Prentice Hall.

NEWELL, A., SHAW, J. C. and SIMON, H. A. (1958) Elements in a theory of human problem solving. *Psychol. Rev.* **65,** 151–66.

NEWELL, A., SHAW, J. C. and SIMON, H. A. (1963) Empirical exploration with the logic theory machine: a case study in heuristics. In: A. FEIGENBAUM and J. FELDMAN (Editors), *Computers and Thought*, McGraw-Hill.

OETTINGER, A. E. (1952) Programming a digital computer to learn. *Phil. Mag.* **1, 43,** 1243–63.

OLDFIELD, R. C. (1954) Memory mechanisms and the theory of schemata. *Brit. J. Psychol.* 14–23.

OLDS, J. A. (1959) High functions of the nervous system. *Ann. Rev. Physiol.* **21,** 381–407.

OLDS, J. A. and MILNER, P. (1954) Positive reinforcement produced by electrical stimulation of septal area and other regions of rat brain. *J. comp. physiol. Psychol.* **47,** 419–27.

OLDS, J. and OLDS, M. (1965) Drives, rewards and the brain. In: *New Directions in Psychology* **2,** 327–410, Holt, Rinehart & Winston, New York.

OLIVER, W. D. (1951) *The Theory of Order*, The Antioch Press.

OSGOOD, C. E. (1949) The similarity paradox in human learning: a resolution. *Psychol. Rev.* **56,** 132–43.

OSGOOD, C. E. (1953) *Method and Theory in Experimental Psychology*, Oxford University Press.

OSGOOD, C. E. and HEYER, A. W. (1952) A new interpretation of figural after-effects. *Psychol. Rev.* **59,** 98–118.

PAP, A. (1949) *Elements of Analytic Philosophy*, Macmillan, New York.

PASCH, A. (1958) *Experience and the Analytic*, Chicago University Press.

PASK, A. G. (1957) Automatic teaching techniques. *Brit. Comm. Elect.* pp. 210–11.

PASK, A. G. (1958) The growth process in a cybernetic machine. *Proc. Second Congress International Association of Cybernetics.*

PASK, A. G. (1959) Organic control and the cybernetic method. *Cybernetica.*

PASK, A. G. (1959) Physical analogues to the growth of a concept. In: *Mechanisation of Thought Processes.* N.P.L. Symposium.

PAVLOV, I. P. (1927) *Conditioned Reflexes*, Oxford University Press.

PAVLOV, I. P. (1928) *Lectures on Conditioned Reflexes*, International Publishers.

PEANO, G. (1894) *Notations de logique mathématique*, Torino.

PEIRCE, C. S. (1931–5) *The Collected Papers of Charles Sanders Peirce*, 6 vols., Harvard University Press.

PENFIELD, W. (1947) Some observations on the cerebral cortex of man. *Proc. Roy. Soc.* **134,** 329–47.

PENFIELD, W. and RASMUSSEN, T. (1950) *The Cerebral Cortex of Man*, Macmillan.

PIERCY, M. F. (1957) Conceptual disorientation in the horizontal plane. *Quart. J. exp. Psychol.* **9,** 65–77.

PITTS, W. and McCULLOCH, W. S. (1947) How we know universals. The perception of auditory and visual forms. *Bull. Math. Biophys.* **9,** 127.

POSTMAN, L. (1947) The history and present status of the law of effect. *Psychol. Bull.* **44,** 489–563.

PRIBRAM, K. H. (1958) Neocortical functions in behavior. In: H. F. HARLOW and C. N. WOOLSEY (Editors), *Biological and Biochemical Bases of Behavior*, University of Wisconsin Press.

PRIBRAM, K. H. (1960) Theory in physiological psychology. *Ann. Rev. Psychol.* **11,** 1–40.

PRICE, H. H. (1953) *Thinking and Experience*, Hutchinson.

PRINGLE, J. W. S. (1951) On the parallel between learning and evolution. *Behaviour* **3,** 174–215.

QUINE, W. V. O. (1953) *From a Logical Point of View*, Oxford University Press.

RABIN, M. O. (1956) Effective computability of winning strategies. In: M. DRESHER, A. W. TUCKER and P. WOLFE (Editors), *Contributions to the Theory of Games.*

RABIN, M. O. and SCOTT, D. (1959) Finite automata and their decision problems. *J. Res. Develop.* **3,** 114–25.

RAMSEY, E. P. (1931) *The Foundations of Mathematics*, Kegan Paul, London.

RAPHAEL, B. (1964) SIR: a computer program for Semantic Information Retrieval. Ph.D. Thesis, M.I.T., Cambridge, Mass.

RAPOPORT, A. (1950a) Contribution to the probabilistic theory of neural nets. I. Randomization of refractory periods and of stimulus interaction. *Bull. Math. Biophys.* **12,** 109–21.

RAPOPORT, A. (1950b) Contribution to the probabilistic theory of neural nets. II. Facilitation and threshold phenomena. *Bull. Math. Biophys.* **12,** 187-97.

RAPOPORT, A. (1950c) Contribution to the probabilistic theory of neural nets. III. Specific inhibition. *Bull. Math. Biophys.* **12,** 317–25.

RAPOPORT, A. (1950d) Contribution to the probabilistic theory of neural nets. IV. Various models for inhibition. *Bull. Math. Biophys.* **12**, 327–37.

RAPOPORT, A. (1952) Ignition phenomena in random nets. *Bull. Math. Biophys.* **17**, 15–33.

RAPOPORT, A. (1955) Application of information networks to a theory of vision. *Bull. Math. Biophys.* **17**, 15–33.

RASHEVSKY, A. (1938) *Mathematical Biophysics*, University of Chicago Press.

REICHENBACH, H. (1938) *Experience and Prediction*, University of Chicago Press.

RIESEN, A. H. (1947) The development of visual perception in man and chimpanzee. *Science* **106**, 107–8.

RIESEN, A. H. (1966) Sensory deprivation. In: E. STELLAR, J. M. SPRAGUE (Editors), *Progress in Physiological Psychology*, **1**, 117–47, Academic Press, New York.

RIGGS, L. A., RATCLIFFE, F., CORNSWEET, J. C. and CORNSWEET, T. N. (1953) Disappearance of a steadily fixated visual test object. *J. Opt. Soc. Amer.* **43**, 495–501.

RIOPELLE, A. J., ALPER, R. G., STRONG, P. N. and ADES, H. W. (1953) Multiple discrimination and patterned string performance of normal and temporal lobectomized monkeys. *J. comp. physiol. Psychol.* **46**, 145–9.

ROBERTS, L. G. (1966) Pattern recognition with an adaptive network. In: L. UHR (Editor), *Pattern Recognition*, Wiley.

ROSEN, R. (1964) Abstract biological systems as sequential machines. *Bull. Math. Biophys.* **26**, 103–111.

ROSENBLATT, F. (1958) The perceptron—a theory of statistical separability in cognitive systems. Cornell Aeronautical Laboratory Inc., Report No. VG-1196-G-1.

ROSENBLATT, F. (1959) Two theorems of statistical separability in the perceptron. In: *Mechanisation of Thought Processes*, N.P.L. Symposium.

ROSENZWEIG, M. R. and LEIMAN, A. L. (1968) Brain functions. In *Ann. Rev. Psychol.* pp. 55-98.

ROSSER, J. B. and TURQUETTE, A. R. (1952) *Many-valued Logics*, North Holland Publishing Co.

RUCH, T. C. and SHENKIN, H. A. (1943) The relation to area 13 on orbital surface of frontal lobes to hyperactivity and hyperphagia in monkeys. *J. Neurophysiol.* **6**, 349–60.

RUSSELL, G. (1957) Learning machines and adaptive control mechanisms. RRE Memo. No. 1369.

RYLE, G. (1949) *The Concept of Mind*, Hutchinson, London.

SAMUEL, A. L. (1963) Some studies in machine learning using the game of checkers. In: A. FEIGENBAUM and J. FELDMAN (Editors), *Computers and Thought*, McGraw-Hill.

SAMUEL, A. L. (1967) Some studies in machine learning using the game of checkers. II. Recent progress. *IBM J. Res. Dev.* **6**, 601.

SAUNDERS, L. (1953) Interfaces between aqueous liquids. *J. Chem. Soc.* **105**, 519–25.

SAUNDERS, L. (1957) Some properties of mixed sols of lecithin and lysolecithin. *J. Pharm. Pharmacol.* **9**, 834–9.

SAUNDERS, L. and THOMAS, I. L. (1958) Diffusion studies with lysolecithin. *J. Chem. Soc.* **85**, 483–5.

SCHADE, J. P. and FORD, D. H. (1965) *Basic Neurology*, Elsevier.

SCOVILLE, W. B. and MILNER, B. (1957) Loss of recent memory after bilateral hippo-campal lesions. *J. Neurol. Neurosurg. Psychiat.* **20,** 11–21.

SELFRIDGE, O. G. (1956) Pattern recognition and learning. In: E. C. CHERRY (Editor), *Information Theory*, Butterworth, London.

SELFRIDGE, O. G. (1959) Pandemonium: A paradigm for learning. In: *Mechanisation of Thought Processes*, N.P.L. Symposium.

SELLARS, W. (1947) Epistemology and the new way of words. *J. Philosophy* **44,** 24.

SEMMES, J. and MISHKIN, M. (1965) Somatosensory loss in monkeys after ipsilateral cortical ablation. *J. Neurophysiol.* **28,** 473–86.

SETTLAGE, P., ZABLE, M. and HARLOW, H. F. (1948) Problem solution by monkeys following bilateral removal of the prefrontal areas. VL. Performance on tests requiring contradictory reactions to similar and to identical stimuli. *J. exp. Psychol.* **38,** 50–65.

SEWARD, P. J. (1949) An experimental analysis of latent learning. *J. exp. Psychol.* **39,** 177–86.

SEWARD, P. J. (1950) Secondary reinforcement as tertiary motivation: a revision of Hull's revision. *Psychol. Rev.* **57,** 362–74.

SEWARD, P. J. (1951) Experimental evidence for the motivating function of reward. *Psychol. Bull.* **48,** 13–49.

SEWARD, P. J. (1952) Delayed reward learning. *Psychol. Rev.* **59,** 200–1.

SEWARD, P. J. (1953) How are motives learned? *Psychol. Rev.* **60,** 99–110.

SHANES, A. M. (1953) Electro-chemical aspects of physiological and pharmacological action in excitable cells. *Pharm. Revs.* **10,** 61–273.

SHANNON, C. E. (1949) Synthesis of two-terminal switching circuits. *Bell Syst. tech. J.* **28,** 656 715.

SHANNON, C. E. (1950) Programming a computer for playing chess. *Phil. Mag.* 356–375.

SHANNON, C. E. (1951) Presentation of a maze-solving machine. In: HEINZ VON FOERSTER (Editor), *Cybernetics*. Transactions of the Eighth Conference of the Josiah Macy Jr. Found., pp. 173–80.

SHANNON, C. E. and WEAVER, W. (1949) *The Mathematical Theory of Communication*, University of Illinois Press.

SHARLOCK, D. P., NEFF, W. D. and STROMINGER, N. L. (1965) Discrimination of tone during and after bilateral ablation of auditory cortical areas. *J. Neurophysiol.* **28,** 673.

SHARPLESS, S. and JASPER, H. H. (1956) Habituation of arousal reaction. *Brain* **79,** 655–80.

SHEFFIELD, F. D. (1949) 'Spread of effect' without reward or learning. *J. exp. Psychol.* **35,** 575–9.

SHEFFIELD, F. D. and ROBY, T. B. (1950) Reward value of a non-nutritive sweet taste. *J. comp. physiol. Psychol.* **43,** 471–81.

SHEFFIELD, F. D. and TENMER, H. W. (1950) Relative resistance to extinction of escape training and avoidance training. *J. exp. Psychol.* **40,** 287–98.

SHEFFIELD, F. D., ROBY, T. B. and CAMPBELL, B. A. (1954) Drive reduction versus consummatory behavior as determinants of reinforcement. *J. comp. physiol. Psychol.* **47,** 349–54.

SHEFFIELD, F. D., WOLFF, J. J. and BACKER, R. (1951) Reward value of copulation without sex drive reduction. *J. comp. physiol. Psychol.* **44**, 3–8.

SHEPHERDSON, J. C. (1959) The reduction of two-way automata to one-way automata, *I.B.M. Journal of Research and Development* **3**, 2, 198–200.

SHERMAN, H. (1959) A quasi-topological method for the recognition of line patterns. *Proc. ICIP*, Paris.

SHERRINGTON, C. S. (1906) *Integrative Action of the Nervous System*, Constable, London.

SHIMBEL, A. (1949) Input–output problems in simple-nerve ganglion system. *Bull. Math. Biophys.* **11**, 165–71.

SHIMBEL, A. (1952) Some elementary considerations of neural models. *Bull. Math. Biophys.* **14**, 68–71.

SHOLL, D. A. (1956) *The Organization of the Cerebral Cortex*, John Wiley, New York.

SIMONS, R. F. (1965) Answering English questions by computer — a survey. *A.C.M. J. of Computing.*

SIMONS, R. F., KLEIN, S. and McCONLOGUE, K. (1964) Indexing and dependency logic for answering English questions. *American Documentation*, **15.**

SKINNER, B. F. (1933) 'Resistance to extinction' in the process of conditioning. *J. gen. Psychol.* **9**, 420–9.

SKINNER, B. F. (1938) *The Behavior of Organisms: An Experimental Analysis*, Appleton-Century-Crofts, New York.

SMITH, K. R. (1952) The statistical theory of the figural after-effect. *Psychol. Rev.* **59**, 401–2.

SOLOMONOFF, R. J. (1957) An inductive inference machine. 1957. Convention Record. I.R.E. Part 2.

SPENCE, K. W. (1947) The role of secondary reinforcement in delayed reward learning. *Psychol. Rev.* **54**, 1–8.

SPENCE, K. W. (1950) Cognitive versus stimulus–response theories of learning. *Psychol. Rev.* **57**, 159–72.

SPENCE, K. W. (1951) Theoretical interpretations of learning. In: S. S. STEVENS (Editor), *Handbook of Experimental Psychology*, John Wiley, New York.

SPENCE, K. W. (1952) Mathematical formulations of learning phenomena. *Psychol. Rev.* **59**, 152–60.

SPENCE, K. W. and LIPPITT, R. (1940) 'Latent' learning of a simple maze problem with relevant needs satiated. *Psychol. Bull.* **37**, 429.

SPERRY, R. W. (1943) The problem of central nervous reorganization after nerve regeneration and muscle transposition. *Quart. Rev. Biol.* **20**, 311–69.

SPERRY, R. W., STAMM, J. S. and MINER, N. (1956) Relearning tests for interocular transfer following division of optic chiasma and corpus callosum in cats. *J. comp. physiol. Psychol.* **49**, 529–33.

SPINELLI, D. N. and PRIBRAM, K. H. (1970) Neural correlation of stimulus response and reinforcement. *Brain Research* **17**, 3, 377–85.

SPINELLI, D. N. and WEINGARTEN, M. (1966) Afferent and efferent activity in single units of the cat's optic nerve. *Exptl. Neurol.* **15**, 347–63.

STANLEY, W. C. and JAYNES, J. (1949) The function of the frontal cortex. *Psychol. Rev.* **56**, 18–33.

STARZL, T. E. and MAGOUN, H. W. (1951) Organization of the diffuse thalamic projection system. *J. Neurophysiol.* **14,** 133–46.

STEIN, L. (1966) Habituation and stimulus novelty: a model based on classical conditioning. *Psychol. Rev.* **73,** 352–6.

STELLAR, E. (1960) *Handbook of Physiology*, Section 1, Neurophysiology III, H. W. FIELD, H. W. MAGORM and V. E. HALL (Editors), Washington, D.C.

STEWART, D. J. (1959) Automata and Behaviour. Ph.D. Thesis, University of Bristol, England.

STEWART, D. J. (1961) *A Bibliography of Cybernetics.* Brunel Monograph 12.

STOUT, G. F. (1896) *Analytic Psychology.*

SUTHERLAND, N. S. (1959) Stimulus analyzing mechanisms. In *Mechanisation of Thought Processes*, N.P.L. Symposium.

TAYLOR, W. K. Computers and the nervous system. In Symposium of Soc. Exp. Biol. on *Models and Analogues in Biology*, vol. 14, pp. 152–68, Cambridge University Press.

THISTLETHWAITE, D. L. (1951) A critical review of latent learning and related experiments. *Psychol. Bull.* **48,** 97–129.

THISTLETHWAITE, D. L. (1952) Reply to Kendler and Maltzman. *Psychol. Bull.* **49,** 61–71.

THORNDIKE, E. L. (1898) Animal intelligence: an experimental study of the associative processes in animals. *Psychol. Rev. Monogr. Suppl* **2,** No 8

THORNDIKE, E. L. (1911) *Animal Intelligence*, Macmillan, New York.

THORNDIKE, E. L. (1932) *The Fundamentals of Learning*, New York: Teachers College.

THORPE, W. H. (1950) The concepts of learning and their relation to those of instinct. Symposium Vol. 4 of Society for Experimental Biology on *Physiological Mechanisms in Animal Behaviour.*

THORPE, W. H. (1956) *Learning and Instinct in Animals*, Methuen, London.

THOULESS, R. H. (1931) Phenomenal regression to the 'real object'. *Brit. J. Psychol.* **21,** 339.

THRALL, R. M., COOMBS, C. H. and DAVIS, R. L. (1954) *Decision Processes*, John Wiley, New York.

TINBERGEN, N. (1951) *The Study of Instinct*, Oxford University Press.

TINKLEPAUGH, O. L. (1928) An experimental study of representative factors in monkeys. *J. comp. Psychol.* **8,** 197–236.

TOLMAN, E. C. (1932) *Purposive Behavior in Animals and Men*, Appleton-Century-Crofts, New York.

TOLMAN, E. C. (1934) Theories of learning. In: F. A. Moss (Editor), *Comparative Psychology*, Prentice-Hall, New York.

TOLMAN, E. C. (1939) Prediction of vicarious trial and error by means of the schematic sowbug. *Psychol. Rev.* **46,** 318–36.

TOLMAN, E. C. (1941) Discrimination versus learning and the schematic sowbug. *Psychol. Rev.* **48,** 367–82.

TOLMAN, E. C. (1952) A cognition motivation model. *Psychol. Rev.* **59,** 389–400.

TOLMAN, E. C. and HONZIK, C. H. (1930) 'Insight' in rats. *Univ. Calif. Publ. Psychol.* **4,** 215–32.

TOLMAN, E. C. and BRUNSWICK, E. (1935) The organism and the causal texture of the environment. *Psychol. Rev.* **42,** 43–77.

Tower, D. B. (1958) The neurochemical substrates of cerebral function and activity. In: H. F. Harlow and C. N. Woolsey (Editors), *Biological and Biochemical Bases of Behavior*, University of Wisconsin Press.

Trotter, J. R. (1957) The timing of bar-pressing behaviour. *Quart. J. exp. Psychol.*, **9**, 78–87.

Turing, A. M. (1937) On computable numbers, with an application to the Entscheidungs problem. *Proc. Lond. Math. Soc.*, ser. 2, **42**, 230–65.

Turing, A. M. (1950) Computing machinery and intelligence. *Mind* **59**, 433–60.

Turing, A. M. (1952) The chemical basis of morphogenesis. *Phil. Trans. Roy. Soc.* 237, 37–72.

Uttley, A. M. (1954) The classification of signals in the nervous system. *Electroenceph. clin. Neurophysiol.* **6**, 479.

Uttley, A. M. (1955) The conditional probability of signals in the nervous system. RRE Mem. No. 1109.

Uttley, A. M. (1955) The probability of neural connexions. *Proc. Roy. Soc.* B **144**, 229.

Uttley, A. M. (1966) The transmission of information and the effect of local feedback in theoretical and neural networks. *Brain Research* **2**, 1, 21–50.

Verbeek, L. (1962) On error minimizing neural nets. In: H. von Foerster and G. W. Zopf (Editors), *Principles of Self-Organization*, Pergamon Press.

Vogt, O. and Vogt, Cécile (1919) Ergebnisse unserer Hurnforschung. *J. Psychol. Neurol.* **25**, 277–462.

von Neumann, J. (1952) *Probabilistic Logics*, California Institute of Technology.

von Neumann, J. and Morgenstern, O. (1944) *Theory of Games and Economic Behaviour*. Princeton University Press.

von Senden, M. (1932) *Raum- und Gestaltauffassung bei operierten Blindgeborenen vor und nach der Operation*, Barth.

Walker, A. E. (1938) *The Primate Thalamus*, Chicago University Press.

Walter, W. G. (1953) *The Living Brain*, Duckworth, London.

Wang, H. (1960) Proving theorems by pattern recognition. *I. Comm. Ass. of Comp. Mach.* **3**, 220–34.

Wang, H. (1964) Towards mechanical mathematics. *IBM J. Res. Dev.* **4**, 2–22.

Ward, A. A. Jnr. (1948) The cingulate gyrus; area 24. *J. Neurophysiol.* **11**, 13–23.

Ward, J. (1918) *Psychological Principles*. Cambridge University Press.

Washburn, M. R. (1908) *The Animal Mind*, Macmillan.

Wason, P. C. and Johnson-Laird, P. N. (1968) *Thinking and Reasoning*, Penguin Books.

Watt, D. A. F. (1970) Management decision-making and 'real' games. *Int. J. Syst. Sci.* **1**, 2, 99–110.

Werner, H. (1935) Studies on contour. I. Qualitative analysis. *Amer. J. Psychol.* **47**, 40–64.

Werner, H. (1940) Studies in contour: strobostereoscopic phenomena. *Amer. J. Psychol.* **53**, 418–22.

Wertheimer, M. (1912) Experimentelle Studien über das Sehen von Bewegung. *Z. Psychol.* **61**, 161–265.

White, D. J. (1969) *Decision Theory*, George Allen & Unwin.

Whitehead, A. N. and Russell, B. (1910, 1912, 1913) *Principia Mathematica*, Cambridge University Press.

WIENER, N. (1948) *Cybernetics*, The Technology Press of M.I.T. and John Wiley & Sons Inc.

WIENER, N. (1949) *The Extrapolation, Interpolation, and Smoothing of Stationary Time Series*, The Technology Press of M.I.T. and John Wiley & Sons Inc.

WILLSHAW, D. J. and LONGUET-HIGGINS, H. C. (1969) The holophone—recent developments. In: B. MELTZER and D. MICHIE (Editors), *Machine Intelligence*, Vol. 4.

WILMER, E. N. (1946) *Retinal Structure and Colour Vision: A Restatement and an Hypothesis*, Cambridge University Press.

WILSON, J. A. (1966) *Information, Entropy and the Development of Structure in Behaviour*, Doctoral Thesis, University of Bristol.

WITTGENSTEIN, L. (1953) *Philosophical Investigations*, Blackwell, Oxford.

WOHLGEMUTH, A. (1911) On the after-effects of seen movement. Monograph (1946) to the *Brit. J. Psychol.*, Cambridge University Press.

WOLPE, J. (1950) Need-reduction, drive-reduction and reinforcement: a neurophysiological view. *Psychol. Rev.* **59**, 8–18.

WOODGER, J. H. (1937) *The Axiomatic Method in Biology*, Cambridge University Press.

WOODGER, J. H. (1939) Technique of theory construction. *Encyclopaedia of Unified Science*, Vol. II, No. 5, Chicago.

WOODGER, J. H. (1951) Science without properties. *Brit. J. Phil. Sci.* **2**, 193–216.

WOODGER, J. H. (1952) *Biology and Language*, Cambridge University Press.

WOODWORTH, R. S. (1938) *Experimental Psychology*, Holt, New York.

YERKES, R. M. (1916) The mental life of monkeys and apes; a study of ideational behaviour. *Behav. Monogr.* **3**, 12.

ZANGWILL, O. L.: There are various references throughout the literature.

AUTHOR INDEX

SUBJECT INDEX